Emergency Radiology

Guest Editor

JORGE A. SOTO, MD

RADIOLOGIC CLINICS OF NORTH AMERICA

www.radiologic.theclinics.com

Consulting Editor
FRANK H. MILLER, MD

January 2012 • Volume 50 • Number 1

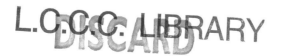
SAUNDERS an imprint of ELSEVIER, Inc.

W.B. SAUNDERS COMPANY
A Division of Elsevier Inc.

1600 John F. Kennedy Boulevard • Suite 1800 • Philadelphia, Pennsylvania 19103-2899

http://www.theclinics.com

RADIOLOGIC CLINICS OF NORTH AMERICA Volume 50, Number 1
January 2012 ISSN 0033-8389, ISBN 13: 978-1-4557-3927-1

Editor: Sarah Barth
Developmental Editor: Eva Kulig

Radiologic Clinics of North America (ISSN 0033-8389) is published bimonthly by Elsevier Inc., 360 Park Avenue South, New York, NY 10010-1710. Months of issue are January, March, May, July, September, and November. Periodicals postage paid at New York, NY and additional mailing offices. Subscription prices are USD 421 per year for US individuals, USD 659 per year for US institutions, USD 202 per year for US students and residents, USD 491 per year for Canadian individuals, USD 827 per year for Canadian institutions, USD 606 per year for international individuals, USD 827 per year for international institutions, and USD 290 per year for Canadian and foreign students/residents. To receive student and resident rate, orders must be accompanied by name of affiliated institution, date of term and the signature of program/residency coordinatior on institution letterhead. Orders will be billed at individual rate until proof of status is received. Foreign air speed delivery is included in all *Clinics* subscription prices. All prices are subject to change without notice. **POSTMASTER:** Send address changes to *Radiologic Clinics of North America*, Elsevier Health Sciences Division, Subscription Customer Service, 3251 Riverport Lane, Maryland Heights, MO63043. **Customer Service: Telephone: 1-800-654-2452** (U.S. and Canada); **1-314-447-8871** (outside U.S. and Canada). **Fax: 1-314-447-8029. E-mail: journalscustomerservice-usa@ elsevier.com** (for print support); **journalsonlinesupport-usa@elsevier.com** (for online support).

Reprints. For copies of 100 or more of articles in this publication, please contact the Commercial Reprints Department, Elsevier Inc., 360 Park Avenue South, New York, New York 10010-1710. Tel.: (+1) 212-633-3812; Fax: (+1) 212-462-1935; E-mail: reprints@elsevier.com.

Radiologic Clinics of North America also published in Greek Paschalidis Medical Publications, Athens, Greece.

Radiologic Clinics of North America is covered in *MEDLINE/PubMed (Index Medicus), EMBASE/Excerpta Medica, Current Contents/Life Sciences, Current Contents/Clinical Medicine, RSNA Index to Imaging Literature, BIOSIS, Science Citation Index,* and *ISI/BIOMED.*

Printed in the United States of America.

Contributors

CONSULTING EDITOR

FRANK H. MILLER, MD
Professor of Radiology; Chief, Body Imaging
Section and Fellowship Program and GI
Radiology, Medical Director MRI, Department
of Radiology, Northwestern University
Feinberg School of Medicine, Chicago, Illinois

GUEST EDITOR

JORGE A. SOTO, MD
Professor of Radiology, Department
of Radiology, Boston University School
of Medicine, Boston, Massachusetts

AUTHORS

STEPHAN W. ANDERSON, MD
Assistant Professor, Department of Radiology,
Boston University School of Medicine, Boston,
Massachusetts

MARK P. BERNSTEIN, MD
Department of Radiology, NYU Langone
Medical Center/Bellevue Hospital and Trauma
Center, New York, New York

ALEXIS BOSCAK, MD
Assistant Professor, Trauma/Emergency
Section, Department of Radiology, University
of Maryland Medical Center, University
of Maryland, Baltimore, Maryland

PARAG BUTALA, MD
Institute of Reconstructive Plastic Surgery,
NYU Langone Medical Center, New York,
New York

FALGUN H. CHOKSHI, MD
Assistant Professor of Radiology, Department
of Radiology, Emory University School
of Medicine, Emory University Hospital,
Atlanta, Georgia

MARK FOLEY, MB, BCh
Radiology Resident, Department of Radiology,
Jackson Memorial Hospital, University of
Miami Miller School of Medicine, Miami, Florida

GEORGE GANSON, MD
Department of Radiology, Winthrop-University
Hospital, Mineola, New York

ALDO GONZALEZ-BEICOS, MD
Department of Radiology, Hospital of Saint
Raphael, Yale School of Medicine, New Haven,
Connecticut

MARTIN L. GUNN, MBChB, FRANZCR
Department of Radiology, University
of Washington, Seattle, Washington

JOHN J. HINES, MD
Department of Radiology, Long Island Jewish
Medical Center, New Hyde Park, New York

JAMLIK-OMARI JOHNSON, MD
Assistant Professor of Radiology and Imaging
Sciences, Division of Emergency Radiology,
Department of Radiology and Imaging
Sciences, Emory University Hospital Midtown,
Atlanta, Georgia

DOUGLAS S. KATZ, MD
Department of Radiology, Winthrop-University Hospital, Mineola, New York

MICHELE A.I. KLEIN, MD
Department of Radiology, Winthrop-University Hospital, Mineola, New York

WAYNE S. KUBAL, MD
Professor of Clinical Radiology, Department of Radiology, University of Arizona Health Sciences Center, Tucson, Arizona

CHRISTINA A. LEBEDIS, MD
Assistant Professor, Department of Radiology, Boston University School of Medicine, Boston, Massachusetts

NISHA MEHTA, MD
Department of Radiology, NYU Langone Medical Center/Bellevue Hospital and Trauma Center, New York, New York

FELIPE MUNERA, MD
Associate Professor of Radiology, Medical Director, Radiology Department, University of Miami Hospital and University of Miami Hospital and Clinics; Director, Patient Safety and Image Quality, Radiology Department,

Jackson Memorial Hospital, University of Miami Miller School of Medicine, University of Miami Medical System; Ryder Trauma Center, Miami, Florida

DIEGO NUNEZ, MD, MPH
Department of Radiology, Hospital of Saint Raphael, Yale School of Medicine, New Haven, Connecticut

KATHIRKAMANTHAN SHANMUGANATHAN, MD
Professor, Trauma/Emergency Section, Department of Radiology, University of Maryland Medical Center, University of Maryland, Baltimore, Maryland

AARON SODICKSON, MD, PhD
Section Head of Emergency Radiology, Department of Radiology, Brigham and Women's Hospital; Assistant Professor of Radiology, Harvard Medical School, Boston, Massachusetts

JORGE A. SOTO, MD
Professor of Radiology, Department of Radiology, Boston University School of Medicine, Boston, Massachusetts

Contents

Many tools and strategies exist to enable the reduction of radiation exposure from computed tomography (CT). The common CT metrics of x-ray output, $CTDI_{vol}$ and DLP, are explained and serve as the basis for monitoring radiation exposure from CT scans. Many strategies to dose optimize CT protocols are explored that, in combination with available hardware and software tools, allow robust diagnostic quality CT scans to be performed with a radiation exposure appropriate for the clinical scenario and the size of the patients. Specific emergency department example protocols are used to demonstrate these techniques.

Computed tomography (CT) and magnetic resonance (MR) play important roles in the evaluation of traumatic brain injury. Modern CT scanners allow for rapid and accurate diagnosis of intracranial hemorrhage and mass effect and allow the efficient implementation of emergent CT angiography. Newer sequences, such as gradient recalled echo, susceptibility-weighted imaging, and diffusion-weighted imaging, can provide greater sensitivity for specific types of diffuse posttraumatic brain injury. MR spectroscopy can provide additional chemical information, and diffusion tensor imaging can provide information about white matter injury. Patient treatment can be optimized using the diagnostic and prognostic information derived from current imaging techniques.

Maxillofacial skeletal injuries account for a large proportion of emergency department visits and often result in surgical consultation. Although many of the principles of detection and repair are basic, the evolution of technology and therapeutic strategies has led to improved patient outcomes. This article aims to provide a review of the imaging aspects involved in maxillofacial trauma and to delineate its relevance to management.

Blunt cerebrovascular injury (BCVI) is uncommon but potentially catastrophic; 80% are caused by vehicle collisions. Ischemic events secondary to untreated BCVI are common, with high injury-specific mortality. This has led to implementation of screening programs based on mechanism of injury, clinical presentation, and injury patterns identified on noncontrast computed tomography (CT) imaging. The standard of reference for diagnosis is four-vessel digital subtraction angiography. Given its availably in trauma service institutions, use of multidetector CT angiography has increased. This article presents the evidence and the controversies surrounding its use. Available protocols, injury description, and grading, as well as potential pitfalls are reviewed.

Aldo Gonzalez-Beicos and Diego Nunez

Tonsillar infection is the most common cause of infections of the neck in children and young adults whereas odontogenic infection is the most common cause in older population groups. Other sources of neck infection include the salivary glands, nasal sinuses, middle ear and mastoids, cervical lymph nodes, and trauma. Computed tomography and magnetic resonance imaging have excellent sensitivity for the recognition of deep infections, particularly for the identification of abscess formation and its precise location and extension of disease. A careful assessment of potential severe complications, such as vascular compromise, osteomyelitis, and airway narrowing, should be performed routinely.

Martin L. Gunn

Although infrequently encountered in busy trauma centers, injuries to the aorta and branch vessels remain an important cause of trauma-related mortality. Advances in the diagnosis and management of these injuries have led to more accurate and timely imaging, and improved patient outcomes. Despite these advances, several challenges in evaluating the severely injured trauma patient remain. This review provides an overview of current concepts in the imaging of aortic and branch vessel injuries, and provides pointers to improve detection and interpretation of more challenging injuries.

Alexis Boscak and Kathirkamanthan Shanmuganathan

Evaluation for splenic injury is an important component of patient assessment after blunt abdominal trauma. Key imaging modalities include ultrasound, particularly for rapid identification of hemoperitoneum, and computed tomography (CT), which permits a more detailed and accurate determination of splenic integrity. Specific findings at contrast-enhanced multidetector CT (MDCT) should prompt the consideration of catheter angiography with arterial embolization as an adjunct to nonsurgical management. This article reviews the roles of imaging in the management of splenic trauma, illustrates the MDCT appearance of various splenic injuries, and discusses imaging-based indications for operative and angiographic intervention.

Christiana A. LeBedis, Stephan W. Anderson, and Jorge A. Soto

Delayed diagnosis of a bowel or mesenteric injury resulting in hollow viscus perforation leads to significant morbidity and mortality from hemorrhage, peritonitis, or abdominal sepsis. The timely diagnosis of bowel and mesenteric injuries requiring operative repair depends almost exclusively on their early detection by the radiologist on computed tomography examination, because the clinical signs and symptoms of these injuries are not specific and usually develop late. Therefore, the radiologist must be familiar with the often-subtle imaging findings of bowel and mesenteric injury that will allow for appropriate triage of a patient who has sustained blunt trauma to the abdomen or pelvis.

GOAL STATEMENT

The goal of the *Radiologic Clinics of North America* is to keep practicing radiologists and radiology residents up to date with current clinical practice in radiology by providing timely articles reviewing the state of the art in patient care.

ACCREDITATION

The *Radiologic Clinics of North America* is planned and implemented in accordance with the Essential Areas and Policies of the Accreditation Council for Continuing Medical Education (ACCME) through the joint sponsorship of the University of Virginia School of Medicine and Elsevier. The University of Virginia School of Medicine is accredited by the ACCME to provide continuing medical education for physicians.

The University of Virginia School of Medicine designates this enduring material activity for a maximum of 15 *AMA PRA Category 1 Credit*(s)™ for each issue, 90 credits per year. Physicians should only claim credit commensurate with the extent of their participation in the activity.

The American Medical Association has determined that physicians not licensed in the US who participate in this CME enduring material activity are eligible for a maximum of 15 *AMA PRA Category 1 Credit*(s)™ for each issue, 90 credits per year.

Credit can be earned by reading the text material, taking the CME examination online at http://www.theclinics.com/home/cme, and completing the evaluation. After taking the test, you will be required to review any and all incorrect answers. Following completion of the test and evaluation, your credit will be awarded and you may print your certificate.

FACULTY DISCLOSURE/CONFLICT OF INTEREST

The University of Virginia School of Medicine, as an ACCME accredited provider, endorses and strives to comply with the Accreditation Council for Continuing Medical Education (ACCME) Standards of Commercial Support, Commonwealth of Virginia statutes, University of Virginia policies and procedures, and associated federal and private regulations and guidelines on the need for disclosure and monitoring of proprietary and financial interests that may affect the scientific integrity and balance of content delivered in continuing medical education activities under our auspices.

The University of Virginia School of Medicine requires that all CME activities accredited through this institution be developed independently and be scientifically rigorous, balanced and objective in the presentation/discussion of its content, theories and practices.

All authors/editors participating in an accredited CME activity are expected to disclose to the readers relevant financial relationships with commercial entities occurring within the past 12 months (such as grants or research support, employee, consultant, stock holder, member of speakers bureau, etc.). The University of Virginia School of Medicine will employ appropriate mechanisms to resolve potential conflicts of interest to maintain the standards of fair and balanced education to the reader. Questions about specific strategies can be directed to the Office of Continuing Medical Education, University of Virginia School of Medicine, Charlottesville, Virginia.

The faculty and staff of the University of Virginia Office of Continuing Medical Education have no financial affiliations to disclose.

The authors/editors listed below have identified no financial or professional relationships for themselves or their spouse/partner:

Stephan W. Anderson, MD; Sarah Barth, (Acquisitions Editor); Mark P. Bernstein, MD; Alexis Boscak, MD; Parag Butala, MD; Falgun H. Chokshi, MD; Mark Foley, MB, BCh; George Ganson, MD; Aldo Gonzalez-Beicos, MD; Martin L. Gunn, MBChB, FRANZCR; John J. Hines, MD; Jamlik-Omari Johnson, MD; Douglas S. Katz, MD; Michele A.I. Klein, MD; Wayne S. Kubal, MD; Christina A. LeBedis, MD; Nisha Mehta, MD; Frank H. Miller, MD (Consulting Editor); Felipe Munera, MD; Diego Nunez, MD, MPH; Kathirkamanthan Shanmuganathan, MD; and Jorge A. Soto, MD (Guest Editor).

The authors/editors listed below have identified the following financial or professional relationships for themselves or their spouse/partner:

Klaus D. Hagspiel, MD (Test Author) is an industry funded research/investigator for Siemens Medical Solutions.
Aaron Sodickson, MD, PhD is a consultant for Siemens CT and Toshiba CT.

Disclosure of Discussion of Non-FDA Approved Uses for Pharmaceutical Products and/or Medical Devices

The University of Virginia School of Medicine, as an ACCME provider, requires that all faculty presenters identify and disclose any off-label uses for pharmaceutical and medical device products. The University of Virginia School of Medicine recommends that each physician fully review all the available data on new products or procedures prior to clinical use.

TO ENROLL

To enroll in the Radiologic Clinics of North America Continuing Medical Education program, call customer service at 1-800-654-2452 or sign up online at http://www.theclinics.com/home/cme. The CME program is available to subscribers for an additional annual fee USD 245.

Radiologic Clinics of North America

THE CLINICS ARE NOW AVAILABLE ONLINE!

Access your subscription at:
www.theclinics.com

Preface
Emergency Radiology

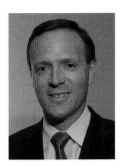

Jorge A. Soto, MD
Guest Editor

It is no secret that technological advances in medical imaging have modified substantially the way that health care is provided to acutely ill patients. In many instances, findings on imaging tests performed as emergency procedures provide the decisive information that directly determines the best management options. In other cases, appropriate triaging of patients initially admitted through the emergency room is performed almost exclusively on the basis of results of imaging examinations. Not surprisingly, the last decade has seen an almost exponential increase in the number and complexity of emergency imaging tests, especially CT. The practice of Emergency Radiology has undergone the same rapid change: as imaging procedures are increasingly performed within short periods of time after the arrival of patients to the emergency room, the expectation for near real-time interpretations (often by subspecialists) has gained popularity. Larger emergency centers provide 24-hour onsite coverage by well-trained radiologists, while others rely on the services of equally well-trained radiologists located off-site, taking advantage of modern universal interconnectivity. Either way, radiologists' input is increasingly affecting the immediate outcome of patients presenting with acute symptoms.

There has also been a growing interest and awareness among health care providers and the public in general about the potentially harmful consequences of the indiscriminate use of ionizing radiation, which must be weighed against the innumerable and significant benefits of properly performed imaging tests. Additionally, changes in the economic landscape have brought increased scrutiny to the use of CT for many indications, including emergency applications. This is an ongoing debate, but radiologists have embraced the challenge to protect patient safety by seeking evidence-based data to support the proper utilization of CT (including the use of alternative imaging modalities) and radiologists and CT manufacturers together have worked intensely to find optimal methods to deliver the inevitable radiation.

This issue of the *Radiologic Clinics of North America* addresses these challenges. As the guest editor, I had the difficult job of selecting topics that are relevant and helpful to the readers in some of the most important areas of Emergency Radiology today. I am indebted to the contributing authors, all of whom are very well known and respected in the field of Emergency Radiology. They understood the importance and timeliness of this issue and found the time in their complex schedules to complete the articles well within schedule. Their

Radiol Clin N Am 50 (2012) xi–xii
doi:10.1016/j.rcl.2011.10.002
0033-8389/12/$ – see front matter © 2012 Elsevier Inc. All rights reserved.

radiologic.theclinics.com

expertise and thoughtfulness are evident in every article. I also want to thank Frank Miller (Consulting Editor for *Radiologic Clinics*), who selected me for this task, and Barton Dudlick and the Elsevier staff, who made my job much easier than I anticipated. Finally, I would like to thank my wife, Ana, and my children, Andrea and Alejandro, for their love and continuous support; their company adds fun and meaning to my work.

Jorge A. Soto, MD
Department of Radiology
Boston University School of Medicine
FGH Building, 3rd Floor
820 Harrison Avenue
Boston, MA 02118, USA

E-mail address:
Jorge.Soto@bmc.org

Strategies for Reducing Radiation Exposure in Multi-Detector Row CT

Aaron Sodickson, MD, PhD[a,b],*

KEYWORDS

- Computed tomography • Radiation exposure • CTDIvol
- DLP • Protocols • Strategies

Radiation exposure has received much attention of late in the medical literature and lay media. As all practicing physicians know, computed tomography (CT) has tremendously advanced our diagnostic capabilities in the emergency department (ED) and broadly throughout medicine. These diagnostic benefits have combined with the widespread availability and rapidity of scanning to produce marked increases in CT use, currently estimated at approximately 69 million CT scans per year in the United States.[1] However, rapidly increasing use has heightened concerns about the collective radiation exposure to the population as a whole and about the high levels of cumulative exposure that may occur in patients undergoing recurrent imaging for chronic conditions or persistent complaints.[2–4]

CT has received the greatest scrutiny because of its relatively high radiation dose per examination; although it accounts for about 17% of all medical imaging procedures, it produces approximately half of the population's medical radiation exposure, with nuclear medicine contributing approximately one-quarter of the collective dose to the population and fluoroscopy and conventional radiograph examinations accounting for the remainder.[5,6]

There are many possible strategies to reduce cumulative radiation exposure to the population as a whole and to individual patients.[7] Once the decision is made to perform a CT scan, many imaging strategies can reduce the radiation dose while maintaining appropriate diagnostic quality for the clinical task at hand. There have been tremendous advances in CT technology in recent years that allow high-quality examinations to be performed at progressively lower radiation doses. The common practice of porting CT protocols from older to newer scanners often fails to take maximal advantage of these new technologies. Routine optimal scan acquisition requires that radiologists invest the effort to understand their technology and to implement dose-optimized protocols, ideally in collaboration with CT manufacturers, CT technologists, and medical physicists. This task is admittedly daunting for many radiologists who often view their primary role as diagnosticians and interpreters of images and often have little detailed training in CT technology.

This article describes several practical opportunities to reduce radiation exposure from CT, with emphasis on how CT protocols can be modified to reduce the dose while maintaining diagnostic quality. Specific implementation of these strategies is highly dependent on the available technology, and there is no replacement for hands-on training at the scanner.

Financial Disclosures: The author serves as a paid consultant to Siemens Medical Solutions and Toshiba America Medical Systems.

[a] Department of Radiology, Brigham and Women's Hospital, 75 Francis Street, Boston, MA 02115, Boston, MA, USA
[b] Harvard Medical School, Boston, MA, USA
* Brigham and Women's Hospital, 75 Francis Street, Boston, MA 02115.
E-mail address: asodickson@partners.org

Radiol Clin N Am 50 (2012) 1–14
doi:10.1016/j.rcl.2011.08.006

REDUCING RADIATION EXPOSURE: BEFORE THE SCAN

The most effective way to reduce radiation exposure is to not perform the examination. Before a scan is performed, many measures can be taken to control use, with the goal of reducing low-yield examinations that will not contribute significantly to the care of the patient. Admittedly, it is often challenging to prospectively determine which examinations these will be. Nonetheless, scrutiny of examination appropriateness is vital. In optimal circumstances, this can rely on well-validated clinical decision rules, such as those for pulmonary embolus or for head or cervical-spine imaging in trauma.[8–10] These rules may be integrated into predefined imaging algorithms in the effort to standardize the imaging approach in specific clinical scenarios or patient populations. Alternatively, these algorithms and expert panel appropriateness criteria may be incorporated into decision support advice during computerized physician order entry.[11,12]

Duplicative imaging and recurrent imaging are natural targets for radiation dose reduction.[13,14] Ordering physician awareness of duplicate imaging may be achieved via review of the medical record or in automated fashion as part of decision support tools. In certain circumstances, interventions to eliminate unnecessary repeat imaging can be highly effective in reducing utilization. As an example, importation of outside hospital imaging examinations from CD to the Picture Archive and Communication System (PACS) has been found to reduce CT utilization by 16% within the first 24 hours of an ED transfer, primarily by eliminating unnecessary repeat scans.[15]

Defensive medicine and self-referral of diagnostic imaging have both been implicated as significant contributors to imaging utilization.[16,17] Effectively addressing these systemic issues will require higher-level attention in our health care delivery system.

UNDERSTANDING THE X-RAY TUBE OUTPUT METRICS, VOLUME CT DOSE INDEX AND DOSE-LENGTH PRODUCT

To understand and monitor radiation exposures from CT scans, a basic understanding is first needed of the radiation exposure metrics commonly used in CT. The volume CT dose index ($CTDI_{vol}$) and the dose-length product (DLP) are well-calibrated and standardized measures of x-ray tube output.[18,19] They are measured in cylindrical acrylic phantoms of standard diameter, either a 16-cm head phantom or a 32-cm body phantom. A 100-mm long ionization chamber connected to an electrometer is placed inside a hole in either the center or periphery of the CTDI phantom, and measurements are made (with the CT table stationary) under a particular CT exposure to yield $CTDI_{100}$ measurements. The $CTDI_{vol}$ is a weighted sum of these central and peripheral measurements, along with a geometric correction to account for the pitch of a helical scan:

$$CTDI_{vol} = \left(\frac{2}{3}CTDI_{100,\ periph} + \frac{1}{3}CTDI_{100,\ center} \right) \Big/ pitch$$

The $CTDI_{vol}$ reported by the CT scanner is most commonly the average value over the length of the scan (although some scanner models report the maximum value). DLP is simply the average $CTDI_{vol}$ times the z-axis extent of the CT exposure from head to foot, so that a doubling in z-axis coverage at a fixed $CTDI_{vol}$ will result in a doubling of the DLP.

$CTDI_{vol}$ and DLP depend heavily on the selected scan parameters, including the peak kilovoltage (kVp) and the tube current-time product mAs = mA × rotation time/pitch, where mA is the tube current in milliamperes. They capture intrinsic scanner factors, including x-ray source efficiency and filtration and collimation of the x-ray source. As such, they are reliable metrics of x-ray tube output or x-ray flux but do not accurately represent the radiation dose to a particular patient, primarily because they do not take into consideration the size of patients.[20]

Limitations of Patient Dose Estimates from $CTDI_{vol}$ and DLP

$CTDI_{vol}$ (measured in milligray [mGy]) is commonly used to approximate patient organ doses. However, this is accurate only for a narrow range of patient sizes closely approximating the size of the CTDI phantom, and the actual organ dose a patient receives depends greatly on the size of the patient.[21–23] $CTDI_{vol}$ overestimates organ dose to large patients because subcutaneous soft tissues attenuate the incident x-rays, essentially shielding the internal organs. Conversely, $CTDI_{vol}$ underestimates organ dose to small patients because more of the incident x-rays reach the internal organs. There are several methods to correct these dose estimates by incorporating patient size information.[23]

The DLP is often used to estimate the overall effective dose to patients through the use of multiplicative conversion "k-factors" derived by Monte Carlo simulations.[19,24] In this approach, the DLP for a particular anatomic region is multiplied by the k-factor derived for the same anatomic region to arrive at an estimated effective dose in millisieverts. The effective dose is a single number intended to reflect the uniform whole-body exposure that would be expected to produce the same overall risk of radiation-induced cancer as the partial-body exposure of the CT scan. It is calculated as a weighted sum of the absorbed doses to the exposed organs where the weighting factors depend on the relative sensitivity of the organs to develop radiation-induced cancer. However, effective dose has substantial limitations in accuracy when applied to individual patients because the weighting factors used represent population averages and do not incorporate the known dependence of radiation sensitivity on age or gender.[25] Further, the commonly used k-factor method assumes a typical-sized patient and does not incorporate the substantial impact of patient size.[26]

Review CTDI_vol and DLP on Every Scan

Current CT scanners have the ability to produce a "patient protocol" or "dose report screen capture" and to include these as a separate series in each examination. Although formats and content vary between manufacturers and scanner models, all at minimum contain the $CTDI_{vol}$ and DLP. Some contain additional scan parameters and some specify whether the 16-cm head phantom or the 32-cm body phantom is used for the reporting.

California has recently enacted legislation to require inclusion of such information in the radiology report,[27] and other regulatory efforts are underway.[28] Regardless of reporting practices or requirements, however, it is crucially important for radiologists to review the $CTDI_{vol}$ and DLP for every scan they interpret. This review allows radiologists to gain familiarity with typical values and to develop a sense of how these metrics ought to vary with patient size. Identification of outliers is important for quality-control efforts to direct CT protocol modifications or to target technologist training as needed. In addition, diagnostic reference levels are becoming more commonplace and represent recommended values of $CTDI_{vol}$ or DLP expected to be adequate for diagnostic quality examinations in most patients (to be exceeded only in the largest of patients).[29,30] Radiologists, technologists, and medical physicists should all have a sense of how their scans compare with these reference values.

REDUCING RADIATION EXPOSURE: DURING THE SCAN

During the scan, the key intervention is to design dose-optimized CT protocols that find the sweet spot between the lowest exposure appropriate for the particular clinical scenario while still providing a robust, diagnostic, quality examination. These measures are the primary focus of this article.

CT Protocol Strategies to Reduce Radiation Exposure

Once the decision has been made to perform a CT scan, there are many available strategies to reduce radiation exposure.[31,32]

Use size-dependent protocols

CT images are created from the small fraction of incident x-rays that successfully pass through the body and reach the detector array, with image noise varying as the square root of the x-ray flux. Large patients absorb more of the incident x-rays than small patients, so to maintain the desired image quality, greater x-ray tube output is needed in large patients compared with small patients. As a result, CT protocols should vary the technique according to the size of the patient. The pediatric radiology community was the leader in the concept of child-sizing CT protocols to avoid excessive pediatric exposures, but the general principle also holds for adult patients, and many methods exist to rationally adjust scan parameters to patient size.[33,34]

Understand and enable scanner dose-reduction tools

The most widely available and the most important technique to adjust CT technique for patient size is automated tube current modulation (TCM), also called dose modulation. TCM techniques adjust the x-ray tube output to the patient's anatomy in order to maintain a desired level of image noise, as shown in **Fig. 1**.[35,36] In longitudinal or z-axis TCM, the x-ray tube output is varied along the z axis (from head to foot) of the patient, with greater mAs used in areas with more tissue to penetrate, such as the shoulders or the pelvis, and lower mAs used in regions of relatively little attenuating material, such as the lungs. All of the CT manufacturers use either 1 or 2 CT projection radiographs (named the scout, surview, scanogram, or topogram depending on the manufacturer) to plan the TCM by measuring the patient's attenuation as a function of position.

Axial or in-plane modulation adjusts the x-ray tube output as the gantry rotates around the patient, typically increasing mAs for lateral projections where there is more tissue to penetrate and decreasing mAs for frontal projections where there is less tissue to penetrate. Depending on the manufacturer, this in-plane mAs variation can be derived using orthogonal scout views, using

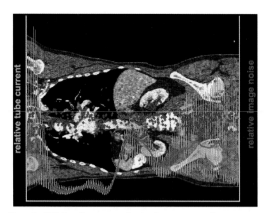

Fig. 1. TCM schemes adjust the x-ray tube output (*green*) as a function of position to maintain a desired image quality, in this case a relatively constant level of image noise (*red*). Longitudinal TCM (*thick green line*) adjusts x-ray flux along the craniocaudal z axis. Note the lower tube current through the lungs compared with the more attenuating shoulders and pelvis. Axial or in-plane TCM adjust tube current as the gantry rotates around the patient (*light green line*). Note the much greater tube current required to penetrate through the shoulders in a lateral versus a frontal projection. (*Modified from* Kalendar WA. Computed tomography. 3rd edition. Erlangen (Germany): Publicis Publishing; 2011; with permission.)

heuristic estimation methods from a single scout view, or online using the angular variation of attenuation observed during the previous gantry rotation to determine the mAs variation during the next rotation.

Electrocardiogram-modulation TCM schemes are used for cardiac-gated scans with x-ray tube output that is substantially decreased or eliminated during portions of the cardiac cycle where data is not needed. Typically, full x-ray tube output is used during the relatively motion-free diastolic portions of the cardiac cycle and is decreased during the more motion-prone systolic phases of the cardiac cycle.

Appropriate use of automatic TCM results in substantial decreases in $CTDI_{vol}$ and DLP for smaller patients as compared with larger patients. Large patients require more x-ray tube output to yield enough x-rays passing all the way through the patients to reach the detectors and create a diagnostic quality scan. **Fig. 2** shows an example of the clinical effects of TCM.

For scans of the abdomen and pelvis in adult patients, $CTDI_{vol}$ varies by approximately a factor of 4 between the largest and smallest adult patients. However, as illustrated in the schematic of **Fig. 3**, the actual patient doses vary by a smaller factor because of the shielding effect of the soft

tissues.[37] Additional techniques are needed to size correct the $CTDI_{vol}$ to obtain reasonably accurate patient doses.[23,38]

The detailed implementations of the CT manufacturers' TCM schemes are quite varied but all involve the user selecting a desired measure of image quality as a starting point. Because of the variable approaches, it is vitally important that radiologists, technologists, and medical physicists be well educated about the exact operations of their particular scanners' TCM methods to realize the desired dose-saving and image-quality benefits. If used incorrectly, such as by selecting an inappropriate image quality constraint, these techniques can paradoxically result in undesired and inappropriate increases to the patient dose. This incorrect usage is thought to have played a role in some of the recent high-profile medical errors in CT perfusion for stroke.[39]

Reduce the number of passes

It is important to critically examine the value of each pass in a given CT protocol. For example, for routine contrast-enhanced scans of the abdomen and pelvis for undifferentiated abdominal pain, many practices have historically performed additional pyelographic phase scans of the kidneys with the rationale that this provides additional free information. Although some radiologists have anecdotally discovered a small number of incidental transitional cell carcinomas, this additional pass typically adds approximately 30% of the radiation dose of the full abdomen/pelvis scan (because it covers approximately 30% of the full scan range) for very low incremental clinical yield. This scan phase should be eliminated in routine use unless there is a compelling clinical reason to keep it in a particular case.

The development of rapid multi-detector scanners in the mid 1990s led to a proliferation of multiphase CT applications incorporating imaging at different time points during intravenous (IV) contrast administration to provide additional information about the enhancement characteristics of certain organs or lesions. Depending on the specific clinical question, it is often possible in these protocols to eliminate one of the phases, such as an initial noncontrast or a delayed postcontrast phase. In protocols for mesenteric ischemia or gastrointestinal bleeding, for example, one may argue to eliminate the noncontrast phase, thereby diverting this additional radiation exposure.

In certain circumstances it may also be possible to combine different contrast phases. For example, CT urography may be performed with a split bolus technique whereby a portion of the IV contrast is administered and allowed enough

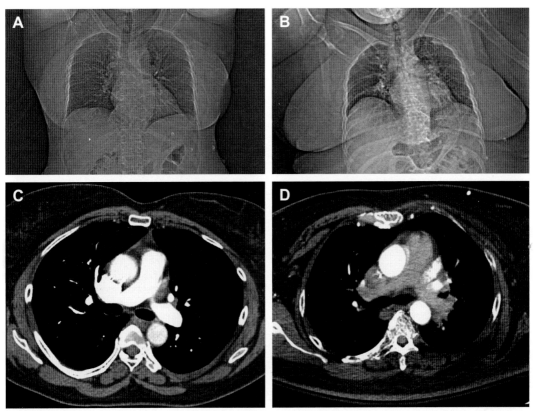

Fig. 2. Clinical effect of automatic TCM (CareDose4D, Siemens AS+ scanner, Forchheim, Germany). A 180-pound patient (*A*) underwent a CT pulmonary angiogram (*C*) and a 325-pound patient (*B*) underwent a dissection CTA (*D*), both with the same quality reference mAs value of 200 (but with different contrast timing delays for the different clinical indications). For the smaller patient, the average effective mAs was automatically adjusted to 276, for a CTDI$_{vol}$ of 18.7 mGy, whereas for the larger patient, the average effective mAs was adjusted to 628, for a CTDI$_{vol}$ of 42.4 mGy. To maintain comparable image quality for both patients, automatic TCM appropriately varied the x-ray tube output by a factor of 2.3 between the two patients.

time to pass into the renal collecting system before the remainder of the contrast is administered with usual nephrographic phase timing resulting in combined nephrographic and excretory phase imaging.[40]

One of the highest-dose examinations common in the ED is for aortic dissection. Traditional aortic dissection CT angiography (CTA) examinations often include 3 passes. First is a noncontrast scan of the chest to assess for intramural hematoma by demonstrating crescentic peripheral high attenuation against the less dense blood pool. This scan is often followed by a cardiac-gated contrast-enhanced CTA of the chest, which is then followed by a delayed scan of the chest, abdomen, and pelvis to assess for branch vessel involvement. Although this approach was designed to answer all possible questions about the aorta and, thus, makes sense for complex aortas, it is worth reconsidering the approach for ED use.

In an ED setting, dissection CTA may be considered a screening examination typically performed to exclude a low pretest probability of this potentially fatal condition. As a result, the yield for acute aortic dissection is often quite low (1%–2% at the author's institution). Of the positive scans a small minority demonstrates isolated intramural hematoma without a visible intimal flap. In addition, these are often tachycardic patients in whom cardiac gating works poorly but typically results in a higher dose than a nongated scan.

As a result, the author's institution has adopted the ED imaging algorithm for aortic dissection shown in **Fig. 4**. Most patients undergo a nongated contrast-enhanced CT angiogram of the chest alone. Elimination of the initial noncontrast chest scan and of the delayed scan through the chest, abdomen, and pelvis yields typical dose savings exceeding 75%.

In this algorithm, a multi-pass protocol may be performed for patients with a high pretest

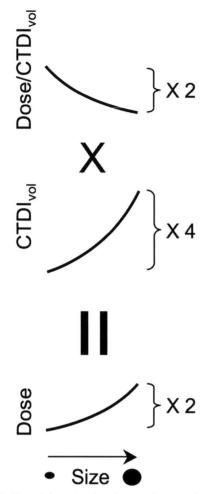

Fig. 3. X-ray tube output and organ dose as a function of patient size for a typical range of adult sizes during abdomen/pelvis scans. For a given x-ray tube output $CTDI_{vol}$, internal organ doses decrease with increasing patient size because of shielding effects (*top*). However (*middle*), appropriately used automatic tube current modulation schemes vary $CTDI_{vol}$ with patient size to maintain desired image quality. The result (*bottom*) of these competing geometric factors is that organ doses are larger for larger patients but to a lesser degree than the raw $CTDI_{vol}$ would predict. (*From* Sodickson A, Turner AC, McGlamery K, et al. Variation in organ dose from abdomen-pelvis CT exams performed with tube current modulation (TCM): evaluation of patient size effects. Radiographic Society of North America 2010 annual meeting. Chicago (IL); with permission.)

probability of disease, such as those with known aortic dissection and concern for extension. However, most patients in the low pretest probability category have the single pass protocol, including a nongated chest CTA. If this scan is normal, the work-up ends. If dissection is present, the scan is extended through the abdomen and pelvis to assess visceral extension. Continuous emergency radiologist availability at the author's ED CT scanner allows this decision to be made instantaneously during real-time monitoring of the scan, so that the extended scan range can be included with the same contrast injection. In a different practice model where a radiologist is not immediately available to make this decision, patients may be subsequently reinjected with a small amount of additional contrast material to assess the distal extent of dissection.

If the single-pass protocol is indeterminate, additional steps may be taken depending on the cause of the indeterminate result. If crescentic peripheral soft tissue along the wall of the aorta raises concern for isolated intramural hematoma without a defined intimal flap, a delayed postcontrast chest CT may be performed 10 to 15 minutes later, after the iodine has cleared the circulating blood pool, as demonstrated in **Fig. 4**. In general, aortic root pulsation artifact can be readily differentiated from aortic root dissection, but when it is truly impossible to differentiate or there is concern for a type A dissection extending into the coronary arteries, a repeat injection may be performed for cardiac-gated chest CTA.

Reduce duplicate coverage
When scanning adjacent body regions, there is often substantial overlap in coverage regions, which results in unnecessary additional radiation exposure. In the example of **Fig. 5**, a patient undergoing a trauma pan-scan has substantial coverage overlap between the head and cervical spine scans, the cervical spine and chest scans, and the chest and abdomen/pelvis scans. It should be understood that there is also additional unseen overlap caused by z overscanning in which the CT scanner exposes an additional area at each end of the prescribed range in order to acquire enough data to reconstruct the top and bottom images. This additional exposure can be substantial but can be significantly reduced on some newer scanners equipped with adaptive collimation systems that minimize the unnecessary additional irradiation.[41]

These areas of prescribed duplicate coverage may be greatly reduced with technologist training or eliminated entirely with combined protocols that image adjacent body regions with a single helical acquisition. The greatest overlap typically occurs between the chest and the abdomen/pelvis scans because chest scans traditionally extend below the posterior costophrenic sulci or adrenal glands and abdominal scans typically extend above the diaphragm, often with additional buffer

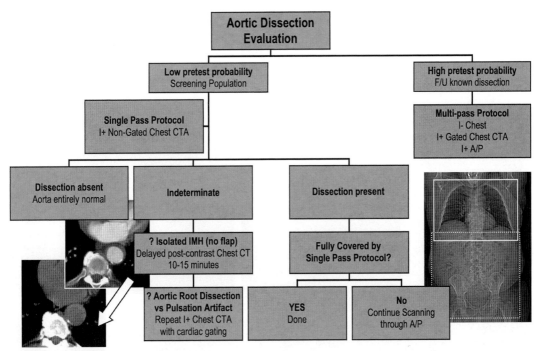

Fig. 4. Dose-reducing aortic dissection imaging algorithm: Most patients undergo the single pass protocol, with negative results. If dissection is present during real-time monitoring, the scan is immediately extended through the abdomen and pelvis (A/P) to assess distal extent (*dotted box* on planning topogram at *right*). Any concern for isolated intramural hematoma (IMH) prompts a delayed postcontrast scan (images at *left*). Pulsation artifact can typically be differentiated from type A dissection, but if needed, a repeat injection of IV contrast could theoretically be performed. F/U, followup.

to ensure full scan coverage. In the trauma setting, it is not necessary to image this overlap region twice. A simple improvement is to instruct the technologists to end the chest scan above the diaphragm, with only enough overlap to ensure complete coverage. Another solution is to perform adjacent scan parts in a single continuous acquisition, although in this situation care must be taken to ensure timing for the appropriate phase of contrast.[42,43] For example, a portal venous phase is considered most sensitive for solid abdominal organ injuries, whereas an earlier arterial phase is preferable to assess aortic injury in the chest. With rapid scanners, a single-pass acquisition may, thus, require a compromise in scan timing or a larger bolus of IV contrast.

Reduce mAs when possible

Image noise requirements and, thus, radiation exposure requirements depend on the diagnostic task at hand and the clinical question to be answered. It is possible to tolerate increased levels of image noise when assessing intrinsically high-contrast structures for which the tissue or pathologic condition of interest is of substantially different attenuation than the surrounding

structures. Evaluations of the lung, CTA, and renal stones are the prototypical examples in which reduced mAs may be used, allowing the radiologist to differentiate a high-density structure of interest from the background despite an increase in image noise. Conversely, low-dose imaging may be detrimental in inherently low-contrast applications, such as liver lesion detection in which the target lesion is of similar density to the background.

Pulmonary nodules stand out against the background air-filled lungs, so scans performed specifically for this reason may be performed at a substantially lower dose than those for a detailed assessment of mediastinal soft tissues. In CTA, successful IV contrast administration creates high-density vascular enhancement against a soft tissue or air background. In ureter CT, high-density renal stones are easy to visualize against the soft tissue density background even at a greatly reduced dose.[44] However, it is important to clearly define the scope of the desired scan; The author's group has not reduced the mAs in routine ED ureter CT scans because it is common to find alternate diagnoses accounting for symptoms when no stones are found.

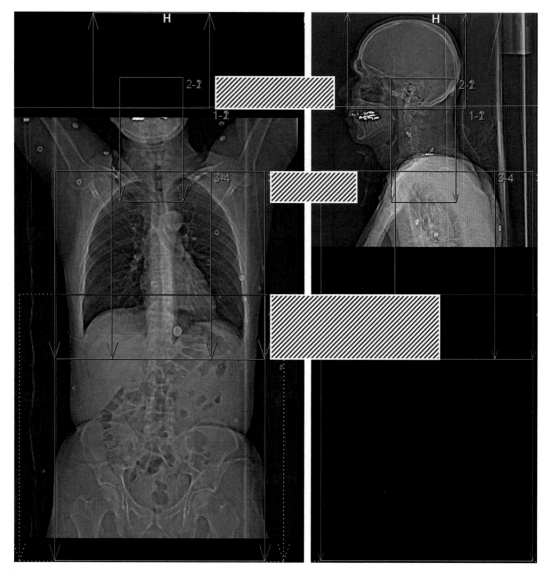

Fig. 5. Overlap between adjacent scan regions in a trauma pan-scan of the head, cervical spine, chest, abdomen, and pelvis. Thin-line boxes denote separately prescribed scan parts, with arrows indicating the direction of scanning. Crosshatched regions indicate areas of overlap that may be reduced with technologist directives or protocol modifications that combine adjacent parts into a single scan.

As a general strategy, practices may systematically reduce radiation dose by incrementally decreasing mAs for select protocols or clinical indications to gradually approach the threshold at which diagnostic confidence is maintained despite noisier images. In seeking the lower end of this comfort zone, incremental 10% to 20% reductions in mAs are reasonable step sizes because these will result in minor increases in image noise by approximately 5% to 10%.

Optimize IV contrast infusions
Any intervention that increases the inherent contrast-to-noise ratio between the target and the background can enable further x-ray tube output reduction by offsetting the increased noise with an increase in the inherent image contrast. For vascular examinations, careful attention to optimizing IV contrast infusion parameters[45] may routinely increase vascular enhancement, thus, increasing the inherent contrast-to-noise ratio and enabling subsequent reduction in x-ray tube output.

Reduce kVp for CTA
Iodine attenuates lower-energy x-rays far more strongly than higher-energy x-rays, resulting in higher Hounsfield units (HU) at lower kVp for

the same underlying concentration of iodine, as shown in **Fig. 6**. At the same time, lowering kVp substantially reduces radiation exposure if mAs is unchanged. This combination of increased enhancement at a lower dose is an ideal synergy for contrast-enhanced CTA examinations and, in patients who are small enough, it may be used to improve image quality, reduce radiation exposure, reduce administered IV contrast volume, or any combination of the 3.

Fig. 7 demonstrates the use of these methods to optimize CT pulmonary angiograms. For patients below an approximate size threshold of 175 pounds, the author uses 100 kVp and a reduced volume and flow rate of IV contrast material. To maintain constant image noise, one would technically need to increase x-ray tube output (mAs) at lower kVp because a greater fraction of the lower-energy x-rays are absorbed. However, the author instead leaves the TCM reference mAs unchanged and tolerates the associated increase

in image noise in these scans, relying on the kVp reduction to preserve or increase vascular enhancement despite a concurrent reduction in total IV contrast volume.

It is important to note that low kVp imaging should not be performed indiscriminately for patients of all sizes because the increase in image noise is simply too great in very large patients. Attempting to correct for this noise increase by increasing mAs is only possible to a point because inherent engineering system limits come into play in the form of a maximum achievable x-ray tube current. When performing CTA examinations with reduced kVp, appropriate size thresholds will depend on the scanner capabilities. A threshold may be chosen based on patient weight or body mass index, physical dimensions, or measures of patient attenuation.[46,47] A new development is the automated selection of kVp by the CT scanner based on the topogram-measured attenuation of the patient (in analogy to TCM adjustment of mAs

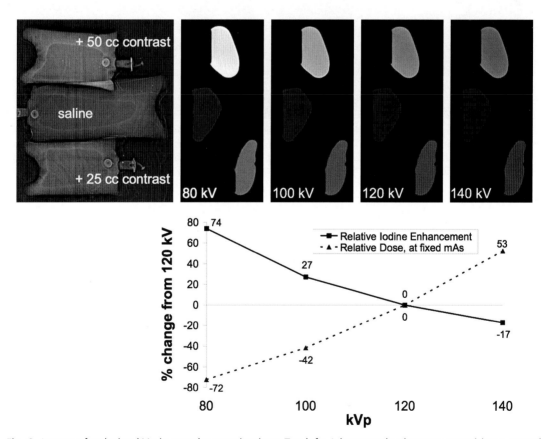

Fig. 6. Impact of reducing kVp in vascular examinations. Top left: A homemade phantom comprising a central bag of saline and 2 peripheral bags of saline containing different iodine concentrations. Top right: Images were obtained with fixed mAs at different kVp values from 80 to 140 on a Sensation 64 scanner (Siemens, Forchheim, Germany). The graph at bottom shows relative iodine enhancement (*solid line*) at each kVp and relative changes in CTDI$_{vol}$ (*dashed line*) normalized to the values at 120 kVp. For vascular examinations in small enough patients, lowering kVp increases iodine enhancement while decreasing dose.

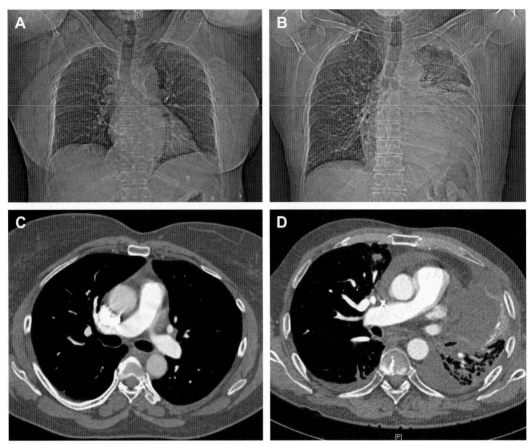

Fig. 7. CT pulmonary angiography examinations at different kVp in 2 patients of comparable size, both performed using automated TCM (CareDose4D, Siemens, Forchheim, Germany) with reference mAs of 200 on a Siemens AS+ scanner. Patient (*A, C*) was scanned at 120 kVp using an IV contrast infusion of 75 mL iopromide 370 (Bayer, Berlin, Germany) at 5 mL/s, followed by a 40-mL saline flush at 5 mL/s. Patient (*B, D*) was scanned at 100 kVp using an IV contrast infusion of 50 mL iopromide 370 at 4 mL/s, followed by a 40-mL saline flush at 4 mL/s. Automated TCM detects similar attenuation for both patients, resulting in an average effective mAs of 276 (*C*) and 272 (*D*). However, the decrease to 100 kVp results in a 42% reduction in $CTDI_{vol}$ from 18.6 to 10.7 mGy. Although (*D*) is slightly noisier than (*C*), image quality remains excellent despite the 33% decrease in administered IV contrast. These high flow-rate contrast infusions work well for breath-hold scan durations less than 9 to 10 seconds but require accurate triggering at the beginning of the contrast enhancement curve. The author uses automated bolus tracking with a region of interest in the main pulmonary artery and a trigger value of 80 HU above unenhanced blood.

values), which has the advantages of directly detecting patient attenuation and adjusting the CT technique to maintain an image quality criterion of choice while ensuring that fundamental CT system limits are respected.[48,49]

External shielding: should it be used?
A common question is whether bismuth breast shields should be used to reduce dose to these radiation-sensitive organs. Proponents point to substantive dose reduction to the breast from the use of overlying shields, whereas opponents argue that the shields introduce noise and artifacts and

that similar dose reduction and image quality can be achieved by lowering the overall scan mAs.[50] Regardless, if overlying shields are used, it is vitally important to use them correctly. The shields must be placed after the planning scout views. Because all manufacturers use the scout images to plan TCM, the placement of shields before the scouts cause the scanner to compensate by increasing x-ray output to penetrate the additional detected attenuation. For the same reason, shields should not be used on scanners with real-time adjustments of the axial TCM because this too will result in an undesired increase in exposure to the patient.

REDUCING RADIATION EXPOSURE: AFTER THE SCAN
Postprocessing Methods to Decrease Noise

There are a variety of postprocessing methods that can be used to reduce image noise. These methods can be used to improve image quality for a given acquisition. Conversely, the scans may be performed with reduced radiation exposure using postprocessing techniques to bring image noise back to desired levels, assuming the postprocessed images are considered of adequate quality when judged on features beyond simply noise levels. In this way, these postprocessing methods may be used in synergy with the acquisition strategies listed previously.

Reconstruct with Smoother Kernels

The use of smoother kernels reduces image noise, as in the noticeable difference between images reconstructed using a soft tissue algorithm versus a bone algorithm. The inevitable tradeoff is in the loss of fine edge detail. Nonetheless, this may be a helpful strategy to salvage noisy images, such as those obtained in patients who are obese.[51]

Reconstruct at Larger Slice Thickness

Image noise is proportional to the square root of the number of x-rays contributing to image creation. Because the number of x-rays scales with slice thickness, image noise is proportional to the square root of the slice thickness if all other parameters are unchanged in image acquisition and reconstruction. For this reason, 1-mm thick images will contain twice as much noise as 4-mm thick images if reconstructed from the same raw data and with the same reconstruction algorithm. For this reason, one should use caution in moving to thinner and thinner slices if they are not truly needed for the diagnostic task at hand.

Iterative Reconstruction

There has been substantive recent effort from all of the major CT manufacturers to develop a class of advanced postprocessing methods loosely grouped under the name iterative reconstruction. Theoretically, iterative reconstruction transforms back and forth between the raw data projection space and the image domain with successive steps of filtered back projection (converting raw data to images) and forward projection (converting images back to raw data). During each iteration, the newly simulated raw data is compared with the acquired raw data, and nonlinear processing is used to correct differences related to image noise and artifacts until a close enough match is achieved.[52]

However, most manufacturers have implemented more rapid shortcut algorithms designed to achieve similar ends because this theoretical approach would require tremendous computer processing power. Implementation details vary between manufacturers but generally involve a variety of algorithms to shift some of the iterative correction steps purely into the raw data or image domains, combined with advanced modeling of the CT acquisition system, and nonlinear image filtering to reduce noise in homogeneous regions while attempting to preserve anatomic edge information.

The somewhat different texture of the resultant images may require some acclimatization on the part of radiologists. However, if resultant image quality is deemed satisfactory, the noise-reduction effect may enable substantial reductions in radiation exposure, with initial reports suggesting possible dose reductions of 30% to 50%.[53]

AFTER THE SCAN: CAPTURING AND MONITORING RADIATION DOSES

The commonly available dose-screen reports are helpful for scan-by-scan monitoring but are not routinely database accessible for large-scale quality improvement and dose-monitoring efforts.[54] Ongoing implementations of standardized Digital Imaging and Communication in Medicine Radiation Dose Structured Reports[55] and other components of the Integrating the Health care Enterprise Radiation Exposure Monitoring Profile[56] promise to help these efforts prospectively after widespread adoption. In the meantime, efforts are underway in many institutions to extract patient- and examination-specific exposure information from historical examinations available on PACS through the use of optical character recognition techniques.[57]

Combining radiation exposure magnitudes with the knowledge of the anatomic region scanned and of the size of the patient will ultimately enable patient-centric longitudinal dose monitoring and radiation risk estimation. The integration of this information into the electronic medical record or incorporation into point-of-care decision support tools may ultimately prove beneficial in risk/benefit decision making and in improving the understanding of the magnitude of risk both by physicians and patients.

SUMMARY

Many tools and strategies exist to enable the reduction of radiation exposure from CT. Available hardware and software tools continue to evolve, and it is vitally important to learn exactly what tools are available on one's CT system and how to configure these tools properly to achieve safe and effective results. Numerous CT protocol optimization strategies have been outlined that may be used in synergy with one another and with the available technology to create robust, high-quality CT protocols with radiation exposure appropriate for the clinical setting and the size of the patient. Successful implementation requires primary engagement from the radiologist, ideally in collaboration with CT manufacturers, CT technologists, and medical physicists.

REFERENCES

1. Benchmark report CT 2007. IMV Medical Information Division. Des Plaines (IL): IMV Medical Information Division; 2007.
2. Brenner DJ, Hall EJ. Computed tomography–an increasing source of radiation exposure. N Engl J Med 2007;357(22):2277–84.
3. Sodickson A, Baeyens PF, Andriole KP, et al. Recurrent CT, cumulative radiation exposure, and associated radiation-induced cancer risks from CT of adults. Radiology 2009;251(1):175–84.
4. Berrington de Gonzalez A, Mahesh M, Kim KP, et al. Projected cancer risks from computed tomographic scans performed in the United States in 2007. Arch Intern Med 2009;169(22):2071–7.
5. Mettler FA, Bhargavan M, Faulkner K, et al. Radiologic and nuclear medicine studies in the United States and worldwide: frequency, radiation dose, and comparison with other radiation sources–1950-2007. Radiology 2009;253(2):520–31.
6. Fazel R, Krumholz HM, Wang Y, et al. Exposure to low-dose ionizing radiation from medical imaging procedures. N Engl J Med 2009;361(9):849–57.
7. Amis ES, Butler PF, Applegate KE, et al. American College of Radiology white paper on radiation dose in medicine. J Am Coll Radiol 2007;4(5):272–84.
8. Wells PS, Anderson DR, Rodger M, et al. Excluding pulmonary embolism at the bedside without diagnostic imaging: management of patients with suspected pulmonary embolism presenting to the emergency department by using a simple clinical model and d-dimer. Ann Intern Med 2001;135(2):98–107.
9. Stiell IG, Wells GA, Vandemheen K, et al. The Canadian CT head rule for patients with minor head injury. Lancet 2001;357(9266):1391–6.
10. Stiell IG, Wells GA, Vandemheen KL, et al. The Canadian C-spine rule for radiography in alert and stable trauma patients. JAMA 2001;286(15):1841.
11. Khorasani R. Can radiology professional society guidelines be converted to effective decision support? J Am Coll Radiol 2010;7(8):561–2.
12. American College of Radiology. ACR appropriateness criteria. Available at: http://www.acr.org/secondarymain menucategories/quality_safety/app_criteria.aspx. Accessed June 8, 2011.
13. Griffey RT, Sodickson A. Cumulative radiation exposure and cancer risk estimates in emergency department patients undergoing repeat or multiple CT. AJR Am J Roentgenol 2009;192(4):887–92.
14. Birnbaum S. Radiation safety in the era of helical CT: a patient-based protection program currently in place in two community hospitals in New Hampshire. J Am Coll Radiol 2008;5(6):714–718.e5.
15. Sodickson A, Opraseuth J, Ledbetter S. Outside imaging in emergency department transfer patients: CD import reduces rates of subsequent imaging utilization. Radiology 2011;260(2):408–13.
16. Massachusetts Medical Society. Investigation of defensive medicine in Massachusetts. 2008. Available at: www.massmed.org/defensivemedicine. Accessed September 9, 2011.
17. Levin DC, Rao VM. The effect of self-referral on utilization of advanced diagnostic imaging. AJR Am J Roentgenol 2011;196(4):848–52.
18. McNitt-Gray MF. AAPM/RSNA physics tutorial for residents: topics in CT. Radiation dose in CT. Radiographics 2002;22(6):1541–53.
19. American Association of Physicists in Medicine. The measurement, reporting and management of radiation dose in CT. Report 96. AAPM task group 23 of the diagnostic imaging council CT Committee. College Park (MD): American Association of Physicists in Medicine; 2008.
20. McCollough CH, Leng S, Yu L, et al. CT dose index and patient dose: they are not the same thing. Radiology 2011;259(2):311–6.
21. Turner AC, Zhang D, Khatonabadi M, et al. The feasibility of patient size-corrected, scanner-independent organ dose estimates for abdominal CT exams. Med Phys 2011;38(2):820–9.
22. Huda W, Vance A. Patient radiation doses from adult and pediatric CT. AJR Am J Roentgenol 2007; 188(2):540.
23. AAPM task group 204. AAPM report 204: size-specific dose estimates (SSDE) in pediatric and adult body CT examinations 2011.
24. Shrimpton P. Assessment of patient dose in CT. Chilton, NRPB-PE/1/2004, 2004.
25. National Research Council (U.S.). Committee to Assess Health Risks from Exposure to Low Level of Ionizing Radiation. Health risks from exposure to low levels of ionizing radiation: BEIR VII, Phase 2. Palo Alto (CA); 2006.

26. McCollough CH, Christner JA, Kofler JM. How effective is effective dose as a predictor of radiation risk? AJR Am J Roentgenol 2010;194(4): 890–6.

27. Padilla A, Alquist EK. California senate bill 1237. 2010. Available at: http://info.sen.ca.gov/pub/09-10/bill/sen/sb_1201-1250/sb_1237_bill_20100929_chaptered.html. Accessed September 9, 2011.

28. Center for Drug Evaluation and Research. Radiation dose reduction - white paper: initiative to reduce unnecessary radiation exposure from medical imaging. Available at: http://www.fda.gov/Radiation-EmittingProducts/RadiationSafety/RadiationDoseReduction/ucm199994.htm. Accessed December 24, 2010.

29. Bongartz G, Golding SJ, Jurik AG, et al. European guidelines for multislice computed tomography; 2004. Available at: http://www.msct.eu/CT_Quality_Criteria.htm. Accessed June 8, 2011.

30. The American College Of Radiology. ACR Practice Guideline for Diagnostic Reference Levels in Medical X-Ray Imaging. 2008. Available at: www.acr.org/SecondaryMainMenuCategories/quality_safety/guidelines/med_phys/reference_levels.aspx. Accessed September 9, 2011.

31. Kalra MK, Maher MM, Toth TL, et al. Strategies for CT radiation dose optimization. Radiology 2004; 230(3):619.

32. McCollough CH, Primak AN, Braun N, et al. Strategies for reducing radiation dose in CT. Radiol Clin North Am 2009;47(1):27–40.

33. The alliance for radiation safety in pediatric imaging. Image gently. Available at: http://www.pedrad.org/associations/5364/ig/index.cfm?page=614. Accessed May 26, 2011.

34. Strauss KJ, Goske MJ, Kaste SC, et al. Image gently: ten steps you can take to optimize image quality and lower CT dose for pediatric patients. AJR Am J Roentgenol 2010;194(4):868.

35. Kalendar WA. Computed tomography. 3rd edition. Erlangen (Germany): Publicis Publishing; 2011.

36. McCollough CH, Bruesewitz MR, Kofler JM, et al. CT dose reduction and dose management tools: overview of available options. Radiographics 2006; 26(2):503–12.

37. Sodickson A, Turner AC, McGlamery K, et al. Variation in organ dose from abdomen-pelvis CT exams performed with tube current modulation (TCM): evaluation of patient size effects. Radiographic Society of North America 2010 annual meeting. Chicago (IL).

38. Israel GM, Cicchiello L, Brink J, et al. Patient size and radiation exposure in thoracic, pelvic, and abdominal CT examinations performed with automatic exposure control. AJR Am J Roentgenol 2010;195(6):1342.

39. FDA. Safety investigation of CT brain perfusion scans: update 11/9/2010. 2010. Available at: http://www.fda.gov/medicaldevices/safety/alertsandnotices/ucm185898.htm. Accessed June 6, 2011.

40. Chow LC, Kwan SW, Olcott EW, et al. Split-bolus MDCT urography with synchronous nephrographic and excretory phase enhancement. AJR Am J Roentgenol 2007;189(2):314.

41. Deak PD, Langner O, Lell M, et al. Effects of adaptive section collimation on patient radiation dose in multisection spiral CT. Radiology 2009; 252(1):140.

42. Ptak T, Rhea JT, Novelline RA. Radiation dose is reduced with a single-pass whole-body multi–detector row CT trauma protocol compared with a conventional segmented method: initial experience. Radiology 2003;229(3):902.

43. Nguyen D, Platon A, Shanmuganathan K, et al. Evaluation of a single-pass continuous whole-body 16-MDCT protocol for patients with polytrauma. AJR Am J Roentgenol 2009;192(1):3.

44. Poletti PA, Platon A, Rutschmann OT, et al. Low-dose versus standard-dose CT protocol in patients with clinically suspected renal colic. AJR Am J Roentgenol 2007;188(4):927.

45. Bae KT. Intravenous contrast medium administration and scan timing at CT: considerations and approaches. Radiology 2010;256(1):32.

46. Menke J. Comparison of different body size parameters for individual dose adaptation in body CT of adults. Radiology 2005;236(2):565.

47. Luaces M, Akers S, Litt H. Low kVp imaging for dose reduction in dual-source cardiac CT. Int J Cardiovasc Imaging 2009;25(S2):165–75.

48. Grant K, Schmidt B. CARE kV - Automated Dose-Optimized Selection of X-ray Tube Voltage. White Paper. Siemens; 2011. Available at: http://www.medical.siemens.com/siemens/en_US/gg_ct_FBAs/files/Case_Studies/CarekV_White_Paper.pdf. Accessed September 9, 2011.

49. Yu L, Li H, Fletcher JG, et al. Automatic selection of tube potential for radiation dose reduction in CT: a general strategy. Med Phys 2010;37(1): 234–43.

50. RSNA News. Research fuels debate over bismuth breast shields. 2011. Available at: http://www.rsna.org/Publications/rsnanews/May-2011/breast_shields_feature.cfm. Accessed June 9, 2011.

51. Modica MJ, Kanal KM, Gunn ML. The obese emergency patient: imaging challenges and solutions. Radiographics 2011;31(3):811–23.

52. Grant K, Flohr T. Iterative reconstruction in image space (IRIS). White Paper; 2010. Available at: http://www.medical.siemens.com/siemens/en_US/gg_ct_FBAs/files/brochures/IRIS_WhitePaper_v3.pdf. Accessed September 9, 2011.

53. Hara AK, Paden RG, Silva AC, et al. Iterative recon-struction technique for reducing body radiation dose at CT: feasibility study. AJR Am J Roentgenol 2009; 193(3):764.

54. Sodickson A, Khorasani R. Patient-centric radiation dose monitoring in the electronic health record: what are some of the barriers and key next steps? J Am Coll Radiol 2010;7(10):752–3.

55. Digital imaging and communication in medicine (DI-COM) supplement 127: CT radiation dose reporting (Dose SR). 2007. Available at: ftp://medical.nema. org/medical/dicom/final/sup127_ft.pdf. Accessed September 9, 2011.

56. Integrating the Healthcare Enterprise. IHE Radiology, Technical Framework Supplement: Radiation Expo-sure Monitoring (REM). 2010. Available at: http://www.ihe.net/Technical_Framework/upload/IHE_RAD_Suppl_REM_Rev2-1_TI_2010-11-16.pdf. Accessed September 9, 2011.

57. Cook TS, Zimmerman S, Maidment AD, et al. Auto-mated extraction of radiation dose information for CT examinations. J Am Coll Radiol 2010;7(11):871–7.

Updated Imaging of Traumatic Brain Injury

Wayne S. Kubal, MD

KEYWORDS

- Traumatic brain injury • Computed tomography
- Magnetic resonance imaging • Diffusion tensor imaging
- Magnetic resonance spectroscopy

Computed tomography (CT) is usually the initial imaging study performed on a patient with traumatic brain injury (TBI). Subsequent imaging with CT and magnetic resonance (MR) are also important for patient management. This article reviews the classic imaging findings in TBI and examines the impact of newer imaging modalities on the care of patients with TBI. The epidemiology of TBI is reviewed. We will then introduce the imaging modalities currently in use to evaluate TBI and to apply these modalities to the various forms of TBI. This discussion focuses on injuries to the brain and does not comment on injuries to the face, neck, or spine that are often present in the patient with TBI.

EPIDEMIOLOGY

TBI is a leading cause of death and disability in the United States. Each year in the United States 1.1 million patients are treated and released from an emergency department and approximately 50,000 die. Every year, 235,000 Americans are hospitalized for nonfatal TBI. Approximately 43% of patients with TBI discharged from acute hospitalizations develop TBI-related long-term disability.[1] Both the direct and indirect economic impacts of these traumatic brain injuries on society are considerable, because those at greatest risk are typically young.

Major risk factors for TBI in the United States are age, gender, and low socioeconomic status. Children and the elderly have the highest rates: 900 per 100,000 for those younger than 10 years and 659 per 100,000 for those older than 74 years.

The rate among men is nearly twice that of women. The propensity for men to incur TBI could be attributed to risk-taking behavior and high-risk activities commonly engaged in by men. Generally, injury occurs more often among persons with low socioeconomic status.[1]

The mortality from TBI is related to the severity of brain injury as determined by the initial Glasgow Coma Scale (GCS) score. The GCS score is the sum of 3 components: the best eye opening response, the best motor response, and the best verbal response. A GCS score of 7 or less represents severe injury, requiring emergent imaging and possible emergent neurosurgery. A score between 8 and 14 represents a moderate injury, also requiring emergent imaging, and a normal GCS score of 15 represents a mild injury that may be managed conservatively.[2] In a large, traumatic coma databank study, patients with severe injury had approximately 36% mortality, whereas, in another study, patients with moderate injury showed a mortality of approximately 2% to 3%.[3,4] Persistent morbidity is also related to the severity of the TBI. A study of patients with moderate injury showed that 96% had symptoms after 3 months, the most common symptoms being headache and memory difficulty.[4] In a different group of patients with mild injury, 84% had persistent symptoms after 3 months.[5] New imaging modalities have provided new prognostic information, but it remains difficult to predict the functional outcome of an individual following TBI.

Approximately 52,000 deaths each year in the United States are attributed to TBI. During

The author has nothing to disclose.
Department of Radiology, University of Arizona Health Sciences Center, Room 1369, 1501 North Campbell Avenue, PO Box 245067, Tucson, AZ 85724, USA
E-mail address: wkubal@email.arizona.edu

Radiol Clin N Am 50 (2012) 15–41
doi:10.1016/j.rcl.2011.08.010

the last few decades, the incidence and mortality for TBI have declined.[6] The decline in incidence may in part be caused by improved safety equipment and its increased usage. The mortalities are heterogeneous and are significantly influenced by local factors such as the nature of the traumatic event, the care in the field provided by emergency medical services, and the hospital care provided. The mortality associated with TBI has declined because of improved imaging and improved treatment. In the 1950s, monitoring of intracranial pressure showed that a sustained pressure increase was correlated with a poor outcome. In the 1970s, emergent CT revolutionized early diagnosis in patients with TBI. CT helps to define the primary injury and, if necessary, to guide surgical intervention.

No good set of clinical criteria has been firmly established to predict which patients will have intracranial abnormalities. Some patients with mild injury by GCS triage may have significant injuries requiring neurosurgical intervention. In one study of patients with minor head trauma and normal GCS score, researchers evaluated the usefulness of 4 risk factors: severe headache, nausea, vomiting, and depressed skull fracture. They found CT abnormalities, judged to be clinically insignificant, in 3.7% of patients with no risk factors; all patients requiring neurosurgery had at least 1 risk factor.[7] In another review, investigators reached a different conclusion: "no set of clinical predictors have yet been put together that is capable of identifying all patients who are safe to be discharged without a CT scan."[8]

The goals of emergent imaging of TBI are, in order of acuity, to allow life-threatening injuries to be rapidly diagnosed and treated, to explain the findings on neurologic examination, and, if possible, to establish prognosis for the patient. CT fulfills the first imaging goal in most cases. MR is indicated when CT fails to fulfill the second imaging goal of explaining neurologic findings. Clinical findings, CT, MR, and, in some cases, advanced imaging each contribute to help to establish patient prognosis.

Emergent CT provides essential information for guiding clinical management, especially in the acute phase of TBI. However, cellular injury, which is likely to be associated with neuropsychological dysfunction, cannot be directly visualized with CT imaging. The goals of follow-up imaging are to aid in the management of the complications of the initial traumatic injury and to provide prognostic information regarding the long-term status of the patient.

IMAGING MODALITIES

CT uses the principle of differential x-ray beam attenuation. The CT scanner x-ray beam is rotated over multiple angles to acquire differential attenuation patterns across the various tissues through a single axial slice through a patient's body. The data is mathematically analyzed to obtain the attenuation value for each pixel within a CT slice. CT is widely available, fast, and is sensitive for the detection and evaluation of injuries requiring acute neurosurgical intervention.[9] It is the primary imaging modality for deciding whether a patient requires surgical or medical treatment. Modern CT scanners use multiple rows of detectors (multi-row-detector CT [MDCT]) and are able to obtain multiple axial slices with 1 rotation of the gantry. The multidetector technology has increased the speed of imaging, so that a patient's entire head can be scanned within a few seconds. Special dose-reduction algorithms should be implemented for pediatric patients. Decreasing the radiation dose is achievable, theoretically decreases the cancer risk, and, if properly done, does not increase the missed injury rate.[10]

The CT data sets can be postprocessed to yield two-dimensional (2-D) or three-dimensional (3-D) reformatted images. 2-D reformatted images in the coronal and/or sagittal planes have become standard in many emergency departments. 3-D surface-rendered images are particularly useful for the detection and characterization of skull and facial fractures.

The rapid speed of modern MDCT scanners has made possible CT angiography (CTA). Iodinated contrast is injected intravenously at a rate of 3 to 5 mL/s. Thin, typically overlapping, CT sections are obtained through the vessel of interest following the contrast bolus. 2-D and 3-D reformatted images are a standard part of the evaluation. CTA has been shown to be useful in the diagnosis of suspected vascular injuries such as pseudoaneurysm, dissection, fistula, and thrombosis.

CT perfusion (CTP) allows the noninvasive evaluation of the tissue perfusion. Rather than following the bolus of intravenous contrast through a vascular territory, continuous scanning of a single slice or contiguous slices can yield time-density curves for each pixel within the image. The passage of the contrast bolus through the brain is analyzed to measure the time to peak density (TTP), the mean transit time (MTT), the cerebral blood volume (CBV), and the cerebral blood flow (CBF). The contrast dose is typically less than that used for CTA. Limitations of this technique include limited coverage and a high radiation dose. CTP is widely used for the evaluation of stroke and intracranial neoplasm. It can provide prognostic information about patients with severe TBI, but it has not found widespread usage for the evaluation of acute TBI.[11]

MR uses the response of protons within biologic tissues to an applied magnetic field. The response is a faint electromagnetic signal of much lower energy than that of x-rays. A major advantage of MR is the lack of ionizing radiation. The signal is received by a coil and is mathematically analyzed to obtain an image. Although CT is the initial imaging study of choice in the evaluation of acute TBI, MR may be indicated if the patient's neurologic status is not explained by the findings on CT. MR may not be available in all trauma centers at all times of the day or night. Other limitations include longer scan times and incompatibility with pacemakers and metallic foreign bodies within the brain or the orbit. Standard sequences such as T1-weighted, T2-weighted, and fluid-attenuated inversion recovery (FLAIR) are usually performed as part of the examination.

Gradient recalled echo (GRE) sequences are sensitive to multiple blood breakdown products. These blood products cause a magnetic susceptibility artifact within the tissue of interest and show the blood products as a blooming focus of low signal intensity. Because of its sensitivity to magnetic susceptibility artifact, these sequences are limited by the presence of metal, such as dental hardware (**Fig. 1**), and are limited by the susceptibility artifact at tissue-air interfaces. Signals from substances with different magnetic susceptibilities compared with their neighboring tissue become out of phase with these tissues. Thus, the phase information offers a means of enhancing contrast in MR.[12] This technique is called susceptibility-weighted (SW) imaging. SW imaging has been shown to be more sensitive than GRE for detection of hemorrhage. A limitation is that SW imaging sequences take longer to perform than GRE.

MR angiography (MRA) creates intensity differences between moving (ie, flowing) protons and stationary tissue protons through the use of specialized gradients. The data can be reformatted in either 2-D or 3-D representations of vascular structures.

Diffusion-weighted (DW) imaging is based on the Brownian motion of water molecules. DW imaging can detect changes in the rate of microscopic water motion. Water molecules within the ventricles diffuse freely, whereas water molecules within the cells have their diffusion restricted by cell membranes, organelles, and macromolecules. Water molecules within the extracellular space have an intermediate diffusion. When there is movement of water from the extracellular space to the intracellular space, the overall diffusion within that volume of tissue becomes more restricted. This restricted diffusion correlates with cytotoxic edema and allows for the early detection of acute stroke, acute diffuse axonal injury (DAI), and acute contusion.

Diffusion tensor imaging (DTI) is based on the way microscopic water diffusion in white matter tracts tends to occur preferentially in 1 direction rather than equally in all directions. This directionality phenomenon is called anisotropy. For example, diffusion is less restricted along the direction of white matter tracts and is more restricted in a direction perpendicular to white matter tracts. The diffusion within white matter tracts is anisotropic, that is, the diffusion differs depending on direction. The degree of anisotropy in a white matter tract indicates the degree of structural integrity and health of the white matter.[9] The most commonly used measurement of anisotropy is fractional anisotropy (FA). The diffusion within the ventricles and within the gray matter is isotropic. The diffusion is independent of direction, there is little or no anisotropy, so the FA value is near zero. In normal, healthy white matter, diffusion is dependent on direction; there is high anisotropy, so the FA is high (**Fig. 2**). When it is damaged, white matter suffers a loss of integrity and a corresponding decrease in FA. Using a computational process called fiber tracking, the diffusion tensor data also allow major white matter tracts to be traced, and whether they are displaced or interrupted by TBI can be assessed (**Figs. 3** and **4**).

MR spectroscopy allows the chemical environment of the brain to be examined noninvasively. A voxel of tissue is selected and the spectrum obtained shows the relative abundance of various metabolites within the selected voxel. At least 3 main metabolites should be evaluated in any spectrum. The metabolites are identified by their individual chemical shift as measured in parts per million (ppm) relative to a reference standard. At 2.0 ppm N-acetyl aspartate (NAA) is a marker for neuronal health and integrity. The creatine peak at 3.0 ppm creatine consists of protons involved in the creatine kinase reaction, which is basic to cellular energy metabolism. At 3.2 ppm, the choline peak consists of protons found in the phospholipid bilayer of cell membranes (**Fig. 5**). The heights of the various peaks correspond with their relative abundance in the selected voxel. When interpreting the MR spectrum, comparisons are made with the creatine peak because it tends to be the most stable in a variety of conditions.

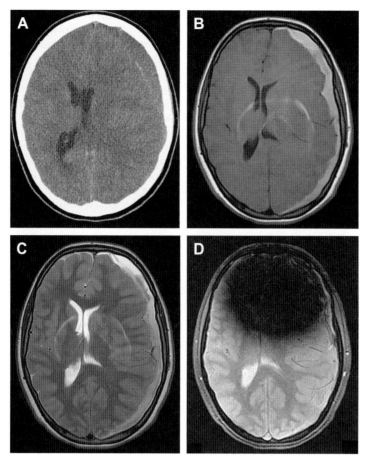

Fig. 1. Isodense subdural hematoma (SDH), artifact from dental hardware. (*A*) Noncontrast CT shows shift of midline structures toward the right. There is an isodense extra-axial collection in the left frontoparietal region consistent with a subacute SDH. It can be recognized by the displacement of cranium matter away from the inner table of the skull. (*B*) Noncontrast and axial T1-weighted MR shows the extent of the extra-axial collection better than does CT. Note the artifact within the center of this image it is from the patient's dental hardware. (*C*) Axial T2-weighted MR shows mild heterogeneity within the panhemispheric SDH. Also noted are cortical veins traversing the subdural space. (*D*) Axial GRE shows a large bifrontal artifact from the patient's dental hardware. GRE sequences are very sensitive to the susceptibility artifact from a metal or blood breakdown products.

The normal NAA peak is nearly twice the height of the creatine peak, whereas the normal choline peak is only slightly smaller than the creatine peak. In brain injury, the NAA peak is typically decreased. There may also be an increase in the choline peak (**Fig. 6**).

Primary and Secondary Brain Injury

Primary brain injury results from the direct application of an external force to the cranium and intracranial contents. When these forces strain the cerebral tissue beyond its structural tolerance, injury results. The injury pattern often reflects the type of strain, which may be compressive, tensile, or shear in nature. Brain contusion occurs at the point of impact as a result of compressive strain.

A subdural hematoma (SDH) may present as a contrecoup injury opposite the point of impact because of a tensile strain placed on the cortical veins. DAI usually occurs at the junction of gray and white matter and is caused by shear strains resulting from rotational acceleration.[13]

Secondary brain damage results from the post-traumatic pathophysiologic cascade that follows the initial injury and contributes to delayed tissue injury and neuronal loss.[14] The initial mechanical disruption of the brain and its vasculature is followed during the first week by cellular damage, the development of edema, and the liquefaction of the hematoma if one is present. Understanding of these processes has been enhanced by recent studies using MR spectroscopy. MR spectroscopy allows the noninvasive measurement of the

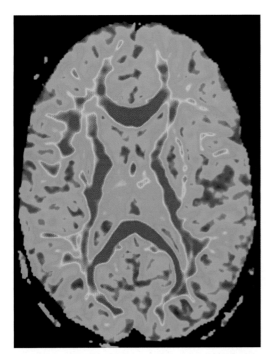

Fig. 2. Normal fractional isotropy. Axial image from an FA map shows normal white matter. The FA is coded by color; portions of the brain with high anisotropy such as white matter tracts appear red, whereas areas of the brain with low anisotropy appear blue. Note that the corpus callosum and internal capsule appear red whereas the cerebrospinal fluid within the ventricles and the gray matter appear blue.

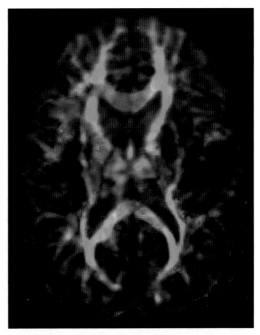

Fig. 3. Normal DTI. DTI shows the major white matter tracts as regions of high anisotropy within the brain. The direction of the white matter tracts is coded by color. White matter tracts running transversely are colored red; white matter tracts running anterior-posterior are colored green; white matter tracts running superior-inferior are colored blue.

concentrations of metabolites in the brain. The most common MR spectroscopy abnormality noted in patients with TBI is a decrease in NAA. Because NAA is a metabolite that marks activity in both neurons and axons, NAA depletion within gray matter is interpreted as evidence of neuronal injury, whereas NAA depletion within white matter is interpreted as evidence of axonal injury.[15] Another common MR spectroscopy finding is the increase of choline. This compound is one of the breakdown products of myelin and cellular membranes.[9] Several studies have shown that MR spectroscopy findings, such as decreased NAA, help to predict long-term neurologic outcomes in both pediatric and adult patients with TBI.[16,17] A longitudinal MR spectroscopy study conducted in patients with mild to moderate TBI showed decreased NAA on the initial examination performed 1 week after injury. Subsequent examination at 1 month following injury showed improvement in the NAA. The regions of brain sampled for the MR spectroscopy were normal on imaging sequences.[18]

During the last several years, multiple articles have appeared in the popular press about concussion. Concussion is poorly defined, but is thought to be associated with posttraumatic physical, cognitive, and sleep alterations. These symptoms comprise the so-called postconcussive syndrome, which usually resolves spontaneously within 7 to 10 days after injury. By GCS triage,

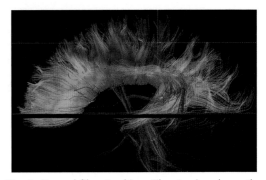

Fig. 4. Normal fiber tracking. Fiber tracing shows the corpus callosum. The direction of the white matter tracts is coded by color as in the DTI. Tracts running transversely are colored red; tracts running anterior-posterior are colored green; tracts running superior-inferior are colored blue. (*Courtesy of* GE Medical Systems, Waukesha, WI; with permission.)

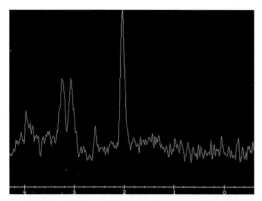

Fig. 5. Normal MR spectroscopy. A normal MR spectroscopy obtained in a normal area of brain. Note that the NAA peak at 2.0 ppm is twice the height of the creatine peak at 3.0 ppm. The choline peak at 3.2 ppm is the same height as the creatine peak.

these patients are considered as having mild TBI. Many of the popular press articles focused on sports-related concussive injury, with good reason. It is estimated that 20% of mild TBI is sports related.[19] Athletes represent a population at greater risk for recurrent concussive episodes. After the first traumatic episode, the probability of recurrence of concussion in athletes increases threefold.[20] This phenomenon is the so-called second-impact syndrome. Recently, MR spectroscopy performed both in laboratory animals and in clinical populations has given quantifiable metabolic validity to the second-impact syndrome. Following any concussive episode,

a period of metabolic abnormality occurs within brain tissue. During this transient period of altered brain metabolism, a second concussive episode of even modest intensity may cause a significant addition to the metabolic abnormality or cause even more extensive brain damage. Identification of this vulnerable period is important when deciding when athletes may safely return to action.

A population of rodents was divided into multiple groups. One group served as a control. One group received a single mild TBI. Another group received 2 mild TBIs separated by 5 days, and another group received 2 mild TBIs separated by 3 days. All of the rodents were sacrificed and their brains were analyzed to measure the level of NAA. Each of the traumatized groups showed decreased NAA compared with the control. The group with a single trauma showed 27% decreased NAA compared with control; the group with multiple traumas separated by 5 days showed a similar decrease in NAA. The group that received multiple traumas separated by 3 days showed 58% decrease in NAA compared with control.[21] These data support the hypothesis that the severity of the biochemical abnormality within brain tissue in a double TBI depends on the interval between traumatic events. The data also confirm the presence of a metabolically vulnerable period. Following TBI, the rodents were able to recover within 5 days so that the second injury had no additive or synergistic effect. The vulnerable period for this rodent population seems to be between 3 and 5 days.

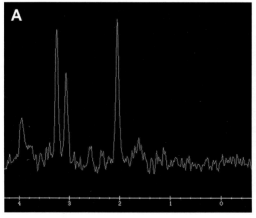
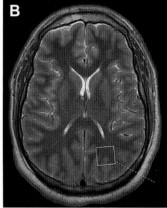

Fig. 6. Subacute TBI, MR spectroscopy. (A) MR spectroscopy was obtained 12 days following TBI. The NAA peak at 2.0 ppm is mildly depressed. A normal NAA peak would be approximately twice the height of the creatine peak seen at 3.0 ppm. The most striking abnormality of this spectrum is the increased choline peak seen at 3.2 ppm. A normal choline peak would be slightly shorter than the creatine peak. (B) The axial T2-weighted image indicates the voxel sampled for the MR spectroscopy. Note the normal appearance of the brain in the left occipital lobe. MR spectroscopy often shows metabolic abnormalities in portions of the brain that are structurally normal.

A cohort of athletes was studied with MR spectroscopy at 3 days, 15 days, and 30 days after concussive head injury. Athletes with a single concussive event showed a decrease in NAA of approximately 19% at 3 days after concussion. At 15 days, NAA was still decreased approximately 15%, and at 30 days the NAA had returned to normal. The athletes in this cohort self-declared complete resolution of symptoms within the first 3 days. A smaller subset of athletes suffered a second concussive injury between 3 and 15 days after the first. Their brains did not show a recovery of NAA but a further diminution of 22% compared with normal. Results of this study show that, in humans as well as laboratory animals, a concussive brain injury opens a temporal window of metabolic abnormality. The closure of this window does not coincide with the resolution of clinical symptoms, and the recovery of brain metabolism is nonlinear. The investigators suggest that noninvasive NAA measurement by MR spectroscopy may be a valid tool in assessing full cerebral metabolic recovery after concussion and may be useful in helping to decide when to allow athletes to return to full activity after TBI.[22]

Histology studies have also shown that repair also begins during the first week after injury. New blood vessels begin to proliferate at the margins of the injury. This neovascularity does not have an intact blood-brain barrier; therefore, contrast enhancement is seen on CT or MR. During the subacute period, microglial cells enter the areas of focal injury, phagocytize the blood products and damaged tissue, and remove them. If the area of injured brain is large, a cavitary area of cystic encephalomalacia lined by glial tissue may result; smaller areas of injury are likely to heal with a glial scar. Quantitative studies performed during the chronic period following moderate to severe TBI show widespread volume loss. These changes have been documented even in the absence of focal lesions. Clinically, these patients have decreased performance on standard neuropsychological tests.[23]

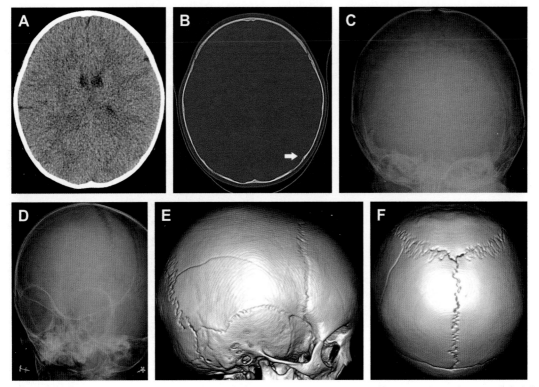

Fig. 7. Subtle linear skull fracture. (*A, B*) Noncontrast axial CT scans at brain and bone windows show a subtle left parietal region linear skull fracture. The fracture is seen just anterior to the left lambdoid suture (*arrow*). The underlying brain appears normal. This fracture could be missed on the axial CT. (*C, D*) Anteroposterior and oblique plain films of the skull show the fracture. (*E, F*) Lateral and top-down 3D surface-rendered projections of the skull are obtained from the CT data set removing the need for additional patient irradiation. They clearly show the linear fracture and its relationship to the normal sutures.

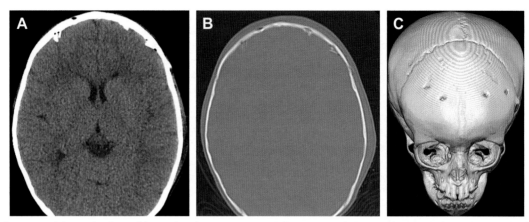

Fig. 8. Dog bite to the frontal bone. (*A, B*) Noncontrast axial CT scans at brain and bone windows show multiple small, depressed fractures involving the frontal bone with minimal underlying brain injury. (*C*) 3-D reformatted image shows the canine pattern of the 4 small depressed skull fractures. Further history revealed that the patient had been bitten by a dog. 3-D reformatted images can be useful in defining skull and facial fractures.

Extra-axial Injuries: Calvarial Fractures

The 3 main types of fractures are linear, depressed, and basilar fractures. Linear fractures are the most common and have the lowest incidence of associated intracranial injury. Linear fractures in the axial plane can easily be missed on axial CT examination. They may be better seen on plain film examination of the skull, but a better alternative is to obtain 3-D surface-rendered views from the CT data set (**Fig. 7**). The identification of nondisplaced linear fractures is aided by knowledge of the location and appearance of normal cranial sutures and synchondroses.

Depressed fractures are more commonly associated with intracranial injuries including contusions and dural tears. These injuries are typically surgically explored to diminish the risk of infection, to ascertain whether a dural tear is present, to remove bone fragments, and to elevate the fracture.[24] To produce a good cosmetic result, presurgical planning is enhanced by 3-D surface-rendered views (**Figs. 8** and **9**).

Basilar fractures are important because of associated injuries to cranial nerves and vessels adjacent to the skull base. Basilar skull fractures can be difficult to detect unless thin sections are obtained. When a basilar skull fracture is diagnosed, further imaging, typically with CTA, is worth considering to evaluate for a possible dissection, thrombosis, or pseudoaneurysm (**Fig. 10**).

Extra-axial Injuries: Anatomy of Fluid Spaces

The imaging appearance of posttraumatic fluid collections is best understood in relation to the

meningeal layers covering the brain. The pia is the deepest layer, covering the brain surface and lining the cortical gyri. It also lines the perforating vessels, forming a perivascular space, the Virchow-Robin space, which communicates with the subarachnoid space.[25] The subarachnoid space is the space between the arachnoid and

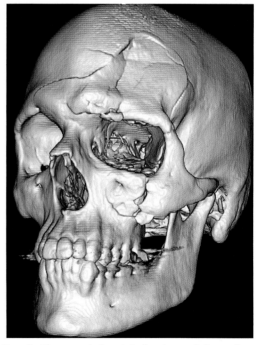

Fig. 9. Depressed frontal fracture. 3-D surface-rendered images of the skull and face are useful for depicting displaced fractures before repair.

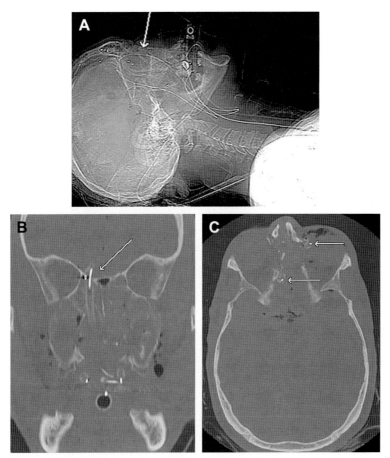

Fig. 10. Basilar skull fracture. (A) Lateral scout view of the head and neck shows malposition of an oral gastric tube (*arrow*). The tube extends above the skull base. (B) Coronal reformatted CT shows extensive injury including comminuted skull base fracture secondary to a self-inflicted gunshot wound. The orogastric tube extends intracranially through a defect in the skull base (*arrow*). (C) Axial CT shows a loop of the malpositioned tube within the left orbit and within the right frontal lobe (*arrows*). The patient's skull base fractures create an increased risk for malpositioning of orogastric or nasogastric tubes.

pia. In normal patients, this is a thin space containing a small amount of cerebrospinal fluid (CSF). The arachnoid is attached to the pia and to the brain surface by fine arachnoid trabeculations. The arachnoid follows the general contour of the brain, but does not extend into the sulci.

The subdural space lies between the inner layer of the dura and the underlying arachnoid. The subdural space normally contains a small amount of fluid, which differs only slightly from CSF. Bridging cortical veins traverse the subdural space. Because the dura is firmly attached to the skull and the arachnoid is attached to the cerebrum, most brain motion occurs across the subdural space, placing the bridging cortical veins at risk for tear.

The dura is a fibrous, 2-layer membrane that is peripheral to the arachnoid. The inner meningeal layer and outer periosteal layer are tightly bound to each other and to the skull. The 2 leaves of dura separate to enclose the venous sinuses. The falx and the tentorium are reflections of the dura. The meningeal layer has a rich capillary network that is responsible for the organization and resolution of SDH.[25] The potential space between the periosteal layer of the dura and the inner table of the skull is the epidural space. Running within the epidural space are branches of the middle meningeal artery. The periosteal layer is tightly adherent to the margins of the cranial sutures; therefore, most epidural fluid collections do not cross the suture margins.

This article divides posttraumatic hemorrhage into categories according to their location: subdural, epidural, subarachnoid, intraventricular, and intraparenchymal.

Extra-axial Injuries: SDH

SDHs are serosanguineous fluid collections within the subdural space. They are caused by rupture of the bridging veins (**Fig. 11**). The elderly and infants are particularly susceptible to this injury because their bridging veins are stretched. The elderly are likely to suffer from age-related volume loss, whereas, children less than 2 years of age may have benign enlargement of the subarachnoid spaces. Low-pressure venous bleeding separates the arachnoid from the dura, stretching the remaining intact veins, which may result in further venous rupture and enlargement of the hematoma. A SDH may be located at the point of direct impact, (ie, a coup injury) or opposite the point of direct impact, (ie, a contrecoup injury). Hemorrhage in these locations can be understood by considering the motion of the brain with respect to the skull and the subsequent rupture of the cortical veins. After initial impact, the brain moves back and forth with respect to the skull. This motion alternately stretches and compresses the cortical veins, leading to bleeding in coup and/or contrecoup locations.

Because of the loose connection between the arachnoid and the dura, a SDH spreads over a considerable area and usually has a crescent configuration overlying the convexity of the brain. SDH can also form along dural reflections such as the falx and the tentorium. Acutely, these collections usually have a uniform high density on CT, although approximately 40% have a heterogeneous density. Causes of the low-density regions within an SDH include unclotted blood in an early stage of hematoma development, serum extruded into the early phase of clot retraction, and CSF within the subdural space because of an arachnoid tear.[26]

The evolution of the CT appearance of SDH may vary depending on multiple patient factors. Within the first week, most are hyperdense on CT.[27] Their subsequent evolution is more complex, with most becoming isodense compared with brain within the second week and then showing a slow decrease in density (**Fig. 12**). Isodense SDHs may be more difficult to visualize on a CT scan; look for the inward buckling of the gray-white interface. Contrast enhancement can improve visualization on CT by showing displacement of cortical veins away from the inner table of the skull. SDHs are well seen by MR. MR can also indicate SDHs of varying age by showing blood in different oxidation states. This application is particularly useful in the evaluation of suspected nonaccidental trauma in a child. The identification of SDHs of differing densities on CT or differing signal intensities on MR do not meet the strict medical legal definition of traumatic events separated in time, but do suggest child abuse (see **Fig. 1**; **Fig. 13**).

The prognosis for patients with SDH is variable and is related to the extent of the primary underlying brain injury rather than the subdural clot itself. The volume of the SDH does not correlate with the patient's preoperative neurologic condition or the 6-month outcome.[28] Another study showed that the ability to control the intracranial pressure was more critical to patient outcome than the timing of the SDH removal.[29] A European study of patients with SDH attempted to correlate mass effect, brain swelling, and patient outcome. Comparing the amount of midline shift with the SDH thickness gave a rough quantitative measure of brain swelling. If the midline shift exceeded the SDH thickness by 3 mm, survival was 50%, but, when the midline shift exceeded the SDH thickness by 5 mm, survival was 25%.[30]

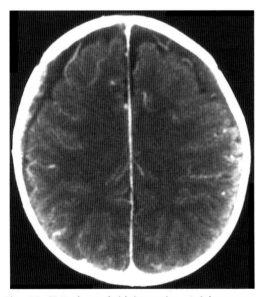

Fig. 11. SDH shows bridging veins. Axial contrast-enhanced CT shows bifrontal, low-density, extra-axial fluid collections compatible with chronic SDH. A more acute component is also present on the right. Note the enhancing bridging veins.

Extra-axial Injuries: Epidural Hematomas

Epidural hematomas (EDH) lie in the space between the inner table of the skull and the periosteal layer of dura. These layers are normally fully attached, but may be forcibly separated by direct traumatic impact, especially if there is an associated fracture. Most commonly, EDHs occur in the temporal and parietal regions where they arise from injuries to branches of the middle

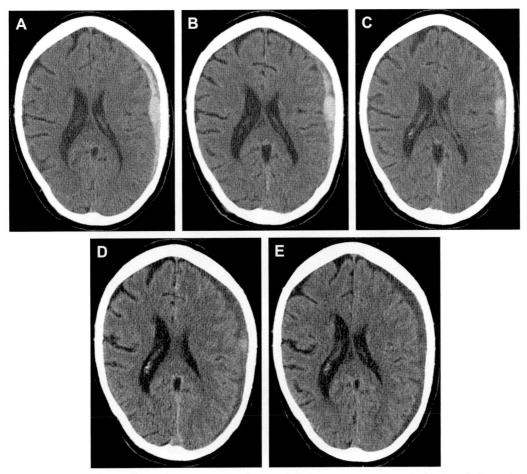

Fig. 12. Evolving SDH. (*A*) Initial noncontrast CT shows a mildly heterogeneous but predominantly hyperdense left SDH. (*B*) CT obtained 4 days after the initial study shows the SDH to be slightly less dense. (*C*) CT obtained 7 days after the initial study showed that portions of the SDH are now isodense to brain. (*D*) CT obtained 13 days after the initial study shows only a small focus of hyperdensity within the subdural collection. (*E*) CT obtained 19 days after the initial study shows the entire subdural collection to be hypodense compared with brain.

meningeal artery. This artery lies in a groove in the inner table of the skull and is thus vulnerable to injury, especially when a fracture is present.[8] EDHs generally result from severe head trauma and are found most commonly in young adults. The compliance of the skull in children, the firm attachment of the dura to the skull in the elderly, and the increased incidence of severe head trauma in young adults are factors contributing to this distribution of injury.

A venous EDH can occur when there has been disruption of a major venous sinus. Venous EDHs often involve a basilar fracture extending to the torcular Herophili or the transverse sinus. These hematomas are uncommon (15%) compared with the arterial EDH (85%) (**Fig. 14**).[24]

The CT appearance of both arterial and venous EDHs is that of a high-attenuation, biconvex, extra-axial collection. The biconvex shape results from the firm attachment of the dura to the inner table of the skull. The margins of the hematoma are limited by the bony sutures. Unlike SDHs, EDHs are not limited by the falx and tentorium. Careful examination of the CT at bone windows allows identification of a skull fracture in 90% or more of adults with an arterial EDH.[31] When acute, an EDH may have a heterogeneous appearance, which is a sign of active bleeding (**Fig. 15**). The low attenuation within the collection represents hyperacute, unclotted blood. Because of their high density, acute EDHs are usually well seen on CT. MR can also show these collections; however, MR is probably less sensitive for the identification of subtle associated skull fractures. MR can be useful for evaluation of other forms of brain injury that may be associated with epidural hematoma.

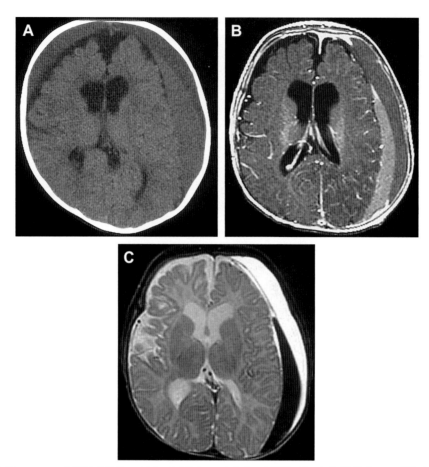

Fig. 13. Multicomponent SDH. (*A*) Noncontrast CT shows bilateral SDHs; the left SDH shows differing densities between 2 components. (*B*) T1-weighted contrast-enhanced MR obtained at a slightly different angle than the CT shows a multicomponent left extra-axial fluid collection compatible with SDH. (*C*) Axial noncontrast T2-weighted MR shows a multicomponent left SDH. SDHs may form membranes within the collection that separate components of differing ages and differing oxidation states. This information is important to the surgeon attempting to drain the SDH.

The symptoms caused directly by an EDH are from the mass effect of the collection, with the larger collections correlating with a higher incidence of coma. The classic clinical presentation of EDH is a brief initial period of unconsciousness, followed by a lucid interval, followed by rapid deterioration as the EDH increases in size. This classic sequence develops in a minority of patients, probably because of the clinical overlay of other associated brain injuries. Focal neurologic signs, such as ipsilateral pupillary dilatation and contralateral hemiparesis, may help to indicate the location of the hematoma.

Small EDHs may be managed conservatively, but 23% show enlargement within the first few days (**Fig. 16**).[32] Larger EDHs, hematomas associated with active bleeding, and hematomas associated with substantial mass effect are usually evacuated emergently. The goal is to remove the EDH before secondary ischemic changes can occur, but the prognosis is related to the degree of associated brain damage.

Extra-axial Injuries: Subarachnoid Hemorrhage

Subarachnoid hemorrhage (SAH) is common in patients with significant brain injury and can be diagnosed by imaging or lumbar puncture. Small SAHs usually result from injury to small cortical veins passing through the subarachnoid space. Larger SAHs can been seen when intraparenchymal hematomas extend to and dissect into the subarachnoid space. Even in this case, the volume of extravasated blood is rarely as large or as extensive as in aneurysmal SAH. Aneurysmal SAH also tends to be distributed centrally, commonly involving the suprasellar, interpeduncular, and

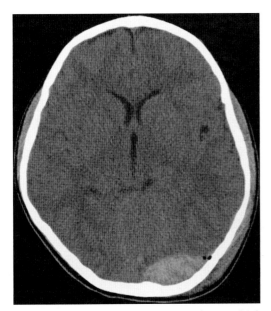

Fig. 14. Venous EDH. Noncontrast CT shows a high-density, biconvex, extra-axial collection in the left occipital region. Two small bubbles of air are noted adjacent to the lateral margin of this collection. The collection represents a venous SDH; the pneumocephalus is secondary to a temporal bone fracture.

prepontine cisterns, whereas posttraumatic SAH has a peripheral distribution.

Acute SAH is seen on CT as areas of high attenuation conforming to the sulcal spaces. Adjacent

contusion is common (**Fig. 17**). CT is more sensitive than spin-echo MR sequences for the detection of small amounts of subarachnoid hemorrhage, although FLAIR MR sequences have been shown to reliably detect acute subarachnoid hemorrhage.[33] If there is a question of SAH arising from an underlying lesion such as an aneurysm or vascular malformation, the patient can be further evaluated with CTA, MRA, or conventional catheter angiography.

SAH does not cause mass effect, but may cause vasospasm and ischemic parenchymal damage, especially in the subacute phase. Later, as the SAH clears, communicating hydrocephalus may result. The blood is phagocytized and transferred to the arachnoid villi. The arachnoid villi become distended and filled with phagocytes. They may become obliterated by the proliferation of connective tissue causing impaired absorption of CSF.

Intra-axial Injuries: Cerebral Contusion

Contusion is bruising of the brain caused by a direct contact and is most often seen at the point of impact. Capillary injury and edema are the result. Approximately 52% of contusions are hemorrhagic on MR,[34] but nearly all have associated microscopic hemorrhage. The hemorrhagic contusions can be seen on CT and MR; the nonhemorrhagic contusions are best seen acutely on DW imaging. When the brain moves relative to

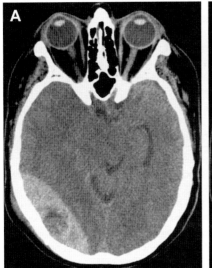
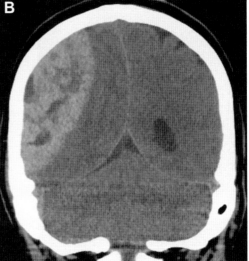

Fig. 15. EDH, subfalcine, and uncal herniation. (*A*) Noncontrast CT shows a high-density, biconvex, extra-axial fluid collection consistent with an acute EDH. The circular area of decreased density within the collection likely represents unclotted blood from active bleeding. Some investigators have termed this finding the swirl sign. There is considerable mass effect with herniation of the uncus of the hippocampus medially into the suprasellar cistern. (*B*) Coronal reformatted CT shows the extent of the EDH and the subfalcine herniation.

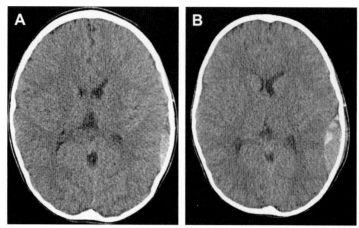

Fig. 16. Enlarging EDH. (*A*) Initial noncontrast CT shows a small left parietal biconvex extra-axial fluid collection compatible with an epidural hematoma. The heterogeneity in this collection may be secondary to active bleeding. (*B*) Noncontrast CT obtained 1 day after the initial CT shows enlargement of the collection, representing an enlarging epidural hematoma.

the skull, the inferior frontal lobes are at increased risk for cortical contusion as they slide over the irregular floor of the anterior cranial fossa (**Fig. 18**). The injury may be limited to the portions of the gyri adjacent to the skull with relative sparing of the underlying white matter. In patients with more severe injury, the volume and depth of tissue injury are greater and the small hemorrhages may coalesce into an intracerebral hematoma. The decision whether to evacuate the hematoma is complex, based in part on the amount of mass effect seen on imaging, the patient's intracranial pressure, and overall condition.

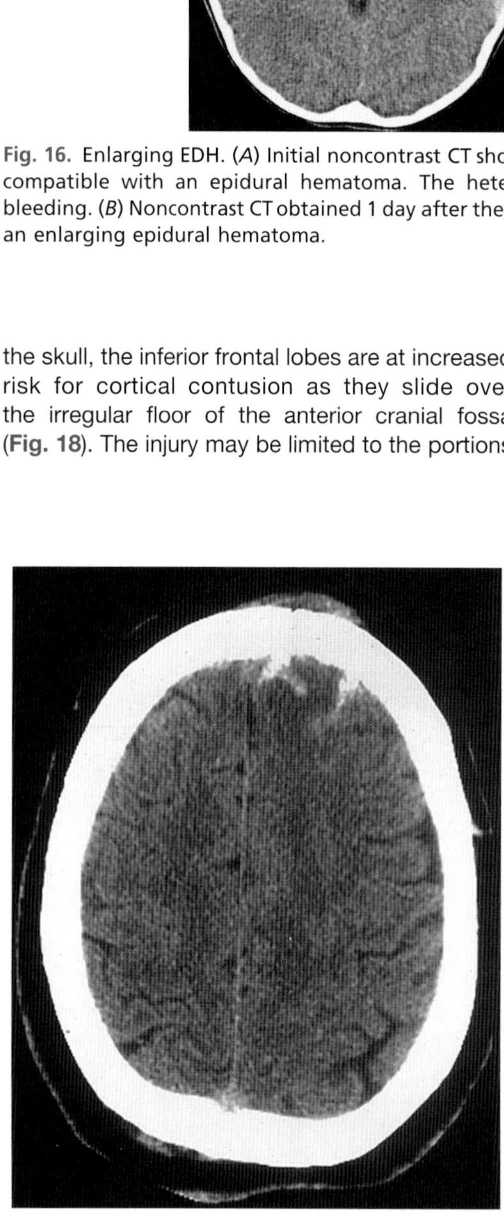

Surrounding the hematoma is an area of edema characterized by markedly decreased cerebral blood flow.[35] Ultrastructural abnormalities described include vascular endothelial swelling and capillary compression.[36] The edema may increase for several days following injury and may contribute to an increase of the intracranial pressure. Healing begins during the first week following injury and, in the next weeks to months, the lesion shrinks to a gliotic scar (**Fig. 19**).

Intra-axial Injuries: Brainstem Injuries

Brainstem injury can occur as a primary or secondary event in TBI. If the brainstem is displaced during trauma, the dorsal lateral aspect of the brainstem may contact the free edge of the tentorium at the tentorial incisura. A small area of either hemorrhagic or nonhemorrhagic contusion may result. The location of the injury is characteristic. The extent of injury depends not only on the nature of the trauma but also on variations in the size and shape of the tentorial incisura (**Fig. 20**).[37]

Secondary brainstem hemorrhage that results from increased intracranial pressure and/or

Fig. 17. Frontal contusion and SAH. Noncontrast axial CT shows a small forehead hematoma, and dense material that conforms to the left frontal cortical sulci. This appearance is typical of CT for posttraumatic, peripheral SAH.

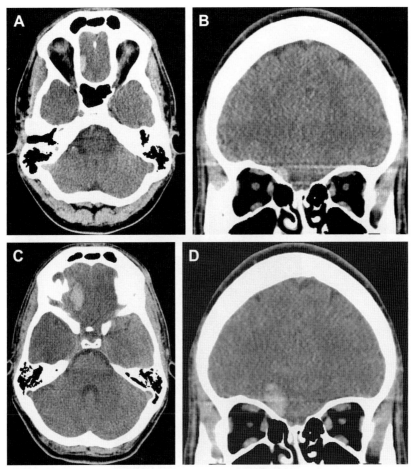

Fig. 18. Enlarging frontal lobe contusion. (*A*, *B*) Initial axial and reformatted coronal CT show a small area of contusion in the inferior right frontal lobe. This contusion was likely caused by the movement of the frontal lobe over the irregular surface of the anterior cranial fossa. (*C*, *D*) Axial and reformatted coronal CT scans obtained 7 hours after the initial CT show enlargement of the right frontal lobe contusion and the development of subtle edema around the hematoma.

descending transtentorial herniation is referred to as Duret hemorrhage. In the late nineteenth century, Henri Duret produced small brainstem hemorrhage in dogs by rapidly increasing their intracranial pressure. Whether those hemorrhages were the same as those seen today in patients with descending transtentorial herniation is not clear. Caudal displacement of the brainstem can produce distortion of blood vessels in the interpeduncular cistern. Injury to these vessels may result in single or multiple secondary hemorrhages currently called Duret hemorrhages.[37] The Duret hemorrhages can be distinguished from direct traumatic brainstem injuries by their location. The Duret hemorrhages are typically in the central pons, whereas direct injuries are located in the dorsal lateral pons (**Fig. 21**).

Intra-axial Injuries: DAI

DAI or shearing injury is an indirect injury. Shearing stress develops within the brain secondary to rotational acceleration as the skull is rapidly rotated. This stress results in axonal stretching, axonal edema, and possibly eventual separation and disruption.[38] A series of patients were studied with DTI within a few days following moderate to severe TBI. As expected, the FA was decreased. Analysis of the decreases in FA showed them predominantly caused by changes in radial diffusion perpendicular to the axon rather than changes in axial diffusion along the axon. These data suggest that early symptoms are likely to be caused by axonal edema rather than axonal separation.[39]

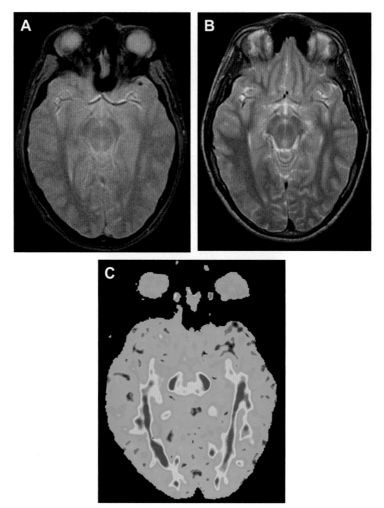

Fig. 19. Temporal contusion with decreased fractional anisotropy. The patient suffered a deceleration injury several months before the MR examination. (*A*) Axial GRE image shows a small focus of hemosiderin in the anterior left temporal lobe. (*B*) Axial T2-weighted image appears nearly normal; there may be a small focus of T2 prolongation within the left anterior temporal lobe. (*C*) FA map shows increased blue signal indicating loss of anisotropy within the left anterior temporal lobe. Note that the extent of white matter abnormality within the temporal lobe is considerably larger than that defined by either the GRE or the T2-weighted sequence.

The severity of the DAI is related to the magnitude of the rotational acceleration. The shear stresses produced by, for example, the head snapping forward in a deceleration injury, are maximal at the periphery, especially at the gray-white junction. More central shear injuries occur when the rotational acceleration is more severe. Thus, injuries at the peripheral gray-white interface may occur with less severe trauma and are more common than injuries of the brainstem or corpus callosum.[40] Although DAI at the gray-white interface is the most common, lesions of the corpus callosum have been found in nearly 50% of patients with significant head injury (**Fig. 22**).[41] Shearing injuries of the brainstem are found only in severe trauma. They are nearly always associated with multiple other white matter hemorrhages.[37]

Classically, patients with DAI present with a history of immediate loss of consciousness. CT in these patients may be normal; to explain the patient's neurologic status, MR is obtained. Because of its greater sensitivity, MR can show injuries in patients who have a depressed level of consciousness and normal findings on CT.[22] The patient may then recover consciousness in an

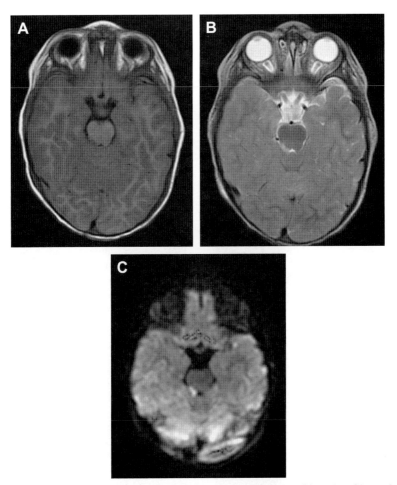

Fig. 20. Brainstem contusion. (*A*) Axial T1-weighted MR shows a subtle area of low signal intensity involving the left posterior lateral aspect of the pons. (*B*) Axial T2-weighted MR shows a small area of high signal intensity involving the left posterior lateral aspect of the pons. (*C*) Axial DW imaging shows a small area of restricted diffusion involving the right posterior lateral aspect of the pons. Findings are compatible with a nonhemorrhagic contusion likely caused by impact against the tentorial incisura.

agitated state. Imaging can help to make the diagnosis of DAI and provide prognostic information based on the location and extent of the lesions. For example, a brainstem injury is associated with a poor clinical prognosis.

CT underestimates the extent of DAI because the punctate hemorrhages resolve quickly and because only a minority (approximately 19%) of diffuse axonal injuries are macroscopically hemorrhagic.[34] For CT to reveal the shearing injuries acutely, the lesion must be hemorrhagic, fairly large, or both. When present, CT findings consist of small areas of hemorrhage, most commonly at the gray-white matter interface, and less commonly in the brainstem and corpus callosum (see **Fig. 22**). The sensitivity of the CT also

decreases following the acute injury as the hemorrhagic products degrade and become isodense with brain. MR is more sensitive than CT because it enables the detection of nonhemorrhagic as well as hemorrhagic lesions.[42,43] Nonhemorrhagic lesions can be detected by FLAIR, proton density, and T2-weighted sequences, but DW imaging is the most sensitive sequence for detection of DAI in the acute setting (**Fig. 23**). Although GRE is sensitive for acute and chronic hemorrhage, DW imaging is sensitive to acute and subacute cytotoxic edema and shows nonhemorrhagic lesions. DW imaging obtained within 2 days after injury correlates with initial GCS and Rankin score at discharge.[44] In the nonacute setting, old hemorrhagic lesions are best identified on GRE or SW

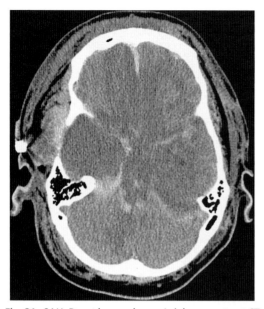

Fig. 21. SAH, Duret hemorrhage. Axial noncontrast CT shows diffuse subarachnoid hemorrhage and a small hemorrhage within the central pons. The central pontine hemorrhage likely represents Duret hemorrhage. Incidentally noted is a right temporal craniotomy.

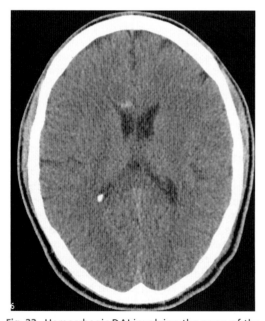

Fig. 22. Hemorrhagic DAI involving the genu of the corpus callosum. Axial noncontrast CT shows a small focus of high density within the genu of the corpus callosum. This finding represents hemorrhagic DAI.

imaging sequences.[45] These sequences have a heightened sensitivity to magnetic field inhomogeneities and therefore are sensitive to the presence of hemosiderin. However, the sensitivity to magnetic field inhomogeneity produces artifact at the skull base and from any metallic devices that may be present.

DTI, a newer technology, performed following DAI has shown good correlation with patient disability. In several clinical series, adult and pediatric patients with chronic DAI who were imaged at least 1 year after injury showed decreased FA (see **Fig. 19**). The changes in FA and fiber tracking correlate with patient outcome; patients with lower FA tend to be more severely disabled than those with mildly decreased FA.[46–49] Patients with acute DAI imaged within 1 week of injury showed decreased FA in the internal capsule and splenium of the corpus callosum. The decreases in FA correlated with the patients' initial GCS and Rankin score at discharge.[49,50]

Intra-axial Injuries: Brain Swelling

Both diffuse and focal cerebral swelling should be carefully monitored in the patient with a TBI (**Fig. 24**). It is one of the most important mediators of secondary brain injury. Severely increased intracranial pressure may produce ischemia as a secondary complication. The cerebral ischemia in turn leads to more edema, even greater increases in intracranial pressure, and results in decreased brain activity. Patients with persistent swelling have a short survival and high mortality.[51] Cerebral swelling is seen on CT as unifocal or diffuse areas of low attenuation. There are signs of mass effect such as effacement of cortical sulci and effacement of cisterns. The ventricles or midline structures may be displaced and there may be loss of normal differentiation between gray and white matter. On MR, the brain shows an increase in edema, which is noted as areas of increased signal intensity on FLAIR and T2-weighted sequences. Subtle, early edema, such as that seen in association with mild contusion, may be not be readily visible in the acute phase on T2-weighted sequences, but is more likely to be visualized on DW imaging. These findings are more easily visualized after a day or two when more significant edema has developed. Using a rat brain percussion injury model, researchers have shown nonhemorrhagic cortical injury as early as 45 minutes following percussion using DW imaging.[52]

On a cellular level, active transport mechanisms at the cell membrane may become disabled. The intracellular calcium is normally maintained at

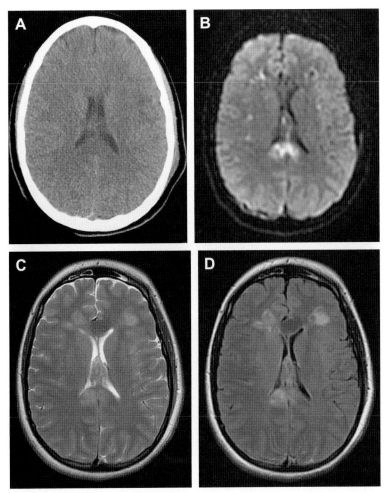

Fig. 23. Nonhemorrhagic DAI involving the splenium of the corpus callosum. (*A*) Axial noncontrast CT is nearly normal but shows subtle subarachnoid hemorrhage within the left sylvian fissure and subtle hypodensity within the corpus callosum. (*B*) Axial DW imaging shows restricted diffusion within the splenium of the corpus callosum and scattered smaller foci of restricted diffusion seen at the gray-white junction. Findings are compatible with DAI. (*C*, *D*) Axial T2-weighted and FLAIR images show T2 prolongation within the splenium of the corpus callosum and scattered foci of T2 prolongation at the gray-white junction of the frontal lobes.

a lower concentration and extracellular calcium by active transport. Following injury, the active transport mechanism can become impaired, allowing influx of calcium. The influx of calcium can lead to secondary cellular injury as well as the release of various neurotransmitters into the extracellular space.[53] The role of calcium channel blockers in the treatment of brain trauma is an area of active research. The blood-brain barrier, which normally restricts the movement of proteins and other solutes into the extracellular space, fails, increasing the vasogenic edema.[53]

Posttraumatic brain swelling and postischemic edema may each contribute toward increasing the intracranial pressure. These 2 processes may be impossible to differentiate on CT or conventional MR. DW imaging is sensitive for showing restricted diffusion characteristic of the cytotoxic edema seen in acute stroke. TBI produces cytotoxic edema as seen in contusions and DAI, but it also results in vasogenic edema with increased water diffusion and net flow toward the ventricles.[54] DW imaging may also be useful in the acute detection of posttraumatic brain swelling

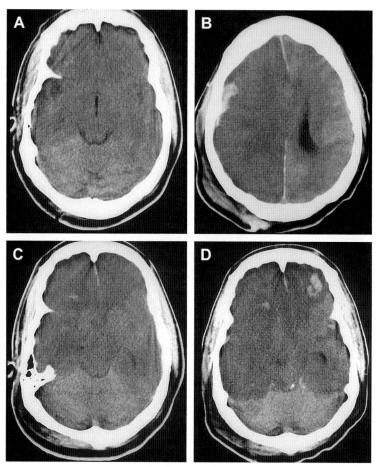

Fig. 24. Delayed hemorrhage and herniation. (*A*) Patient presents with trauma. Initial CT, although mildly degraded by patient motion, appears normal. (*B*, *C*) Patient's clinical condition deteriorated and a second CT was obtained after approximately 24 hours. Two images from the second CT show extensive brain swelling manifested by decreased density within the frontal lobes bilaterally and the right temporal lobe. There is compression of cortical sulci and narrowing of the quadrigeminal plate cistern. Several areas of hemorrhage are also noted in the right frontal lobe. (*D*) Patient's condition continued to deteriorate and another CT was obtained approximately 34 hours after the initial trauma. The CT findings have progressed. The brain swelling has increased to the point at which the quadrigeminal plate cistern is completely effaced. New areas of hemorrhage are now present in the left frontal lobe. The patient expired shortly after this study.

and the differentiation of ischemic tissue from tissue swollen by vasogenic edema, as suggested by animal experiments.[54]

Intra-axial Injuries: Brain Herniation

Either swelling or hematoma can displace a portion of the brain from its normal location, causing a herniation. The common patterns of brain herniation correlate with patterns of compressive and ischemic injury. Subfalcine herniation, seen on imaging as midline shift, describes displacement of the cingulate gyrus beneath the falx, which is rigid. Subfalcine herniation often results from a parietal SDH. As the brain is displaced beneath the falx, branches of the ipsilateral anterior cerebral artery may become trapped, resulting in post-traumatic infarction within the anterior cerebral artery territory (**Fig. 25**).[55]

Temporal lobe mass effect, such as may be caused by an epidural hematoma, may result in medial herniation of the uncus of the hippocampus into the suprasellar cistern or a descending herniation through the tentorial incisura. The posterior cerebral artery may be trapped against the edge of the tentorium at the incisura, resulting in posterior cerebral artery infarction.[56]

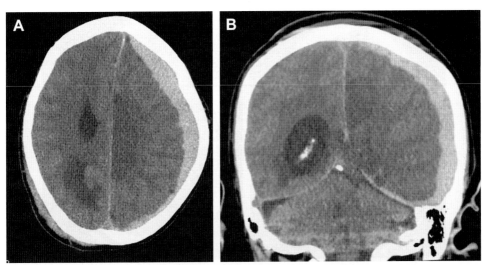

Fig. 25. Acute SDH, subfalcine herniation, anterior cerebral artery infarction. (*A*, *B*) Axial and reformatted coronal CT show a left high-density extra-axial fluid collection compatible with an acute SDH. The hematoma is causing considerable mass effect and causing subfalcine herniation. The low density noted adjacent to the falx represents infarction involving a branch of the left anterior cerebral artery. The artery is compressed against the underside of the falx by the mass effect generated by the SDH.

Descending transtentorial herniation occurs when the upper brainstem is displaced inferiorly through the tentorial incisura. This displacement may occur in the setting of massive supratentorial brain swelling. On imaging, the quadrigeminal plate cistern and other cisterns at the base of the brain are effaced. Both posterior cerebral arteries may be trapped against the edge of the tentorium, resulting in bilateral occipital lobe infarcts.[57] There may also be compression of the distal basilar artery, resulting in brainstem infarct or ischemia in those areas served by the short perforating pontine arterial branches. This mechanism has been suggested as the cause of posttraumatic Duret hemorrhage.[58]

Therapy to prevent brain herniation and subsequent ischemic damage may be directed toward drainage of the posttraumatic hematoma, decompression of the ventricular system via shunt placement, and minimization of brain swelling. When the brain swelling cannot be adequately controlled, a wide craniectomy may be performed, allowing brain to herniate through the wide defect in the skull (**Fig. 26**). This procedure preserves the remaining brain. When the brain swelling diminishes, the brain that has herniated through the defect is evaluated for viability, and a partial lobectomy may be performed before replacement of the bone flap or cranioplasty.

Gunshot injuries

Gunshot wounds to the head, especially penetrating injuries, have a high morbidity and mortality. One group reported an overall mortality of 87% in these patients.[59] The best clinical predictor of overall outcome is the GCS at admission. CT findings of multilobar injury and intraventricular hemorrhage correlate with poor outcome.[59,60] The surgical management of these patients is controversial. Some neurosurgeons favor a surgical approach consisting of minimal local debridement while preserving as much cerebral tissue as possible. Other surgeons are more aggressive and try to remove all bone and any metallic fragments that are reasonably accessible (see **Fig. 26**). In theory, intracranial bone and metallic fragments that are not removed might be associated with a higher rate of infection. In a small group of 13 patients, there was no correlation between the presence of retained fragments and the subsequent development of intracranial infection or epilepsy.[60]

Vascular Injuries

This article discusses some of the mechanisms of vascular compression, which may result from brain herniation and the associated patterns of posttraumatic infarction. In addition to the

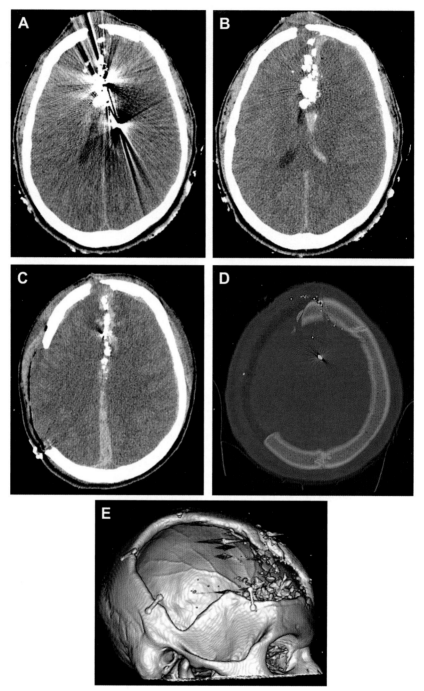

Fig. 26. Gunshot injury to the brain. (*A*, *B*) Noncontrast CT shows gunshot injury to the frontal lobes with extensive intracranial bone and bullet fragments. There is intraventricular hemorrhage and subdural hemorrhage along the falx. (*C*) noncontrast CT obtained 1 day later shows the right craniectomy with brain herniating through the craniectomy defect. There has been brain swelling indicated by loss of cortical sulci and blurring of the gray-white margin. The parafalcine SDH has increased in volume. (*D*) Noncontrast CT shows that, after several additional surgical procedures, many but not all of the bone fragments and bullet fragments have been removed and the patient has received a right cranioplasty. (*E*) 3-D surface-rendered image shows the extent of the cranioplasty, which was performed using a material less radiodense than bone. The multiple remaining bone fragments and bullet fragments can also be appreciated.

extrinsic vascular compression, TBI may cause direct injury to intracranial vessels. The location and nature of the vascular injury are related to the path of penetrating trauma, the points of vascular fixation in relation to osseous structures, and the proximity of vessels to the edges of dural reflections. The bifurcation of the anterior cerebral artery into pericallosal and callosal marginal branches is vulnerable to vascular injury because of its proximity to the inferior margin of the falx. Following trauma, transection or pseudoaneurysm formation can result (**Fig. 27**).

The cavernous segment of the internal carotid artery is vulnerable to injury because of its proximity to the dural reflections making up the cavernous sinus and its fixation at the skull base. Injuries in this region are often associated with basilar fractures and may manifest as transection, occlusion, or pseudoaneurysm.[61] Rapid extravasation of arterial blood into the cavernous sinus caused by transection of the cavernous portion of the internal carotid artery may result in a carotid cavernous fistula. These fistulae often result in

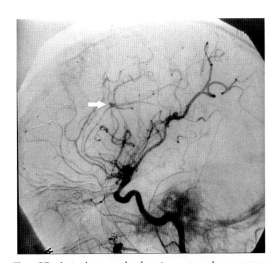

Fig. 27. Anterior cerebral artery pseudoaneurysm. Lateral view from a carotid artery angiogram shows an abnormal triangular collection of contrast arising from the distal anterior cerebral artery (*arrow*). This finding represents a posttraumatic pseudoaneurysm. The distal anterior cerebral artery is at risk because of its proximity to the inflexible inferior margin of the falx.

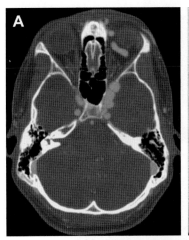

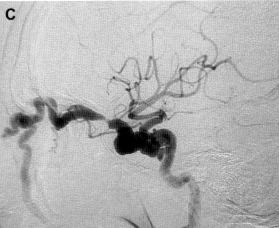

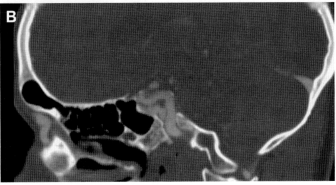

Fig. 28. Carotid cavernous sinus fistula. (*A*) Axial image from a CTA shows prominence of the left cavernous sinus and left superior ophthalmic vein. Findings are compatible with a carotid cavernous sinus fistula. (*B*) Sagittal image from the CTA shows apparent communication between the cavernous segment of the internal carotid and the cavernous sinus. (*C*) A lateral view from a left internal carotid angiogram confirms the fistula. Contrast extravasates from the cavernous segment of the internal carotid; it distends the cavernous sinus, and the cavernous sinus drains via a dilated and tortuous superior ophthalmic vein.

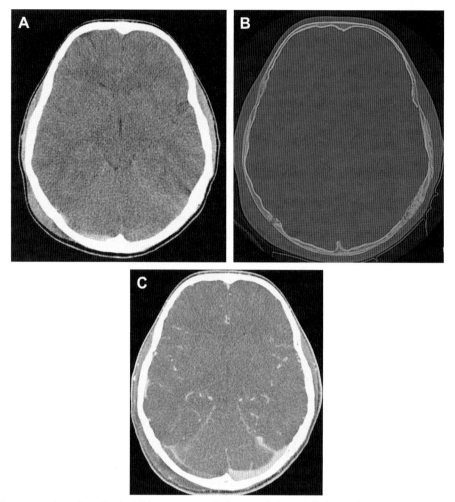

Fig. 29. Transverse sinus thrombosis. (*A*) Noncontrast CT shows a right occipital scalp hematoma and a small, high-density, left occipital extra-axial fluid collection compatible with a venous EDH or clotted blood within the right transverse sinus. (*B*) Noncontrast CT shows a right occipital scalp hematoma and a nondisplaced occipital fracture. (*C*) Contrast-enhanced axial CT from a CT venogram shows a normal and widely patent left transverse sinus and occlusion of the right transverse sinus.

distention of the ipsilateral cavernous sinus and ipsilateral superior ophthalmic vein (**Fig. 28**). Proximal vascular injuries may also serve as foci for thromboemboli, which may migrate distally, causing areas of cerebral infarction.

Patients with basilar fractures are also at increased risk for venous sinus thrombosis. One-hundred and forty patients with basilar fractures extending to a dural sinus or the jugular bulb were evaluated with MDCT venography. Thrombosis was identified in 57 (40.7%) (**Figs. 29** and **30**). Four of the patients with thrombosis had associated hemorrhagic venous infarction.[62]

Vascular injuries may be evaluated with CTA, MRA, or catheter angiography. Each of these modalities has its own advantages. CTA can be performed efficiently as part of the traumatized patient's initial evaluation. The area of evaluation can be suggested by the path of penetrating trauma or by associated fractures. These studies can be performed efficiently using multidetector CT scanners. The patient can move from the initial trauma CT to endovascular or surgical intervention as necessary. MRA is noninvasive; however, it may be most suitable as a follow-up study to monitor the evolution or healing of a vascular injury. Catheter angiography is the only one of the three methods that allows for endovascular treatment as well as diagnosis. It also remains the gold standard for the evaluation of subtle vascular injury.

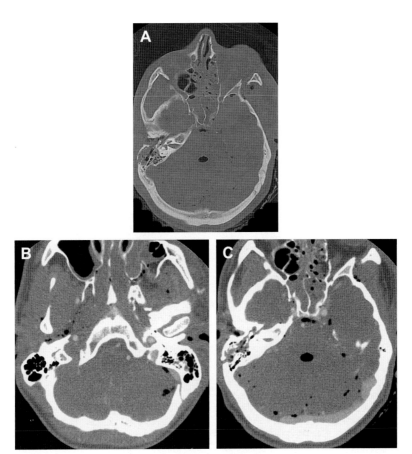

Fig. 30. Skull fractures and venous sinus thrombosis. (*A*) CT viewed at bone windows shows fractures of the right temporal bone and face as well as scattered pneumocephalus. (*B*) Axial postcontrast CT from a CTA shows patency of the left sigmoid sinus but occlusion of the right sigmoid sinus. (*C*) Axial postcontrast CT from a CTA shows patency of the left transverse sinus but occlusion of the right transverse sinus.

SUMMARY

Both CT and MR play important roles in the evaluation of TBI. CT is the mainstay initial imaging procedure. Modern CT scanners allow for rapid and accurate diagnosis of intracranial hemorrhage and mass effect. They also allow the efficient implementation of emergent CTA. MR imaging is more sensitive for the diagnosis of diffuse brain injury. Standard spin-echo and FLAIR imaging provides useful information; however, newer sequences such as GRE, SW imaging, and DW imaging can provide greater sensitivity for specific types of diffuse posttraumatic brain injury. MR spectroscopy can provide additional chemical information and DTI can provide information about white matter injury; both may prove useful in assessing injury severity, guiding patient care, and, most important, predicting patient outcome. Overall patient treatment can be optimized using the diagnostic and prognostic information derived from current imaging techniques.

REFERENCES

1. Corrigan JD, Selassie AW, Orman JA. The epidemiology of traumatic brain injury. J Head Trauma Rehabil 2010;25(2):72–80.
2. Brocker B, Rabin N, Levin A. Clinical and surgical management of head injury. Neuroimaging Clin N Am 1991;1:387–96.
3. Marshall LF, Gautille T, Klauber MR, et al. The outcome of severe closed head injury. J Neurosurg 1991;75:S28–36.
4. Rimel RW, Giodani B, Barth JT, et al. Moderate head injury: completing the clinical spectrum of brain trauma. Neurosurgery 1982;11:344–51.
5. Rimel RW, Giodani B, Barth JT, et al. Disability caused by minor head injury. Neurosurgery 1981;9:221–8.
6. Sosin DM, Sniezek JE, Waxweiler RJ. Trends in death associated with traumatic brain injury, 1979 through 1992. Success and failure. JAMA 1995;273:1778–80.
7. Miller EC, Holmes JF, Derlet RW. Utilizing clinical factors to reduce head CT scan ordering for minor head trauma patients. J Emerg Med 1997;15:453–7.

8. Borczuk P. Mild head trauma. Emerg Med Clin North Am 1997;15:563–79.

9. Provenzale JM. Imaging of traumatic brain injury: a review of the recent medical literature. AJR Am J Roentgenol 2010;194(1):16–9.

10. Arrangoiz R, Opreanu RC, Mosher BD, et al. Reduction of radiation dose in pediatric brain CT is not associated with missed injuries or delayed diagnosis. Am Surg 2010;76(11):1255–9.

11. Wintermark M, van Melle G, Schnyder P, et al. Admission perfusion CT: prognostic value in patients with severe head trauma. Radiology 2004;232(1):211–20.

12. Haacke EM, Xu Y, Cheng YC, et al. Susceptibility weighted imaging (SWI). Magn Reson Med 2004;52(3):612–8.

13. Kubal WS. Imaging of traumatic brain injury. Emergency and trauma radiology categorical course syllabus. ARRS 2000;1–10.

14. Faden AI. Pharmacological treatment of central nervous system trauma. Pharmacol Toxicol 1996;78(1):12–7.

15. Ross BD, Kreis ET, Haseler LJ, et al. IH MRS in acute traumatic brain injury. J Magn Reson Imaging 1998;8:829–40.

16. Holshauser BA, Ashwal S, Luh GY, et al. Proton MR spectroscopy after acute central nervous system injury: outcome prediction in neonates, infants, and children. Radiology 1997;202:487–96.

17. Friedman SD, Brooks WM, Jung RE, et al. Proton MR spectroscopic findings correspond to neuropsychological function in traumatic brain injury. AJNR Am J Neuroradiol 1998;19:1879–85.

18. Nakabayashi M, Suzaki S, Tomita H. Neural injury and recovery near cortical contusions: a clinical magnetic resonance spectroscopy study. J Neurosurg 2007;106(3):370–7.

19. Vagnozzi R, Signoretti S, Cristofori L, et al. Assessment of metabolic brain damage and recovery following mild traumatic brain injury: a multicentre, proton magnetic resonance spectroscopic study in concussed patients. Brain 2010;133(11):3232–42.

20. Cantu RC. Recurrent athletic head injury: risks and when to retire. Clin Sports Med 2003;22(3):593–603.

21. Vagnozzi R, Signoretti S, Tavazzi B, et al. Hypothesis of the postconcussive vulnerable brain: experimental evidence of its metabolic occurrence. Neurosurgery 2005;57(1):164–71.

22. Vagnozzi R, Signoretti S, Tavazzi B, et al. Temporal window of metabolic brain vulnerability to concussion: a pilot 1H-magnetic resonance spectroscopic study in concussed athletes–part III. Neurosurgery 2008;62(6):1286–95.

23. Tate DF, Khedraki R, Neeley ES, et al. Cerebral volume loss, cognitive deficit, and neuropsychological performance: comparative measures of brain atrophy: II. Traumatic brain injury. J Int Neuropsychol Soc 2011;17(2):308–16.

24. Provenzale J. CT and MR imaging of acute cranial trauma. Emerg Radiol 2007;14(1):1–12.

25. Gean AD. Extra-axial collections. In: Gean AD, editor. Imaging of head trauma. New York: Raven; 1994. p. 75–145.

26. Reed D, Robertson WD, Graeb DA, et al. Acute subdural hematomas: atypical CT findings. AJNR Am J Neuroradiol 1986;7:417–21.

27. Lee KS, Bae WK, Bae HG, et al. The computed tomographic attenuation and the age of subdural hematomas. J Korean Med Sci 1997;12:353–9.

28. van den Brink WA, Zwienenberg M, Zandee SM, et al. The prognostic importance of the volume of traumatic epidural and subdural haematomas revisited. Acta Neurochir (Wein) 1999;141:509–14.

29. Wilberger JR Jr, Harris M, Diamond DL. Acute subdural hematoma: morbidity, mortality, and operative timing. J Neurosurg 1991;74:212–8.

30. Zumkeller M, Behrmann R, Heissler HE, et al. Computed tomographic criteria and survival rate for patients with acute subdural hematoma. Neurosurgery 1996;39:708–12.

31. Zimmerman RA, Bilaniuk LT. Computed tomographic staging of traumatic epidural bleeding. Radiology 1982;144:809–12.

32. Sullivan TP, Jarvik JG, Cohen WA. Follow-up of conservatively managed epidural hematomas: implications for timing of repeat CT. AJNR Am J Neuroradiol 1999;20:107–13.

33. Noguchi K, Ogawa T, Inugama A, et al. Acute subarachnoid hemorrhage: MR imaging with fluid-attenuated inversion recovery pulse sequences. Radiology 1995;196:773–7.

34. Gentry LR, Godersky JC, Thompson B. MR imaging of head trauma: review of the distribution and radiopathologic features of traumatic lesions. AJR Am J Roentgenol 1988;150(3):663–72.

35. Schroder ML, Muizelaar JP, Bullock MR, et al. Focal ischemia due to traumatic contusions documented by stable xenon-CT and ultrastructural studies. J Neurosurg 1995;82:966–71.

36. Bullock R, Maxwell WL, Graham DI, et al. Glial swelling following human cerebral contusion: an ultrastructural study. J Neurol Neurosurg Psychiatry 1991;54:427–34.

37. Gentry LR, Godersky JC, Thompson BH. Traumatic brain stem injury: MR imaging. Radiology 1989;171(1):177–87.

38. Johnson MH, Faerber EN. Trauma. In: Faerber EN, editor. CNS magnetic resonance imaging in infants and children. London: MacKeith Press; 1995. p. 98–115.

39. Newcombe VF, Williams GB, Nortje J, et al. Analysis of acute traumatic axonal injury using

diffusion tensor imaging. Br J Neurosurg 2007;
21(4):340–8.

40. Gean AD. White matter shearing injury and brain-stem injury. In: Gean AD, editor. Imaging of head trauma. New York: Raven; 1994. p. 207–48.

41. Gentry LR, Thompson B, Godersky JC. Trauma to the corpus callosum: MR features. AJNR Am J Neuroradiol 1988;9:1129–38.

42. Parizel PM, Özsarlak Ö, Van Goethem JW, et al. Imaging findings in diffuse axonal injury after closed head trauma. Eur Radiol 1998;8:960–5.

43. Mittl RL, Grossman RI, Hiehle JF, et al. Prevalence of MR evidence of diffuse axonal injury in patients with mild head injury and normal head CT findings. AJNR Am J Neuroradiol 1994;15:1583–9.

44. Schaefer PW, Huisman TA, Sorensen AG, et al. Diffusion-weighted MR imaging in closed head injury: high correlation with initial Glasgow Coma Scale score and score on modified Rankin Scale at discharge. Radiology 2004;233(1):58–66.

45. Wardlaw JM, Statham PF. How often is haemosiderin not visible on routine MRI following traumatic intracerebral hemorrhage? Neuroradiology 2000; 42:81–4.

46. Xu J, Rasmussen IA, Lagopoulos J, et al. Diffuse axonal injury in severe traumatic brain injury visualized using high-resolution diffusion tensor imaging. J Neurotrauma 2007;24(5):753–65.

47. Wilde EA, Chu Z, Bigler ED, et al. Diffusion tensor imaging in the corpus callosum in children after moderate to severe traumatic brain injury. J Neurotrauma 2006;23(10):1412–26.

48. Benson RR, Meda SA, Vasudevan S, et al. Global white matter analysis of diffusion tensor images is predictive of injury severity in traumatic brain injury. J Neurotrauma 2007;24(3):446–59.

49. Inglese M, Makani S, Johnson G, et al. Diffuse axonal injury in mild traumatic brain injury: a diffusion tensor imaging study. J Neurosurg 2005;103(2): 298–303.

50. Huisman TA, Schwamm LH, Schaefer PW, et al. Diffusion tensor imaging as potential biomarker of white matter injury in diffuse axonal injury. AJNR Am J Neuroradiol 2004;25(3):370–6.

51. Lobato RD, Sarabia R, Cordobes F, et al. Posttraumatic cerebral hemispheric swelling. Analysis of 55 cases studied with computerized tomography. J Neurosurg 1988;68:417–23.

52. Alsop DC, Hisayuki M, Detre JA, et al. Detection of acute pathologic changes following experimental traumatic brain injury using diffusion-weighted magnetic resonance imaging. J Neurotrauma 1996;13:515–21.

53. Popp JA, Bourke RS. Pathophysiology of head injury. In: Wilkins RH, Rengatchary SS, editors, Neurosurgery, 2. New York: McGraw-Hill; 1985. p. 1536–43.

54. Hanstock CC, Faden AI, Bendall R, et al. Diffusion-weighted imaging differentiates ischemic tissue from traumatized tissue. Stroke 1994;25:843–8.

55. Rothfus WE, Goldberg AL, Tabas JH, et al. Callosomarginal infarction secondary to transfalcial herniation. AJNR Am J Neuroradiol 1987;8:1073–6.

56. Wernick S, Wells RG. Sequelae of temporal lobe herniation: MR imaging. J Comput Assist Tomogr 1989;13:323–5.

57. Mirvis SE, Wolf AL, Numaguchi Y, et al. Posttraumatic cerebral infarction diagnosed by CT: prevalence, origin, and outcome. AJR Am J Roentgenol 1990;154:1293–8.

58. Alexander E Jr, Kushner J, Six EG. Brainstem hemorrhages and increased intracranial pressure: from Duret to computed tomography. Surg Neurol 1982; 17:107–10.

59. Hofbauer M, Kdolsky R, Figl M, et al. Predictive factors influencing the outcome after gunshot injuries to the head-a retrospective cohort study. J Trauma 2010;69(4):770–5.

60. Kim TW, Lee JK, Moon KS, et al. Penetrating gunshot injuries to the brain. J Trauma 2007;62(6): 1446–51.

61. Goodwin JR, Johnson MH. Carotid injury secondary to blunt head trauma: case report. J Trauma 1994; 37:119–22.

62. Delgado Almandoz JE, Kelly HR, Schaefer PW, et al. Prevalence of traumatic dural venous sinus thrombosis in high-risk acute blunt head trauma patients evaluated with multidetector CT venography. Radiology 2010;255(2):570–7.

The Imaging of Maxillofacial Trauma and its Pertinence to Surgical Intervention

Nisha Mehta, MD[a], Parag Butala, MD[b], Mark P. Bernstein, MD[a],*

KEYWORDS

• Maxillofacial trauma • Surgery • Imaging

Maxillofacial skeletal injuries account for a large proportion of emergency department visits and often result in surgical consultation.[1] Although many of the principles of detection and repair are basic, evolving technology and novel therapeutic strategies have led to improved patient outcomes.

The goal of imaging studies in the trauma setting is to define the number and location of facial fractures, with particular attention toward identifying injuries to functional portions of the face and those with cosmetic consequence. By understanding common fracture patterns and the implications for clinical management, radiologists can better construct clinically relevant radiology reports and thus facilitate improved communication with referring clinicians. This article aims to provide a review of the imaging aspects involved in maxillofacial trauma and to delineate its relevance to management.

TECHNOLOGY

Imaging in most emergency departments for significant facial trauma begins with CT scanning. Although plain radiographs were once standard imaging, they do not provide sufficient information to assess injury severity and displacement, two key aspects essential for emergent management and surgical planning. In addition, radiographic positioning is difficult and potentially dangerous for multitrauma patients, in particular patients requiring cervical spine clearance. Modern multidetector CT (MDCT) scanners have revolutionized trauma imaging and provide a fast, safe, cost-effective, and sensitive means for assessing trauma for bone and soft tissue injuries. Furthermore, with the advent of MDCT, facial scans can now be performed contemporaneously with head, thoracic, and abdominal scans, facilitating a rapid assessment for trauma patients with multiple potential injuries.

MDCT offers excellent spatial resolution, which in turn enables exquisite multiplanar reformations, and 3-D reconstructions, allowing enhanced diagnostic accuracy and surgical planning. These reconstructions assist in the assessment of fracture fragment displacement and rotation as well as identification of fracture patterns. For these reasons, MDCT is the imaging technique of choice in maxillofacial trauma.

Although 2-D transaxial and coronal images are more accurate and sensitive than 3-D reconstructions, 3-D imaging is often preferred by surgeons because it simulates a surgeon's process of visualizing fractures in operative planning. Nonetheless, it is important to recognize limitations in 3-D imaging, namely the introduction of artifact during

The authors have no financial support or interests to disclose.
a Department of Radiology, NYU Langone Medical Center/Bellevue Hospital and Trauma Center, 550 First Avenue, New York, NY 10016, USA
b Institute of Reconstructive Plastic Surgery, NYU Langone Medical Center, 550 First Avenue, TCH-169, New York, NY 10016, USA
* Corresponding author.
E-mail address: Mark.Bernstein@nyumc.org

Radiol Clin N Am 50 (2012) 43–57
doi:10.1016/j.rcl.2011.08.005

the reformation process, decreased ability to visualize nondisplaced fractures, the lack of adequate soft tissue evaluation, and difficulty viewing deep fractures on surface views.[2]

At the Bellevue Hospital and Trauma Center currently scans are from the frontal sinus through the hyoid bone to include both the mandible and the facial bones. Scanning is acquired at submillimeter thickness with overlap (0.625 mm × 0.4 mm) to generate high-quality multiplanar reformations and 3-D reconstructions. CT images are reviewed at 2-mm thick reformations oriented parallel and perpendicular to the hard palate to achieve symmetry in both the transverse and coronal planes. Sagittal images are also generated for review. All images are processed using bone and soft tissue algorithms (**Fig. 1**). Additional oblique or curved reformations and 3-D reconstructions are generated according to the area of interest on a case-by-case basis.

MR imaging may occasionally be used to evaluate soft tissue injury with the advantage of avoiding ionizing radiation while providing excellent soft tissue contrast. MR imaging is particularly helpful in assessing cranial nerve deficits. Although MR imaging also offers multiplanar capabilities, it is limited in its ability to assess cortical bone and is often not a feasible modality secondary to accessibility and availability. In addition, it is usually impractical in the trauma setting due to the need to rule out life-threatening injuries promptly and patient inability to remain still during the lengthy examination. Most importantly, metallic fragments must be excluded before imaging with MR imaging.

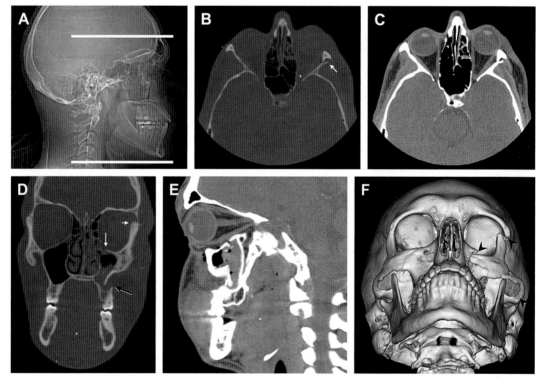

Fig. 1. A 22-year-old man, assaulted, with facial pain. (A) CT scout view shows scan range from top of the frontal sinus to the bottom of the hyoid to include the entire facial skeleton, including the mandible. Transaxial images in bone (B) and soft tissue (C) demonstrate a left lateral orbital wall fracture (*white arrow*) with left periorbital swelling. The globes and lenses are intact. Retrobulbar soft tissues are normal. (D) Coronal reformation reveals fractures of the left zygomaticofrontal suture (*short white arrow*), left orbital floor (*long white arrow*), and left zygomaticomaxillary suture (*black arrow*). Together, with zygomatic arch fracture (not shown), this injury pattern is a ZMC fracture. (E) Oblique sagittal reformation along the plane of the left optic nerve shows the orbital floor fracture to better advantage giving the surgeon an improved understanding of the size and depth of the defect. The optic nerve and superior and inferior rectus muscles are well displayed on this projection. (F) 3-D reconstruction in a Water's projection shows the overall ZMC fracture pattern (*arrowheads*) in a single image and aids in surgical planning.

NASAL FRACTURES
Anatomy

The nasal region consists of bony and cartilaginous portions. Whereas the anterior nasal septum is cartilaginous, the remainder of the nasal septum, consisting of the posterior perpendicular plate of the ethmoid, vomer, nasal crest of the maxilla, and nasal crest of the palatine bone, is bony. The upper third of the nasal region (consisting of the nasal bones proper, the frontal process of the maxilla, and the nasal process of the frontal bone) is bony, whereas the middle and lower thirds of the nasal region (composed of the upper lateral and lower alar cartilages, respectively) are cartilaginous.

Injuries

The nose is the most prominent facial projection. Consequently, nasal bone fractures account for approximately 50% of all facial fractures, with the majority involving the distal third of the nose.[3] Because the diagnosis is usually made clinically and radiologic evaluation is usually unnecessary, there is limited role for dedicated imaging. Radiology reports from head CT scans or imaging directed at detecting other facial fractures, however, often bring a nasal bone fracture to the attention of the emergency department staff and facilitate further evaluation, which can prevent clinical complications, such as a cosmetic deformity or a septal hematoma resulting in saddle nose deformity. In these cases, early reduction prevents bony malunion, thus avoiding the need for osteotomy to anatomically reduce fracture fragments.

Several classification systems exist for nasal and septal fractures, grouping fractures according to whether fractures are unilateral or bilateral, degree of displacement, comminution, midline deviation, and septal and soft tissue injury (**Fig. 2**). Generally, nasal trauma with septal fracture or dislocation causing severe alteration of the nasal midline or with severe soft tissue injury requires an open repair, whereas most others can be treated with closed reduction.[4]

NASO-ORBITAL-ETHMOID FRACTURES
Anatomy

The interorbital space is referred to as the naso-orbital-ethmoid (NOE) region; it represents the bony confluence of the nose, orbit, maxilla, and cranium. The space is defined by the thin medial orbital walls laterally, the sphenoid sinus posteriorly, the cribriform plate superiorly, and the bony pillar (the frontal process of the maxilla, nasal process of the frontal bone, and the thick proximal nasal bones) anteriorly. Several key structures lie within this region, including the olfactory nerves, the lacrimal sac, the nasolacrimal duct, the ethmoid vessels, and the medial canthal tendon.

Injuries

Once an anteriorly directed force is sufficient to fracture the nasal bones, the posterior ethmoid air cells offer little resistance and are easily fractured with impaction and resultant telescoping. The fracture pattern then progresses from simple nasal fracture into the NOE type, which additionally involves the medial orbit, septum, and nasofrontal junction. This pattern is most often seen in blunt trauma directed at the nasal bridge.

CT is essential to identifying the location of the injury, pattern type, degree of comminution and displacement, and associated fractures and soft tissue injury. CT typically demonstrates blood in the ethmoid air cells and impacted fractures in

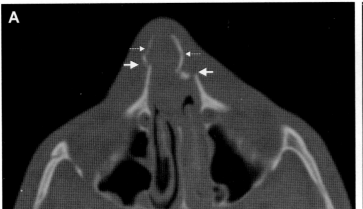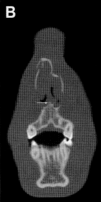

Fig. 2. Nasal fractures. (*A*) Transaxial and (*B*) coronal CT reformations of a 25-year-old male victim of assault shows bilateral comminuted nasal fractures through the frontal processes of the maxillae (*arrows*), displaced to the right. Nasomaxillary sutures lie just anteriorly (*small dotted arrows*). (*B*) Anterior nasal spine identified by the arrow.

the NOE region (**Fig. 3**). Often, with displaced fractures, the nasal septum is buckled on impaction, such that, both clinically and on CT, the nose appears pushed back between the eyes. If left untreated, NOE fractures can result in marked facial deformity with functional and cosmetic implications, including (but not limited to) telecanthus, enophthalmos, ptosis, and obstruction of the lacrimal system. These deformities are extremely challenging to correct secondarily and should be addressed immediately.[5]

NOE fractures are commonly associated with Le Fort II and III fractures; therefore, the pterygoid plates should be carefully evaluated. One study showed that 65% of patients with NOE fractures had concomitant facial fractures, most commonly a Le Fort maxillary or frontal sinus fracture.[6] Disruption of the cribriform plate should be assessed because the olfactory nerves can be disrupted, and more seriously, this injury can lead to cerebrospinal fluid (CSF) leak, pneumocephalus, or tension pneumocephalus after resuscitation efforts. Also, because NOE fractures are associated with high-impact trauma that involve the medial orbital walls, ocular injuries, such as hyphema, vitreous hemorrhage, lens dislocation, and globe rupture, should be excluded.[7]

Radiologically, one of the key segments of the NOE fracture to evaluate is the medial orbital rim where the medial canthal tendon inserts. Because the medial canthal tendon provides medial support to the globe and keeps the eyelid in apposition to the globe, recognizing potential injury is important to ensure appropriate work-up and treatment. Identification of a fracture through the inferomedial orbital rim at the lacrimal fossa implies disruption of the medial canthal tendon insertion (see **Fig. 3**B). Injury of the medial canthal tendon is closely associated to injury of the lacrimal drainage system, which can lead to obstruction and epiphora.[8]

Many NOE classification types have been proposed in the literature. The Markowitz system is among the most common, which categorizes NOE fractures according to the status of the medial canthal tendon along with the degree of comminution of the fragment of bone to which it remains attached.[9] Practically speaking, it is important for surgeons to know whether a fracture is unilateral or bilateral and whether it is simple (a large single segment) or comminuted. This, in combination with identifying associated fractures and assessing the internal orbit, determines the amount of exposure, the type of stabilization, and the number and type of surgical approaches needed.[10] In general, fractures that demonstrate displacement necessitate open reduction and stabilization. Marked comminution of the medial orbital wall, particularly in the region of the lacrimal fossa, where the medial canthal ligament attaches and the nasofrontal ducts are located, can require transnasal fixation. If the nasofrontal ducts are involved, surgical obliteration is often indicated to prevent the formation of a frontal mucocele. NOE fractures may also extend posteriorly to the optic canal or superiorly to the frontal sinus and intracranial structures, and this should also be noted.

FRONTAL SINUS FRACTURES
Anatomy

There is high variability in the frontal sinus, with regards to anatomy and volume: 10% of individuals have a unilateral sinus, 5% have a rudimentary sinus, and 4% have no frontal sinus. The anterior wall is thick and can tolerate as much as 2200 lb of force before fracturing, whereas the posterior wall is thin and relatively delicate. The dura and frontal lobes lie just posterior to the posterior table, and the orbital roof and nasofrontal ducts lie just inferior. The only drainage port from the frontal sinus is the nasofrontal duct, located at the

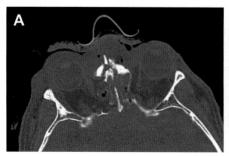
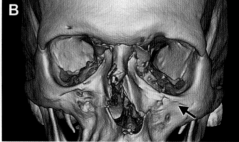

Fig. 3. NOE fracture. A 46-year-old man in a construction accident. (*A*) Transaxial CT image shows comminution of the nasal bones and ethmoid air cells with impaction as the nose is pushed back between the eyes from frontal force. (*B*) 3-D CT reconstruction shows the multiple interorbital fractures seen with the NOE fracture pattern. Note the fracture through the inferomedial orbital rim (*arrow*), implying medial canthal tendon injury.

inferomedial aspect of the frontal sinus, which empties into the middle meatus.

Injuries

Frontal sinus fractures result from direct anterior upper facial impact at the frontal bone and comprise 5% to 12% of all maxillofacial fractures.[11] They are uncommon, because the nasal prominence usually protects the naso-orbital region. Because of the high G force necessary for fracture to occur, these high-energy injuries result in 75% of patients presenting with significant injury, including shock, brain injury, coma, and associated facial fractures. The force of impact propels the head and cervical spine into extension, leading to concomitant intracranial injury in 38% of patients.[12] One-third of injuries are isolated to the anterior table, whereas two-thirds involve both anterior and posterior tables (**Fig. 4**).

Prompt and appropriate management is essential, because complications, such as brain abscesses, meningitis, encephalitis, mucoceles, and mucopyoceles, can occur. MDCT should be used as early as possible to exclude injury to the central nervous system and determine the location and extent of injury. Particular attention should be paid to the anterior and posterior tables and the nasofrontal duct, because injuries to these three structures dictate classification and subsequent treatment.[13] Also, if present, pneumocephalus can indicate dural violation, which may prompt neurosurgical intervention.

Injury to the nasofrontal outflow tract is present in 70% of cases and indicated by (1) anatomic outflow tract obstruction, (2) frontal sinus floor fracture, and (3) medial anterior table fracture. Coronal images are particularly helpful for evaluating the base of the frontal sinus at the site of the ostium of the duct. Fracture fragments within the tract are diagnostic of nasofrontal outflow tract obstruction.[14]

Although treatment goals are similar among surgeons, controversy regarding exact management of frontal sinus fractures exists.[15] As long as the nasofrontal duct is uninjured and there is no CSF leakage, nondisplaced fractures of the anterior and posterior walls of the frontal sinus do not usually require surgical treatment. Because of the possibility of delayed infection, however, many recommend long-term follow-up with CT.[16]

Solitary depressed anterior wall fractures can lead to cosmetic deformities and are treated with anterior wall restoration to obtain aesthetically acceptable contours. Nasofrontal duct injury or posterior wall injury with a dural tear or CSF leak usually requires removal of the sinus mucosa and obliteration of the cavity to prevent mucocele or mucopyocele formation.[17] Displaced posterior wall fractures, particularly when there is more than one table width of displacement, can require cranialization to treat ongoing CSF leaks (see

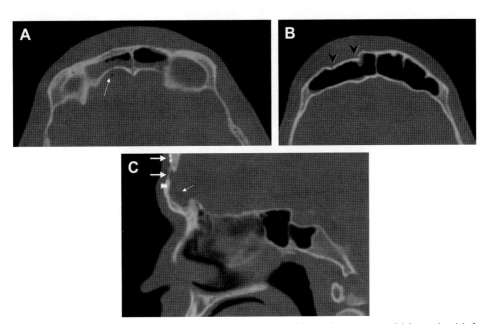

Fig. 4. Frontal sinus fractures. (*A*) Transaxial CT image of 19-year-old man in a motor vehicle crash with fractures of both the anterior and posterior tables of the frontal sinus. Note pneumocephalus (*dotted arrow*). (*B*) Larger frontal sinus in a 45-year-old woman after motor vehicle crash with only fracture of the anterior table (*arrowheads*). (*C*) Sagittal CT reformation of a different patient after cranialization of the frontal sinus with anterior fixation (*white arrows*). Note absence of the posterior table (*dotted arrow*).

Fig. 4C). This involves mucosal stripping, naso-frontal duct obliteration, and removal of posterior table fragments. In surgical procedures where the frontal sinus is preserved, serial CT scans in the postoperative period are often performed to assess for adequate drainage of the sinus, and failure of the sinus to clear is an indication of impaired drainage that may lead to infection.[18] In these cases, aggressive medical therapy and/or endoscopic or open surgical drainage are used.

ORBITAL FRACTURES
Anatomy

Seven bones make up the bony orbit: the frontal bone, zygoma, maxilla, lacrimal bone, ethmoid bone, sphenoid bone, and palatine bone. The optic canal, superior orbital fissure, and inferior orbital fissure are the three openings in the posterior orbit. In trauma imaging, fractures of the orbit are usually referenced in relation to the four orbital walls: the orbital floor, orbital roof, medial orbital wall, and lateral orbital wall.

Injuries

Orbital fractures may be isolated or part of a more complex fracture pattern. They frequently occur in conjunction with zygomaticomaxillary complex

(ZMC), Le Fort fractures, and NOE fractures. There are several typical injury patterns that are seen.

The orbital blow-out fracture typically occurs when an object larger than the bony orbit impacts the orbit with sufficient force to increase intraorbital pressure and fracture the thin orbital floor, medial wall, or both (Fig. 5). Blow-out fractures are considered pure when the thick orbital rim remains intact. The free fragment sign on CT demonstrates an isolated fragment within the maxillary sinus with depressed or displaced orbital floor fractures. With an acute injury, hemorrhage into the adjacent sinus should be present. If the sinuses are clear, the injury is likely remote. Fractures through the medial orbital wall that are not blow-out fractures are rarely isolated and should raise suspicion of NOE or Le Fort II or III fracture patterns.

Common complications include extraocular muscle herniation and enophthalmos (discussed later). Orbital emphysema is another complication, in which floor and medial wall fractures allow the release of adjacent paranasal sinus air into the orbit. Although this is usually a self-limited condition, it warrants comment because it can cause mass effect on the adjacent soft tissues and be a rare cause of decreased vision due to either occlusion of the central retinal artery or optic neuropathy.[19]

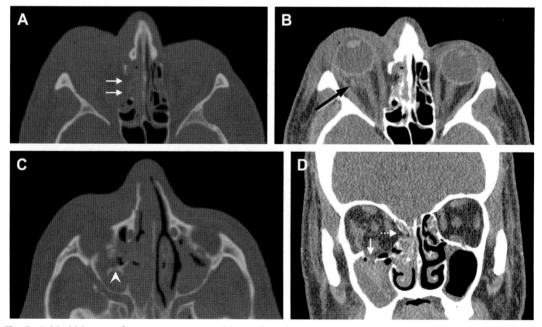

Fig. 5. Orbital blow-out fractures. A 50-year-old man found unconscious. Transaxial CT through the midorbits in bone (A) and soft tissue (B) demonstrate right periorbital soft tissue swelling with blow-out fracture of the right medial orbital wall (white arrows). Irregular appearance to the optic nerve insertion represents optic nerve injury (black arrow). (C) Transaxial image through the upper maxillae shows free fragment on the right (arrowhead) indicating a right orbital floor blow-out fracture as well. (D) Coronal reformation shows medial orbital wall (dotted arrow) and orbital floor (arrow) blow-out fractures.

The blow-in fracture usually results from a high-energy impact to the frontal bone and consists of fracture and depression of the orbital roof into the orbit (**Fig. 6**). Blow-in fractures are often associated with intracranial injury and loss of orbital volume leading to exophthalmos. Associated ocular injuries are reported in 14% to 29% of cases.[20] If the fracture propagates to the orbital apex, the optic nerve can be injured by direct fracture fragment penetration, hemorrhage into the sheath, avulsion from the posterior globe, or ischemia resulting from increased intraorbital pressure. If there is imaging and clinical evidence of optic nerve impingement, emergent surgical treatment is usually indicated because this can be associated with blindness as well as injury to the cavernous portion of the carotid artery.

The blow-up fracture involves cranial displacement of the orbital roof, which increases orbital volume and is strongly indicative of intracranial injury (**Fig. 7**). Isolated lateral orbital wall fractures can occur but are more commonly associated with zygoma fractures with disruption of the zygomaticofrontal suture.

CT imaging plays a key role not only in diagnosis of these fractures but also in determining management. Although indications for surgical repair are controversial, evidence of mechanical entrapment or evidence of enophthalmos includes well-established criteria mandating urgent repair.

Particularly with orbital blow-out fractures, there may be resulting herniation of the intraorbital fat and rectus muscles, which can lead to entrapment of the muscles on a free edge of the fracture fragment causing diplopia. Entrapment is a surgical emergency and lack of evidence of entrapment on

CT does not exclude the condition, and a careful physical examination is critical. Coronal CT is particularly useful for displaying herniation and can suggest entrapment based on kinking of a muscle or isolation of the inferior rectus muscle (**Fig. 8**). The inferior rectus muscle normally appears oval on coronal images; if it appears round, pathology should be suspected. Making the diagnosis of herniation is particularly challenging in the case of trap-door fractures, most common in pediatric patients secondary to more pliable bone. In these cases, the orbital floor is fractured and displaced inferiorly but then snaps back into place; however, the herniated inferior rectus muscle remains trapped across the fracture and is at risk of ischemia. CT findings of this type of herniation are particularly subtle, and the only sign may be the loss of the inferior rectus muscle shadow in the orbit.[21]

Another parameter in determining the need for surgical intervention is the size of the orbital floor defect, because larger defects increase the risk of future enophthalmos. With this condition, the globe sinks posteriorly and inferiorly into the maxillary sinus. Many surgeons opt for repair in any defect greater than 1 cm^2, whereas others use a standard of displacement greater than 50% of the orbital floor. Other surgeons judge by the amount of fat or soft tissue displacement. Some use CT to calculate the increase in orbital volume compared with the uninjured side and then use this to determine the risk for postinjury enophthalmos[22]; however, no firm data exist to support this approach. Because criteria vary among surgeons, the size of each fracture should be estimated in the radiology report.

Surgical repair can consist of either a bone graft from the outer table of the skull or the use of a titanium or resorbable implant. If an implant is used, the patient should be monitored for new-onset diplopia and, if present, emergent CT scan should be performed to ensure there is no mechanical impedance. When evaluating for placement, care should be taken to ensure that floor implants are directed superiorly to simulate the superior incline of the orbital floor (**Fig. 9**).

Globe Injury

Injury to the globe, retrobulbar hematoma, and optic nerve injury are considered more emergent than entrapment or enophthalmos; therefore, these soft tissue injuries should be assessed immediately when approaching a facial CT.[23]

Penetrating ocular injuries can lead to globe rupture secondary to pressure gradients favoring extrusion of the vitreous, because normal intraocular pressure is higher than intraorbital pressure. The flat tire sign, seen on CT as posterior flattening

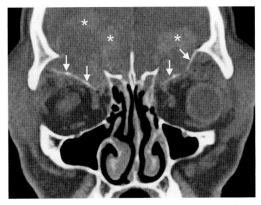

Fig. 6. Bilateral blow-in fractures. A 52-year-old man suffered a knee to the head playing softball. Coronal CT reformation shows bilateral orbital blow-in fractures (*arrows*). Note the significant bilateral frontal lobe contusions (*asterisk*).

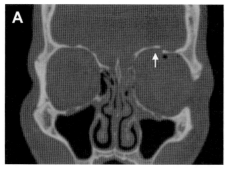

Fig. 7. Orbital blow-up fracture. A 40-year-old man assaulted. Coronal (*A*) and oblique sagittal (*B*) reformations show cranial displacement of left orbital roof fracture fragment (*arrows*). Note pneumocephalus (*dotted arrows*) implying violation of the dura.

of the globe, indicates globe rupture (**Fig. 10**A). Globe hemorrhage can be intravitreous, subscleral, or subretinal (see **Fig. 10**B).

Lens dislocation is diagnosed by a dependent lens lying on the retina (see **Fig. 10**C). In the case of partial tear of the zonular fibers, lens subluxation may be seen on CT as an oblique or vertically oriented lens, supported anteriorly on one side. If one lens appears hypodense relative to the contralateral lens, acute lens edema should be suspected because this may lead to a traumatic cataract. The difference in attenuation is usually approximately 30 Hounsfield units.

Often, it is difficult to evaluate optic nerve function clinically in the emergency room setting. Therefore, CT scan plays an important role in evaluation of the optic nerve. Transaxial and oblique sagittal images are particularly helpful in determining the presence of an optic nerve hematoma (see **Fig. 5**B).

Size and density are important in determining the detectability of foreign bodies. Metallic foreign bodies are readily identified; however, dry wood and plastic appear hypodense on CT, similar to air and fat, respectively. Because it can be difficult to differentiate a foreign body and air, it is helpful to look for a geometric margin. Despite this, at times, a nonmetallic foreign body is difficult to exclude and MR imaging can be helpful, provided that a noncontrast head CT has excluded the presence of a metallic foreign body.[24]

Lastly, a rare condition that requires emergent intervention and must be assessed in the setting of trauma is the presence of a carotid-cavernous fistula. This is done by evaluating the facial CT for the presence of a dilated superior ophthalmic vein, a nonspecific finding that indicates the need for confirmation with CT angiography or conventional angiography.[25]

ZYGOMA
Anatomy

The malar eminence defining the anterolateral cheek projection is formed by the zygoma, which has four principal attachments–the frontal bone, the maxilla, the arch of the temporal bone, and the greater wing of the sphenoid. They therefore

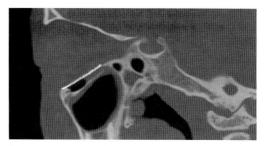

Fig. 8. A 53-year-old woman pedestrian struck by car. Coronal CT reformation shows left orbital floor fracture with herniation of orbital fat. The inferior rectus muscle appears enlarged, compared with right side, and lies up against the free orbital floor edge (*arrow*), raising concern for entrapment.

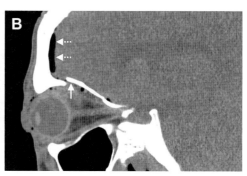

Fig. 9. A 21-year-old woman after repair of orbital floor blow-out fracture. Oblique sagittal CT reformation shows titanium plate across the large orbital floor defect.

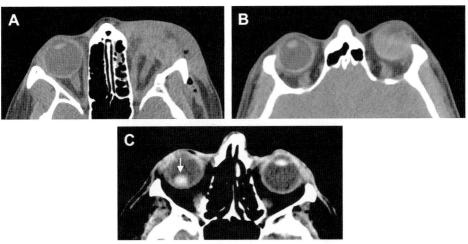

Fig. 10. Globe injuries. (A) Transaxial CT reformation of a left globe rupture in a 16-year-old girl after motor vehicle crash. Flattening of the posterior globe is common, referred to as the flat tire sign. (B) Globe hemorrhage on the left seen in a 38-year-old man after penetrating injury. (C) Right lens dislocation (arrow) in a 77-year-old man after fall.

contribute a large proportion of the orbital floors and lateral orbital walls.

Injuries

The prominent position of the zygoma makes it particularly susceptible to traumatic injury. Although the zygoma itself is a strong bone and contributes to the buttress system of the midface, the surrounding sutures and bones that articulate with the zygoma are weaker. A common resulting fracture pattern is the ZMC fracture pattern, which usually results from an anterolateral impact to the cheek and effectively separates the zygoma along its sutural attachments (see Fig. 1B–D). This pattern represents a spectrum of fractures varying in the degree of bone loss and displacement. Classically referred to as a tripod fracture, the term is a misnomer and should be avoided, because it overlooks the posterior attachments of the zygoma.

Isolated fractures of the zygomatic arch are uncommon, representing only 11% of zygomatic arch injuries.[26] These do not require operative reduction unless there is severe depression causing a cosmetic deformity or inability to completely close the jaw due to impingement of the depressed arch on the coronoid process of the mandible (Fig. 11). Fractures along the zygomaticomaxillary suture often extend across the infraorbital canal and can injure the infraorbital nerve, resulting in malar paresthesia.

CT is crucial in determining operative management of fractures, particularly because swelling often precludes accurate clinical assessment of deformity. Transverse, coronal, and 3-D images are particularly helpful (see Fig. 1D–F). The degree of comminution and displacement is important, because severe comminution affects the preferred surgical approach for exposing and subsequently aligning the arch.[27] Concurrent zygomatic arch fractures are not always obvious on CT, and deformity of the arch is sufficient to suggest a fracture. Another frequently overlooked ZMC fracture occurs in the temporal bone portion of the upper transverse maxillary buttress. This angulation must be reduced before other fractures are addressed or facial width is increased and underprojection of the cheek results.[28]

Mandible fractures are the most commonly associated fracture with fractures of the zygomatic arch, accounting for 21% of coexisting fractures.[29] The orbital floor and orbital apex are also

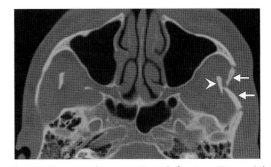

Fig. 11. Depressed zygomatic arch fracture. Transaxial CT image of a 51-year-old man post assault shows a comminuted depressed left zygomatic arch fracture (arrows). Fragments impinge on the coronoid process of the mandible (arrowhead).

commonly injured. As discussed previously with orbital floor fractures, there are multiple criteria for orbital exploration, and CT findings of degree of comminution and displacement should be reported. Some studies report that approximately 30% to 44% of patients with ZMC fractures require an orbital incision. For orbitozygomatic fractures, the lateral orbital wall, in particular, should be assessed on the transaxial images, because this is the location of the articulation of the zygoma with the greater wing of the sphenoid. The large width of this articulation facilitates assessment for degree of displacement and malposition of the fractured fragments. Nondisplaced orbitozygomatic fractures can be managed nonoperatively. If, however, displacement of the greater wing of the sphenoid is medial and into the orbital apex, there is resulting danger to the internal carotid arteries and multiple cranial nerves of the cavernous sinuses.[30] Displaced fractures are almost always treated with operative reduction

and fixation and should be performed as soon as possible, because osteotomies may be necessary after 3 to 4 weeks.

MAXILLARY FRACTURES
Anatomy

The central midface is occupied by the paired maxillae, which form the upper jaw. The maxillae house the maxillary teeth by way of the alveolus and attach laterally to the zygomatic bones. The facial buttress system highlights lines of inherent strength across the midface, with the strongest buttresses vertically oriented and the horizontal buttresses providing secondary support (**Fig. 12**).

Injuries

There are three classic fracture patterns of the maxilla, Le Fort I, II, and III, which by definition detach the maxilla from the skull base via fracture through the pterygoid plates (**Fig. 13**). Most

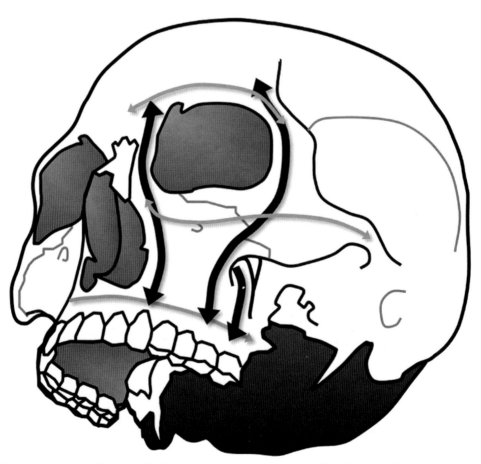

Fig. 12. Facial buttresses. Strong vertical buttresses are shown as curved thick black double arrows. From medial to lateral these are the nasofrontal buttress, zygomatic buttress, and pterygomaxillary buttress. The horizontal buttresses are shown as curved, thinner, double arrows.

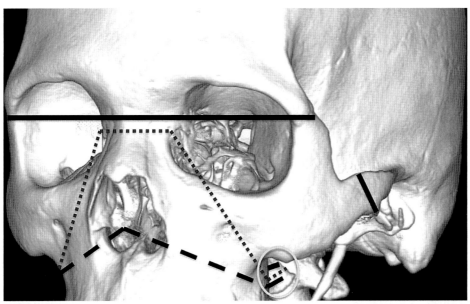

Fig. 13. Le Fort fracture patterns. Le Fort I pattern (*dashed line*) traverses the maxillae and lower nasal septum. Le Fort II pattern (*dotted line*) runs obliquely across the maxillae to the inferior orbital rims and crosses the nasal bridge. Le Fort III pattern transversely crosses the orbits and nasal bridge and involves the zygomatic arches. All Le Fort patterns extend posteriorly to fracture the ptyergoid plates (*circle*).

midface fractures are asymmetric, although Le Fort's initial descriptions outlined symmetric fracture patterns. Therefore, patients often have an asymmetric Le Fort fracture pattern.

A Le Fort I fracture pattern is the result of direct horizontal impact to the upper jaw creating malocclusion with a free-floating hard palate. This results in a transverse fracture through the maxilla passing above the tooth roots, crossing the floor of the maxillary sinus and lower nasal septum, with posterior extension through the pterygoid plates (**Fig. 14**). It does not involve the infraorbital rims.

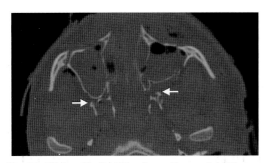

Fig. 14. Bilateral Le Fort I fractures. Transaxial CT image through the maxillae in a 33-year-old woman ejected from motor vehicle shows fractures of the anterior, medial, and posterior maxillary walls bilaterally. Fractures through the bilateral pterygoid plates are present (*arrows*), indicative of the Le Fort fracture pattern.

Direct impact to the central midface results in a Le Fort II fracture, which separates the nasal region from the cranium. It is a pyramidal fracture that crosses the zygomaticomaxillary sutures bilaterally, fracturing the inferior orbital rims medially, and traverses the nasal bridge. Posteriorly, there is fracture of the pterygoid plates (**Fig. 15**).

Complete craniofacial disjunction is referred to as Le Fort III fracture. The fracture is suprazygomatic and transversely extends across the nasofrontal suture and across the medial and lateral orbital walls, separating the zygomaticofrontal sutures and zygomatic arches and terminating through the pterygoid plates (**Fig. 16**).

Because Le Fort fractures usually result in marked damage to both the facial buttresses and the more fragile posterior bones, these fractures cause significant functional and cosmetic deficiencies. Often, similar to NOE fractures, there is backward displacement of the central midface. Additionally, damage to the vertical buttresses can lead of loss of facial height. Given the high incidence of concurrent facial fractures, surgical repair after these injuries is usually complex.

Of particular concern are the highly associated concomitant fractures of the hard palate, dentoalveolar units, and/or mandible, which disrupt occlusion. Reestablishment of normal occlusion must occur before attempting to surgically anchor the upper midface to the maxilla. Similarly, injury to

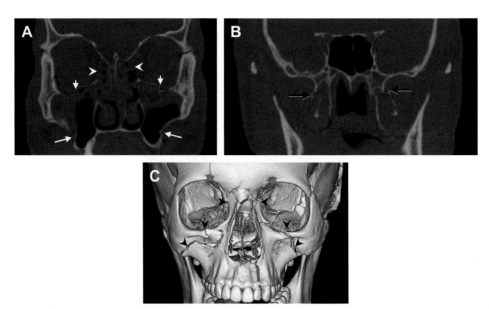

Fig. 15. Bilateral Le Fort II fractures in a 40-year-old man after motor vehicle crash. (*A*) Coronal CT image shows fractures through the lateral maxillary walls (*long arrows*), inferior orbital rims (*short arrows*), and across the medial orbital walls (*arrowheads*), creating a pyramidal fracture characteristic of the Le Fort II pattern. (*B*) Coronal image posteriorly shows comminution of the pterygoid plates (*arrows*). (*C*) 3-D reconstruction shows the Le Fort II fracture pattern in a single projection (*arrowheads*).

the frontal bar from concurrent ZMC, NOE, or frontal sinus fractures requires correction before resuspending the midface from the frontal bar.

Degree of comminution is another important factor, because severe comminution may preclude adequate restoration of facial height and projection, thus necessitating bone grafting.

Unfortunately, many Le Fort fractures can traverse the orbital apex. As discussed previously, the orbital apex is associated with injuries to the carotid canal. Because the surgical repair mechanism for Le Fort fractures generally entails the use of significant manual force on the part of a surgeon, it is important for the surgeon to know preoperatively how close the fracture line extends to the orbital apex and carotid canal so that a more gentle reduction technique can be used.

MANDIBULAR FRACTURES
Anatomy

The mandible is a horseshoe-shaped bone consisting of a curved anterior horizontal portion, the body, with two perpendicular posterior vertical struts, the rami. There is a superior anterior projection from each ramus, the coronoid process, which serves as the attachment for the temporalis muscle, as well as a superior posterior projection from each ramus, the condyle, which articulates with the temporal bone at the temporomandibular joint. The temporomandibular joints are the only mobile segments of the facial skeleton and are complex synovial joints that permit hinge, translation, and rotational movements. The mandible forms the lower jaw and holds the mandibular teeth in place. It contains the inferior alveolar nerve canal, which houses the inferior alveolar nerve as well as serving as an attachment for the muscles of mastication.

Injuries

Mandible fractures represent a large proportion of facial fractures and are typically caused by assault. They are classified according to anatomy (symphysis, parasymphysis, body, angle, ramus, coronoid, subcondylar, and condyle), and at least 50% are associated with a second fracture. The most common 2-part fracture is the parasymphyseal fracture with a contralateral subcondylar fracture (**Fig. 17**). A flail mandible is a symphyseal fracture with bilateral subcondylar fractures that necessitates surgery to restore preinjury facial width and height (**Fig. 18**).

Once a fracture is identified, the primary goal is to restore preinjury occlusion, with management ranging from nonoperative to mandibulomaxillary fixation with arch bars and occlusal wiring, to open reduction and internal fixation or, in the case of a contaminated wound, external fixation.[31]

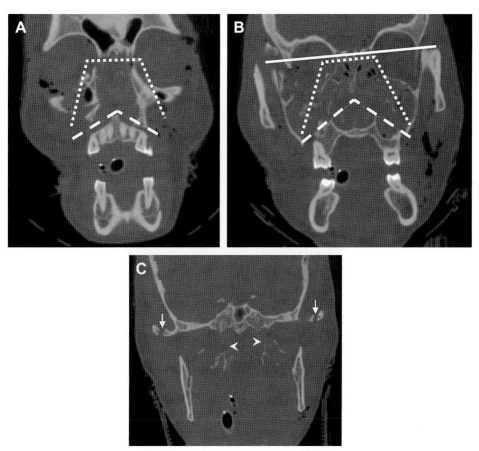

Fig. 16. Bilateral Le Fort I, II, and III fractures in a 30-year-old woman pedestrian struck by truck. Coronal reformations from anterior (*A*) to posterior (*C*). Le Fort I fractures shown by dashed line in (*A*) and (*B*). Le Fort II fractures shown by dotted line in (*A*) and (*B*). Le Fort III fractures shown by transverse solid line (*B*) and arrows through the posterior zygomatic arches in (*C*). (*C*) Pterygoid plates are comminuted (*arrowheads*).

CT is nearly 100% sensitive in detecting fractures of the mandible, which is superior to the 86% sensitivity of curved panoramic (Panorex) radiographs. CT is often insufficient, however, to

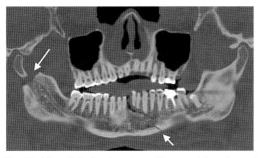

Fig. 17. Mandible fracture in a 19 year old male post assault. Panoramic curved CT reformation shows subcondylar fracture on the right (*long arrow*) and parasymphyseal fracture on the left (*short arrow*).

evaluate dental structures, and the Panorex radiograph can better visualize dental root fractures, particularly when the fracture is located at the angle.[32] Panoramic radiographs are thus often used in conjunction with the CT and particularly helps elucidate the relationship of fractures at the mandibular angle to the surrounding teeth (most importantly, the third molars). Cervical spine clearance is necessary before the acquisition of the Panorex radiograph.

Fractures through the tooth socket and alveolus are open fractures. Acute tooth loss is implied by a radiolucent socket and should prompt further evaluation for aspirated or ingested tooth fragments. Many surgeons consider most mandibular fractures as open fractures, therefore regarding them as contaminated, an indication for antibiotic prophylaxis. Some surgeons recommend tooth extraction if the fracture contains a tooth or if there is evidence of abscess.

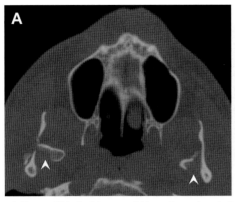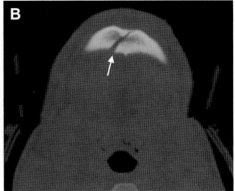

Fig. 18. Flail mandible in 32-year-old intoxicated male intoxicated. Transaxial images show (*A*) bilateral condylar fractures (*arrowheads*) and (*B*) symphyseal fracture (*arrow*).

SUMMARY

Maxillofacial fractures are common, and knowledge of fracture patterns and their implication for management is crucial to facilitating effective and efficient communication between the radiologist and the referring physician. When possible, pertinent details should be delineated in radiology reports.

REFERENCES

1. Pathria MN, Blaser SI. Diagnostic imaging of craniofacial fractures. Radiol Clin North Am 1989;27: 839–53.
2. Saigal K, Winokur RS, Finden S, et al. Use of three-dimensional computerized tomography reconstruction in complex facial trauma. Facial Plast Surg 2005;21(3):214–20.
3. Muraoka M, Nakai Y. Twenty years of statistics and observation of facial bone fracture. Acta Otolaryngol Suppl 1998;538:261–5.
4. Ondik MP, Lipinski L, Dezfoli S, et al. The treatment of nasal fractures: a changing paradigm. Arch Facial Plast Surg 2009;11(5):296–302.
5. Herford AS, Ying T, Brown B. Outcomes of severely comminuted (type III) nasoorbitoethmoid fractures. J Oral Maxillofac Surg 2005;63(9):1266–77.
6. Ellis E 3rd. Sequencing treatment for naso-orbito-ethmoid fractures. J Oral Maxillofac Surg 1993; 51(5):543–58.
7. Shelton D. Nasal-orbital-ethmoid fractures. In: Alling CI, Osbon D, editors. Maxillofacial trauma. Philadelphia: Lea & Febiger; 1988. p. 363–71.
8. Becelli R, Renzi G, Mannino G, et al. Posttraumatic obstruction of lacrimal pathways: a retrospective analysis of 58 consecutive naso-orbitoethmoid fractures. J Craniofac Surg 2004;15(1):29–33.
9. Markowitz BL, Manson PN, Sargent L, et al. Management of the medial canthal tendon in nasoethmoid orbital fractures: the importance of the central fragment in classification and treatment. Plast Reconstr Surg 1991;87(5):843–53.
10. Sargent LA. Nasoethmoid orbital fractures: diagnosis and treatment. Plast Reconstr Surg 2007; 120(7 Suppl 2):16S–31S.
11. May M, Ogura JH, Schramm V. Nasofrontal duct in frontal sinus fractures. Arch Otolaryngol 1970;92:534–8.
12. Brandt KE, Burruss GL, Hickerson WL, et al. 3rd. The management of mid-face fractures with intracranial injury. J Trauma 1991;31:15–9.
13. Yavuzer R, Sari A, Kelly CP, et al. Management of frontal sinus fractures. Plast Reconstr Surg 2005; 115(6):79e–93e [discussion: 94e–5e].
14. Rodriguez ED, Stanwix MG, Nam AJ, et al. Twenty-six year experience treating frontal sinus fractures: a novel algorithm based on anatomical fracture pattern and failure of conventional techniques. Plast Reconstr Surg 2008;122(6):1850–66.
15. Bell RB. Management of frontal sinus fractures. Oral Maxillofac Surg Clin North Am 2009;21(2):227–42.
16. Tiwari P, Higuera S, Thornton J, et al. The management of frontal sinus fractures. J Oral Maxillofac Surg 2005;63(9):1354–60.
17. Tedaldi M, Ramieri V, Foresta E, et al. Experience in the management of frontal sinus fractures. J Craniofac Surg 2010;21(1):208–10.
18. Smith TL, Han JK, Loehrl TA, et al. Endoscopic management of the frontal recess in frontal sinus fractures: a shift in the paradigm? Laryngoscope 2002;112(5):784–90.
19. Key SJ, Ryba F, Holmes S, et al. Orbital emphysema— the need for surgical intervention. J Craniomaxillofac Surg 2008;36(8):473–6.
20. Lawrason JN, Novelline RA. Diagnostic imaging of facial trauma. In: Mirvis SE, Young JWR,

editors. Diagnostic imaging in trauma and critical care. Baltimore (MD): Williams & Wilkins; 1992. p. 243–90.

21. Bansangi ZC, Meyer DR. Internal orbital fractures in the pediatric age group: characterization and management. Opthalmology 2000;107(5):829–36.

22. Kokemueller H, Zizelmann C, Tavassol F, et al. A comprehensive approach to objective quantification of orbital dimensions. J Oral Maxillofac Surg 2008;66(2):401–7.

23. Lee HJ, Jilani M, Frohman L, et al. CT of orbital trauma. Emerg Radiol 2004 Feb;10(4):168–72.

24. Kubal WS. Imaging of orbital trauma. Radiographics 2008;28(6):1729–39.

25. Anderson K, Collie DA, Capewell A. CT angiographic appearances of carotico-cavernous fistula. Clin Radiol 2001;56(6):514–6.

26. Carlin CB, Ruff G, Mansfeld CP, et al. Facial fractures and related injuries: a ten year retrospective analysis. J Craniomaxillofac Trauma 1998;4:44.

27. Hollier LH, Thornton J, Pazmino P, et al. The management of orbitozygomatic fractures. Plast Reconstr Surg 2003;111(7):2386–92 [quiz: 2393].

28. Hopper RA, Salemy S, Sze RW. Diagnosis of midface fractures with CT: what the surgeon needs to know. Radiographics 2006;26(3):783–93.

29. Obuekwe O, Owotade F, Osaiyuwu O. Etiology and pattern of zygomatic complex fractures: a retrospective study. J Natl Med Assoc 2005;97:992.

30. Linnau KF, Hallam DK, Lomoschitz FM, et al. Orbital apex injury: trauma at the junction between the face and the cranium. Eur J Radiol 2003;48(1):5–16.

31. Stacey DH, Doyle JF, Mount DL, et al. Management of mandible fractures. Plast Reconstr Surg 2006; 117(3):48e–60e.

32. Wilson IF, Lokeh A, Benjamin CI, et al. Prospective comparison of panoramic tomography (zonography) and helical computed tomography in the diagnosis and operative management of mandibular fractures. Plast Reconstr Surg 2001;107:1369.

Multi-Detector Row CT Angiography of the Neck in Blunt Trauma

Felipe Munera, MD[a],*, Mark Foley, MB, BCh[b],
Falgun H. Chokshi, MD[c]

KEYWORDS

- BCVI • CT angiography • Trauma • Carotid injury
- Vertebra injury

Blunt cerebrovascular injury (BCVI) is an uncommon, although potentially catastrophic, injury to the carotid or vertebral arteries through their cervical segments, sustained via blunt trauma. The most common cause of BCVI is motor vehicle collision, accounting for 80% of injuries. Ischemic events secondary to untreated BCVI are common (up to 68%),[1] with a high injury-specific mortality rate of 25% to 38%.[2] If BCVI is identified and treated before development of neurologic complications, the incidence of stroke and death is significantly reduced,[3,4] with only a small increased risk of anticoagulation-related complications.

Although previously thought to occur in less than 0.1% of blunt trauma patients,[5] recent studies show a much higher rate of BCVI with an incidence of approximately 1.2% in all blunt trauma patients[6] and up to 2.7% in the severely injured polytrauma patient.[7] With the implementation of aggressive screening programs based on mechanism of injury, clinical presentation and injury patterns identified on initial noncontrast CT imaging, the incidence of BCVI in the screened population can vary from 5.5% to 34%.[6,8]

The current standard of reference for the diagnosis of BCVI remains four-vessel digital subtraction angiography (DSA). DSA is more expensive and has limitations, including logistical constraints and limited availability, particularly off-hours, at some institutions. Furthermore, given its invasive nature, there is an inherent complication risk of approximately 1% related to the procedure itself (hemorrhage, hematoma, and stroke). With multidetector CT angiography (MDCTA) units now widely available in most hospitals with an established trauma service, there has been an increasing use of CT angiography (CTA) for detection of BCVI.

This article presents the evidence and the controversies surrounding the practice of imaging in patients with suspected BCVI. Discussion is centered on the increasing reliance on MDCT in the workup of these patients, but it will also consider the important contributions of clinical criteria in selecting patients for appropriate imaging, based on risk and probability of injury. Available protocols, injury description, and classification, as well as potential pitfalls are reviewed.

PATIENT SCREENING AND RISK FACTORS FOR BCVI

Screening guidelines developed in recent years are mostly derived from research performed by

---

The authors have nothing to disclose.

[a] Radiology Department, Jackson Memorial Hospital, Ryder Trauma Center, University of Miami Miller School of Medicine, University of Miami Medical System, 1611 North West 12th Avenue, West Wing 279, Miami, FL 33136, USA

[b] Department of Radiology, Jackson Memorial Hospital, University of Miami Miller School of Medicine, 1611 North West 12th Avenue, West Wing 279, Miami, FL 33136, USA

[c] Department of Radiology and Imaging Sciences, Division of Neuroradiology, Emory University School of Medicine, Emory University Hospital, 1364 Clifton Road N.E., Atlanta, GA 30322, USA

* Corresponding author.

E-mail address: fmunera@med.miami.edu

doi:10.1016/j.rcl.2011.08.007
0033-8389/12/$ – see front matter © 2012 Elsevier Inc. All rights reserved.

Biffl and colleagues[8] and Cothren and colleagues.[9] They identified a subset of trauma patients at increased risk of suffering from BCVI (**Box 1**). These risk factors are broadly divided into mechanism of injury, clinical findings on initial trauma assessment that would suggest the presence of BCVI, or an injury pattern or abnormalities identified on initial CT scan that would suggest or predispose toward the possibility of presence of an injury to the carotid or vertebral arteries. Although these provide useful screening criteria, it should be noted that 20% to 22% of patients with confirmed BCVI do not have any of these associated risk factors. Therefore, these injuries may be only identified after subsequent clinical deterioration or may be discovered incidentally, as occurs with patients undergoing whole body MDCTA for polytrauma (see later discussion).

Mechanism of Injury

An understanding of the mechanisms causing BCVI allows clinicians to quickly identify a subset of patients who are at a higher risk. This may expedite clinical management decisions in addition to providing the radiologists some critical information that raises the reader's index of suspicion for vessel injury.

Box 1
Modified Denver screening criteria for BCVI

Focal neurologic deficit (not explained by head CT scan)

Infarct on head CT scan

Nonexpanding cervical hematoma

Massive epistaxis

Anisocoria or Horner syndrome

Certain types of cervical spine fractures

Basilar skull fracture

Severe facial fracture (Le Fort type II and III)

Seatbelt sign above clavicle

Cervical bruit or thrill

Glasgow Coma Scale score less than 8

Data from Eastman AL, Chason DP, Perez CL, et al. Computed tomographic angiography for the diagnosis of blunt cervical vascular injury: is it ready for primetime? J Trauma 2006;60:925–9; and Biffl WL, Moore EE, Offner PJ, et al. Optimizing screening for blunt cerebrovascular injuries. Am J Surg 1999;178:517–22.

The primary mechanisms of carotid artery injury are believed to be secondary to direct neck trauma or a hyperflexion or hyperextension injury with a rotational component, which results in stretching of the carotid vessels over the lateral processes of the upper cervical spine. Vertebral arterial injuries, on the other hand, are frequently secondary to cervical spine injuries, with up to 70% of patients who sustain a vertebral arterial injury showing a documented cervical spine injury. Alternatively, in patients with cervical spine injury, the incidence of vertebral arterial injury varies between 17% and 46%.[10] The mechanism causing a vertebral artery injury can be either a direct vessel injury secondary to impingement by a fracture fragment,[11] particularly in foramen transversarium fractures,[12] or excessive traction, as seen in fractures or dislocations. There is a higher incidence of vertebral arterial injury in patients with multilevel foraminal fractures and in comminuted fractures of the foramen transversarium (**Fig. 1**).

Clinical Presentation and Findings Suggestive of BCVI

Clinical presentations that should raise suspicion for possible BCVI include injury patterns such as seatbelt or clothesline injuries to the neck region, near hanging injury, and hyperflexion or hyperextension injuries, particularly when associated with craniofacial injuries.[13]

Clinical findings in the acute trauma setting that suggest the presence of BCVI include active arterial hemorrhage from the mouth or neck, expanding cervical hematoma or a cervical bruit in patients less than 50 years of age, focal neurologic deficits, such as Horner syndrome or hemiparesis, and a neurologic examination that is discordant with CT scan findings.

Injuries predisposing to BCVI

A pattern of injuries identified on initial or secondary CT scans has also been positively associated with BCVI. These include craniofacial injuries such as diffuse axonal injury with a Glasgow coma scale score less than 6, basilar skull fracture with extension to the carotid canal, and Le Fort II and III facial and mandibular fractures (**Fig. 2**). The subsequent development of ischemic stroke on secondary CT scan or MR imaging should immediately raise suspicion for possible BCVI. In the neck, the presence of cervical spine injury, particularly any fracture of the C1-C3 vertebrae, cervical spine subluxations, and transverse foramen fractures at any cervical spine level are associated with BCVI, predominantly of the vertebral artery (**Fig. 3**).[14,15]

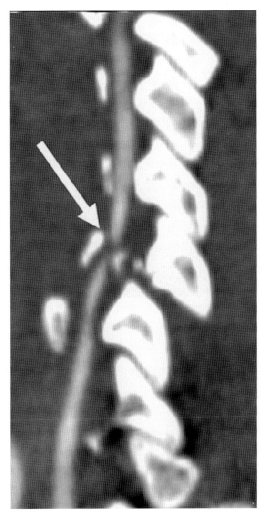

Fig. 1. An 18-year-old male involved in a motor vehicle collision. Right parasagittal oblique maximum intensity projection (MIP) image from a whole body CTA shows a facet fracture and subluxation. Additionally, there is a vertically oriented filling defect in the vertebral artery, representing a dissection (*arrow*).

In a recent study of 9935 blunt trauma patients, Berne and colleagues[14] performed univariate analyses exploring associations between individual risk factors and BCVI to determine which patients should be screened with MDCTA. Factors found to be most predictive of the presence of BCVI were cervical spine fracture (odds ratio [OR] 7.46), mandible fracture (OR 2.59), high Injury Severity Score (ISS) (OR 1.05), and low Glasgow Coma Scale (GCS) score (OR 0.93). Although the investigators reported that the higher the ISS and the lower the GCS score, the greater the risk of

an associated BCVI, no single number of GCS or ISS by itself was found to justify screening for BCVI.

A craniocervical trauma scoring system has been proposed to select blunt trauma patients for MDCTA evaluation. This scoring system assigns one point to each of the following: cervical subluxations or dislocations, fractures lines reaching an arterial structure, and high-impact mechanisms of injury, such as a high-speed motor vehicle accident, struck pedestrian, fall from a height greater than standing, and direct blow to the head or neck. The investigators reported a 21.9% risk of arterial injury for patients with a score of 2 and 52.2% for patients with a score of 3.[16]

MDCTA imaging protocol

Evaluation of the arteries of the neck can either be performed as a dedicated CT angiogram of the neck or as part of a whole-body CT angiogram. At the authors' institution, a busy level 1 trauma center, we typically perform a dedicated CT angiogram of the neck in patients with any of the reported screening criteria for increased risk of injury and in patients presenting with blunt head and neck trauma who received an unenhanced brain and/or cervical spine CT scan as part of their initial trauma evaluation with findings predictive of an increased risk of arterial injury. In our experience, isolated craniocervical trauma necessitating CTA occurs less commonly than multisystem polytrauma. Therefore, whole-body CTA is the routine method for scanning severe blunt polytrauma patients who have an indication for cervical spine imaging and contrast-enhanced body CT scan at our institution.

We perform a dedicated neck CTA on 64-MDCT scanners with 0.6 mm detector configuration. Our region of coverage extends from the aortic arch to the circle of Willis, with an automated triggering device centered in the ascending aorta. The patients receive 50–100 mL of iodinated contrast material (350 mg/mL, ioversol, Mallinckrodt) at 5 mL/sec followed by a 40 mL saline bolus at a similar rate. The images are reconstructed at 0.6 mm and 1.5 mm slices in axial, coronal and sagittal planes. Three dimensional reconstructions are generated by the radiologist at the picture archiving and communication system (PACS) workstation by using incorporated software (thin-client).

We obtain a whole body CTA examination in severely injured polytrauma patients with 64 detector scanners from the circle of Willis to the symphysis pubis, using a continuous acquisition with 0.6 mm collimation with neck images reconstructed at 1.5 mm slices. Our protocol

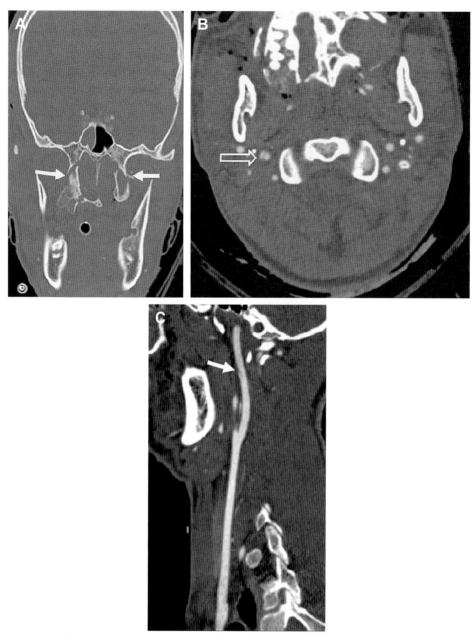

Fig. 2. A 35-year-old man involved in a motor vehicle collision, with coronal and axial images from the CTA (*A* and *B*, respectively). (*A*) There are bilateral pterygoid plates fractures (Le Fort type fractures, *arrows*). (*B*) The right internal carotid artery has a linear filling defect (*open arrow*), indicating a dissection. (*C*) The sagittal curved multiplanar reformatted (MPR) image confirms the dissection (*arrow*).

involves a biphasic injection of 100 mL of iodinated contrast (350 mg/mL, ioversol, Mallinckrodt) at 4 cc/sec for 15seconds, then at a rate of 3 cc/sec followed by a 40 cc saline bolus at 4 cc/sec. Efficiency is improved by using a fixed empiric delay of 20 seconds (or 25 seconds for patients older than 55 years) given a reported mild correlation between age and a delay in the peak arterial enhancement.[17,18] Separate dedicated coronal and sagittal reformations of

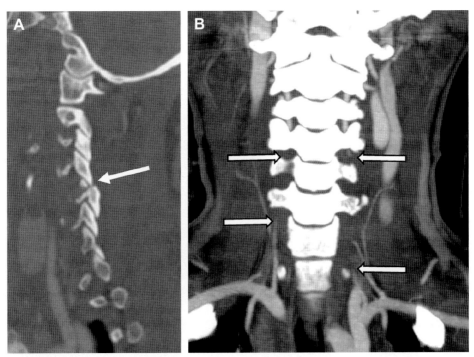

Fig. 3. A 17-year-old man's status after an all-terrain vehicle rollover. (A) Right parasagittal reformatted image from cervical spine CT scan shows a facet fracture dislocations (*arrow*). Similar findings were present on the left side. Coronal MIP from whole body CTA (B) shows abrupt cutoff of the vertebral arteries bilaterally, indicating segmental occlusions (*arrows*). The margins of the occluded segments are demonstrated by the arrows.

the neck in both bone and soft tissue algorithms are generated, with the additional use of incorporated thin client software by the on call radiologist for 3D post-processing and further troubleshooting.

For a dedicated neck CT angiogram, the patient's arms are positioned by the side. However, for whole body CT angiography, the patient's arms may be raised above the head (after initial noncontrast scan of the brain). This reduces streak artifact and radiation exposure to the torso, at the cost of some streak artifact in the neck. Despite some image degradation by this artifact, several studies have shown the performance of dedicated neck CTA and whole body CTA for evaluation of BCVI to be comparable.[19,20] To minimize radiation dose, we use automatic dose modulation in all patients.

MDCTA diagnostic performance

In the early era using 4-slice detector row scanners, CTA was considered inadequate for detection of BCVI, with Miller and colleagues[21] reporting a sensitivity of 47% and 53%. However,

as CT scanner technology advanced to incorporate more detectors in their units, and as these scanners became more disseminated, the sensitivity and specificity of CTA for detecting BCVI seems to be significantly improving. A study performed by Eastman and colleagues[22] using 16 slice MDCTA demonstrated a much higher sensitivity (97.7%) and specificity (100%) with improved detection of low-grade injuries compared with the four-slice technology. Other studies strike a note of caution because they do not replicate a similar sensitivity and specificity,[23] in particular research performed by Goodwin and colleagues[24] comparing 16-slice and 64-slice CTA with angiography showed a less than optimal sensitivity (29% for 16-slice and 54% for 64-slice scanning for real-time interpretation). More recently, research performed by DiCocco and colleagues[25] using 32-slice scanners also showed poor performance of CTA compared with DSA for BCVI. Despite this conflicting evidence, given its widespread availability and multiple advantages, initial screening for BCVI using MDCTA is an established practice at many large institutions, including the authors", and DSA is reserved for definitive treatment or diagnosis in equivocal cases or for patients with a negative CTA and persistent clinical concern.

Types of Vascular Injuries and Injury Grading

A classification system for carotid artery injuries, subsequently adapted for vertebral arterial injuries, has been devised by Biffl and colleagues[26] and is based on the appearance of the vessel, wall, and lumen. Although devised initially for use with DSA, the increasing use of CTA for screening and diagnosis of BCVI led to the extrapolation of the grading system to be used for interpretation of CTAs (**Table 1**). Grade 1 injuries involve any abnormality to the vessel wall (irregularity, intramural hematoma, or dissection) that causes less than 25% of vessel lumen narrowing (**Fig. 4**). Differentiation from artifacts may be difficult and follow-up studies may be necessary. Grade 2 injuries result in greater than 25% of vessel lumen narrowing and include the presence of intraluminal thrombus or a raised intimal flap (see **Fig. 2**). Grade 3 injuries represent pseudoaneurysm formation (**Fig. 5**). Grade 4 injuries are related to vessel occlusion from any cause (**Fig. 6**), and Grade 5 injuries involve vessel transection or arteriovenous fistula (**Fig. 7**).

Grading injuries is important because, in general, the higher the grade of carotid artery injury, the more likely the patient is to suffer from subsequent cerebrovascular ischemic events, ranging from 3% in grade 1 injuries to 100% in grade 5 injuries. Interestingly, the relationship

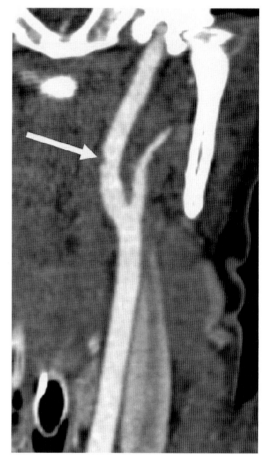

Fig. 4. A 32-year-old woman's status after a motor vehicle collision. Curved multiplanar reformation shows a mild contour irregularity of the right internal carotid artery (*arrow*), compatible with a grade 1 injury. The patient was treated with aspirin and had no further complications.

Table 1
Vessel injury grading and stroke rate

Grade	Description	Carotid Artery Injury Cerebrovascular Accident Rate	Vertebral Artery Injury Cerebrovascular Accident Rate
I	Wall irregularity or intramural hematoma/dissection with resultant luminal stenosis <25%	3%	19%
II	Intraluminal thrombus or raised intimal flap, OR >25% luminal stenosis secondary to intramural hematoma/dissection	11%	40%
III	Pseudoaneurysm	33%	13%
IV	Vessel occlusion	44%	33%
V	Transection OR arteriovenous fistula (hemodynamically significant)	100%	Not reported

Data from Biffl WL, Moore EE, Offner PJ, et al. Blunt carotid and vertebral arterial injuries. World J Surg 2001;25(8):1036–43; with permission.

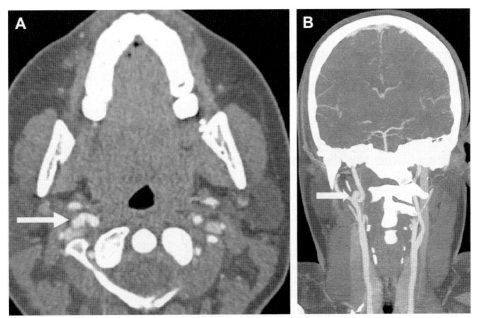

Fig. 5. An 18-year-old man's status after a motor vehicle collision. Axial CTA image (*A*) shows a 3-mm outpouching from the right internal carotid artery (*arrow*), which is confirmed to be a pseudoaneurysm (grade 3 injury, *arrow*) on the MIP reformatted image (*B*). There is no associated luminal compromise and the patient was successfully treated with anticoagulation therapy and the pseudoaneurysm was stable on a follow-up angiogram obtained 8 months later (not shown).

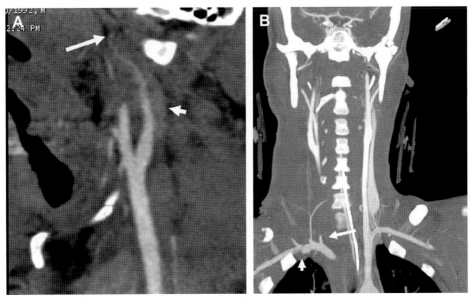

Fig. 6. (*A*) A 17-year-old man's status after a motor vehicle collision. Sagittal reformatted image from CTA shows gradual tapering of the right internal carotid artery terminating in an occlusion (*long arrow*), representing a grade 4 injury. The short arrow shows intramural hematoma (grade 2 injury). (*B*) A 17-year-old man's status after an all-terrain vehicle rollover. Coronal oblique slab MIP image from whole-body CTA shows an abrupt cutoff of the right vertebral artery (*long arrow*), indicating occlusion (grade 4 injury). Also, a linear filling defect in the right subclavian artery (*short arrow*), representing a dissection (grade 2 injury). Vertebral artery occlusions in the setting of BCVI are often abrupt, compared with the gradual tapering often seen with internal carotid artery occlusions. The right internal carotid artery is outside of the plane of the image and was not injured. (*Reproduced from* Chokshi FH, Munera F, Rivas LA, et al. 64-MDCT angiography of blunt vascular injuries of the neck. Am J Roentgenol 2011;196:W309–15; with permission.)

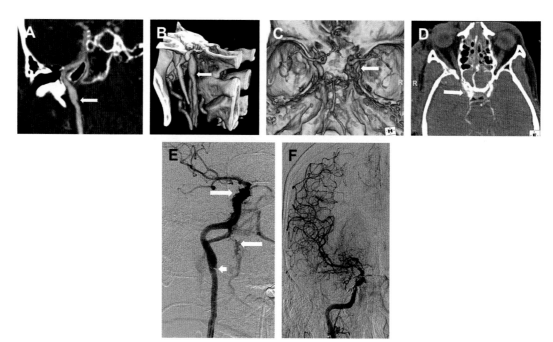

Fig. 7. A 50-year-old man's status after a fall from 12 ft (3.6 m). (*A*) Sagittal oblique reformation and (*B*) three-dimensional volume-rendered images of the right internal carotid artery from a whole-body CTA shows wall thickening (*short arrows*) and a linear filling defect (*arrows*), representing an intramural hematoma and an intimal flap from a dissection, respectively (grade 2 injuries). Injuries to more than one vessel are reported in 18% to 38% of BCVI, so careful inspection for other lesions is important. (*C & D*) Three-dimensional volume-rendered image and axial image of the CTA acquired at the base of the skull show asymmetric enlargement and early enhancement of the right cavernous sinus (*arrows*), suggesting a carotid cavernous fistula. The fistula was of the direct-type due to adjacent skull base fractures. This is a grade 5 injury (hemodynamically significant arteriovenous fistula or transection). (*E*) Digital subtraction angiography image shows a filling defect in the mid to proximal right internal carotid artery (*short arrow*), confirming the intimal flap. Early filling of the right cavernous sinus (*long arrows*), confirming the carotid-cavernous fistula. (*F*) DSA after coiling of the right carotid cavernous fistula, now without early filling of the right cavernous sinus. (*Data from* Sliker CW, Shanmuganathan K, Mirvis SE. Diagnosis of blunt cerebrovascular injuries with 16-MDCT: accuracy of whole-body MDCT compared with neck MDCT angiography. Am J Roentgenol 2008;190:790–9; and Berne JD, et al. Sixteen-slice multidetector computed tomographic angiography improves the accuracy of screening for blunt cerebrovascular injury. J Trauma 2006;60:1204–10.)

between injury grade and subsequent ischemic events for vertebral arterial injury does not seem to be linear, with the highest rate of ischemic events occurring in grade 2 injuries (40%) and a reported overall risk of ischemic stroke in any blunt vertebral injury of 24% (**Fig. 8**). To our knowledge, grade 5 injuries of the vertebral artery have not yet been reported.[10,27]

MDCTA findings of arterial injury

One of the main benefits of CTA compared with conventional angiography is the ability to visualize the arterial wall using multiplanar reconstructed images. With newer MDCTA units, the ability for volumetric acquisition allows for

generation of high quality multiplanar and curved reformatted images, which improves the visualization of previously difficult areas to evaluate, such as the high cervical and intracranial portions of the carotid and vertebral arteries, as well as improving the ability to characterize the types of vessel injury and their relationship to the surrounding tissues.

Vascular lesions following blunt and penetrating trauma have similar imaging features.[28–33] Minimal intimal irregularity (grade 1) is an injury finding described in the literature as an area of nonstenotic luminal irregularity that may be seen only on multiplanar or volume-rendered reconstructions (see **Fig. 4**).

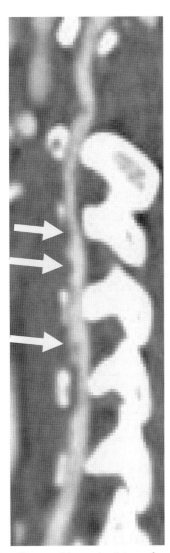

characterized on multiplanar images (see **Figs. 2** and **7**). Grade 2 lesions may be associated with a broad range of luminal narrowing ranging from 25% to near occlusion. Therefore, a more precise quantification is required for adequate treatment planning. Sliker[34] advocated quantifying the degree of luminal narrowing in patients with grade 2 injuries because of the potential hemodynamic consequences associated with lesions causing more severe arterial stenosis (**Fig. 9**).

Pseudoaneurysms (grade 3) describe out-pouching of the vessel beyond the expected caliber of the vessel wall. Secondary luminal narrowing may or may not be present (see **Fig. 5**; **Fig. 10**; **Fig. 11**). Although most BCVIs are at the level of C1-C2, they can occur anywhere, so a careful evaluation of the entire course of each vessel is warranted (see **Fig. 11**).

Vessel occlusions (grade 4) are seen when there is a lack of vessel opacification above a level at which there is enhancement of the surrounding arteries. In the case of carotid artery injuries, the vessel takes a more tapered narrowing, versus vertebral arterial injuries that characteristically have a more abrupt termination (see **Figs 3** and **6**).

In vessel transection with extravasation (grade 5) there is extravascular contrast surrounding the site of vessel injury, more often seen in penetrating than in blunt trauma.

Early venous filling of the adjacent veins with a relative increase in the caliber is compatible with presence of an arteriovenous fistula (grade 5) (see **Fig. 7**). In the authors' experience, as well as that of other authors, the direct arteriovenous communication is usually not visualized following blunt trauma.[34]

Fig. 8. An 18-year-old man's status after a motor vehicle rollover accident. Sagittal reformatted image from a whole-body CTA shows a contour irregularity affecting greater than 25% of the diameter of the right vertebral artery (*arrows*), a grade 2 injury.

An intramural hematoma caused by a dissection (grade 1 or 2) is reported when there is a focal thickening of the vessel wall, which may be either eccentric or concentric in appearance (see **Fig. 6**).

Filling defects within the vessel lumen on CTA may be either secondary to a raised intimal flap or intraluminal thrombus (both grade 2 injuries). In the case of an intraluminal thrombus, the filling defect may be rounded or oblong, whereas an intimal flap typically has a linear configuration that is best identified on axial images and

Patient outcomes and treatment

It is important to identify BCVI early in the patient's hospital course, because asymptomatic patients with documented BCVI have shown to have a significant improvement in neurologic outcome when early treatment with antiplatelet agents, endovascular therapy, or anticoagulation is instituted.[33] Unfortunately, not all patients are asymptomatic at presentation, with established stroke rates at the time of diagnosis ranging between 10% and 51% (see **Fig. 9**).[35,36] Despite this, when treatment was initiated, Stein and colleagues[37] reported a marked decrease in the rate of complicating cerebrovascular accidents, from 26% to 4% ($P = .0003$). A separate study by Eastman and colleagues[38] in 2009, which compared stroke rates from an earlier time when DSA was used for diagnosis to recent data using CTA for diagnosis, the stroke rate dropped from 15% to 4%. Strokes may occur secondary to

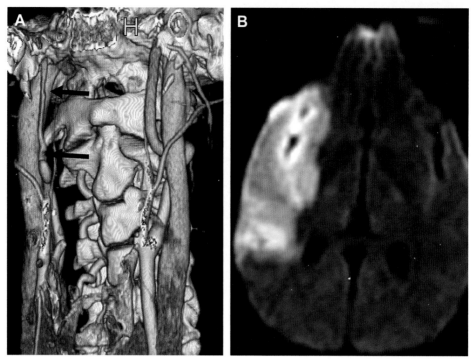

Fig. 9. A 45-year-old man involved in a motor vehicle collision who presented with left hemiplegia. (*A*) Coronal oblique volume-rendered image of the CTA shows a long segment of narrowing with intimal irregularity in the right internal carotid artery, compromising more than 25% of the vessel diameter (*black arrows*), consistent with a dissection (grade 2 injury). (*B*) Axial diffusion-weighted MR image of the brain shows a large area of hyperintensity in the right middle cerebral artery territory, compatible with acute infarction.

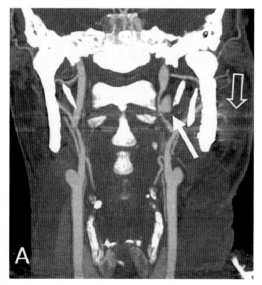

Fig. 10. A 40-year-old man's status after a scooter accident with focal neurologic deficits and suspected neck injury. (*A*) Coronal reformatted image from the CTA shows an outpouching arising from the left internal carotid aneurysm, representing a pseudoaneurysm (*solid arrow*), grade 3 injury. There is associated compression of the arterial lumen. The open arrow shows streak artifact from dental amalgam, which does not significantly limit evaluation of the injuries in this case. The patient was treated successfully with a covered stent.

either vessel occlusion or thrombus formation with distal embolization. Thromboemboli occur more frequently in nonocclusive injuries such as intimal injury, pseudoaneurysm, or dissection. The disrupted intimal layer promotes thrombogenesis in these cases.[5,39,40]

In vertebral arterial injuries, the clinical outcome can be variable, ranging from asymptomatic to vertebrobasilar insufficiency, stroke, or death. Unlike the carotid arteries, there is frequently one-side dominance to the vertebral artery circulation (50% left, 25% right, 25% bilateral) with 15% of the normal population having one vertebral artery that is atretic.[41] Surprisingly, injuries to the dominant vessel would not be expected to have a greater risk for severe neurologic sequelae than injuries to a nondominant or atretic vessel.

For grade 1 and 2 injuries, the current body of evidence supports systemic anticoagulation in the absence of contraindications, with heparin used as a first-line treatment and antiplatelet agents for those patients not considered candidates for full anticoagulation.[3,42] Serious bleeding as a result of this treatment has been recognized as a complication, leading to

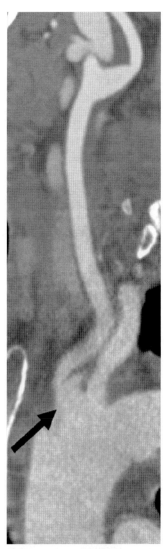

Fig. 11. A 77-year-old man's status after a motor vehicle collision. Curved multiplanar reformation from the whole-body CTA shows an outpouching of contrast at the origin of the left common carotid artery (*black arrow*), indicating a pseudoaneurysm (grade 3 injury). The patient was treated successfully with a covered stent.

patients with grade 3 injuries (pseudoaneurysm), with fewer stents deployed for grade 2 and grade 4 injuries (see **Figs 10** and **11**). These investigators demonstrated equivalent stroke outcomes (after diagnosis stroke rate of 4%) for stenting and medical therapy, although stenting was also performed on higher grade injuries for which a much higher stroke rate is expected.

Follow-Up Imaging

Irrespective of the treatment selected, the current expert opinion recommends that cases of BCVI should undergo routine reevaluation within 7 to 10 days. Biffl and colleagues[43] found that over half of their patients (57%) with grade 1 injuries had undergone interval healing, whereas 8% had progressed to pseudoaneurysm formation (grade 3 injury) necessitating further treatment. For grade 2 injuries, a smaller percentage of injuries (22%) had healed, whereas a higher percentage (46%) had worsened. They determined that follow-up angiography changes management in up to 61% of patients with BCVI, particularly in grade 1 and 2 injuries. For grade 3 injuries, follow-up angiography is routine because many of these lesions are treated with endovascular approaches. Most grade 4 injuries remain unchanged at follow-up.

Imaging pitfalls
An awareness of several potentially misleading artifacts and other pitfalls is essential for accurate interpretation of CTA examinations. As described above, streak artifact can be seen as part of whole-body CTA. Streak artifact from spinal hardware or dental amalgam may result in considerable image degradation; such that assessment of some arterial segments may not be possible (see **Fig. 10**).

In the older population, atherosclerotic disease, such as soft plaque, can mimic vascular injuries, such as intramural hematoma, intimal injury, or occlusion. A close assessment of these areas, with knowledge of the characteristic locations for atherosclerotic disease as well as the presence of associated calcifications may help to distinguish chronic vascular disease from acute injury (**Fig. 12**). Improper bolus timing, too early or late, may also affect image quality by inadequate vessel opacification resulting in poor assessment of the vessel wall as well as venous contamination. In the acute trauma setting, when altered mental status or anxiety are frequently present, motion may affect image quality. Although motion artifact can usually be easily identified by evaluating the adjacent structures, distinguishing motion artifact caused by vessel

recommendations of tight control of activated partial thromboplastin time of between 40 and 50 seconds.[43]

Endovascular therapy is also a recognized treatment option for BCVI. A study reported by DiCocco and colleagues[36] described patients that were treated with endovascular stent placement 7 to 10 days after starting the anticoagulation therapy. Most of these stents were placed on

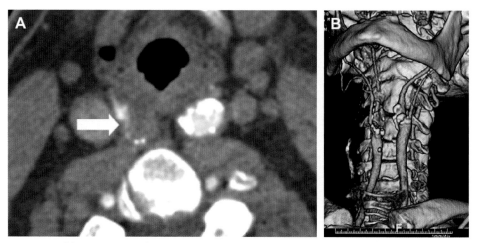

Fig. 12. A 71-year-old man's status after a motor vehicle collision. (*A*) Axial whole-body CTA image shows occlusion of the proximal right internal carotid artery (*arrow*). (*B*) Oblique three-dimensional volume-rendered reconstruction shows severe atherosclerotic disease as the underlying cause, not a BCVI. The patient also had active extravasation of contrast within the mesentery (not shown).

pulsation from true intimal injuries or dissections may be impossible.

Finally, vessel tortuosity, particularly of the high cervical and intracranial portions of the internal carotid arteries, and distal vertebral arteries is a common finding. These tortuous vessels may be best evaluated with curved multiplanar reformatted images or three-dimensional reconstructions (**Fig. 13**).[44,45]

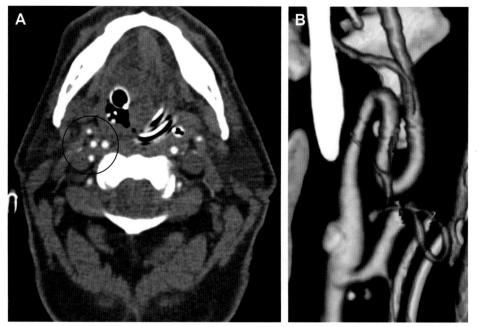

Fig. 13. A 69-year-old man struck by a car who suffered multiple craniofacial injuries. (*A*) Axial whole-body CTA image shows multiple round foci of enhancement within the right carotid space (*circle*). (*B*) Three-dimensional volume-rendered image shows a markedly tortuous right internal carotid artery, without any evidence of BCVI.

SUMMARY

MDCTA is increasingly used as the initial method of diagnosis in patients suspected of having BCVI. This underscores the need for radiologists to acquire considerable knowledge about the various mechanisms of injury, clinical presentation, and injury patterns identified on MDCTA.

ACKNOWLEDGMENTS

The authors would like to thank Gary H. Danton, MD, PhD, for his assistance in obtaining some of the three-dimensional images used in this article. (Gary H. Danton, MD, PhD, Assistant Professor of Clinical Radiology, University of Miami Miller School of Medicine, Jackson Memorial Hospital, and Ryder Trauma Center, Florida).

REFERENCES

1. Schneidereit NP, Simons R, Nicholapu S, et al. Utility of screening for blunt vascular neck injuries with computed tomographic angiography. J Trauma 2006;60:209–15.

2. McKevitt EC, Kirkpatrick AW, Vertesi L, et al. Blunt vascular neck injuries: diagnosis and outcomes of extracranial vessel injury. J Trauma 2002;53:472–6.

3. Cothren C, Moore EE, Biffl WL, et al. Anticoagulation is the gold standard therapy for blunt carotid injuries to reduce stroke rate. Arch Surg 2004;139:540–5.

4. Edwards N, Fabian TC, Claridge JA, et al. Antithrombotic therapy and endovascular stents are effective treatment for blunt carotid injuries: results from long-term followup. J Am Coll Surg 2007;204:1007–13.

5. Biffl WL, Moore EE, Ryu RK, et al. The unrecognized epidemic of blunt carotid arterial injuries: early diagnosis improves neurologic outcome. Ann Surg 1998; 228:462–70.

6. Berne JD, Reuland KS, Villarreal DH, et al. Sixteen-slice multi-detector computed tomographic angiography improves the accuracy of screening for blunt cerebrovascular injury. J Trauma 2006;60:1204–10.

7. Mutze S, Rademacher G, Matthes G, et al. Blunt cerebrovascular injury in patients with blunt multiple trauma: diagnostic accuracy of duplex Doppler US and early CT angiography. Radiology 2005;237:884–92.

8. Biffl WL, Moore EE, Offner PJ, et al. Optimizing screening for blunt cerebrovascular injuries. Am J Surg 1999;178:517–22.

9. Cothren CC, Moore EE, Ray CE Jr, et al. Screening for blunt cerebrovascular injuries is cost-effective. Am J Surg 2005;190:845–9.

10. Biffl WL, Moore EE, Elliott JP, et al. The devastating potential of blunt vertebral arterial injuries. Ann Surg 2000;231:672–81.

11. Fasset DR, Dailey AT, Vaccaro AR. Vertebral artery injuries associated with cervical spine injuries: a review of the literature. J Spinal Disord Tech 2008;21:252–8.

12. Oetgen ME, Lawrence BD, Yue JJ. Does the morphology of foramen transversarium fractures predict vertebral artery injuries? Spine 2008;33:E957–61.

13. Biffl WL, Cothren CC, Moore EE, et al. Western trauma association critical decisions in trauma: screening for and treatment of blunt cerebrovascular injuries. J Trauma 2009;67:1150–3.

14. Berne JD, Cook A, Rowe SA, et al. A multivariate logistic regression analysis of risk factors for blunt cerebrovascular injury. J Vasc Surg 2010;51:57–64.

15. Cothren CC, Moore EE, Ray CE Jr, et al. Cervical spine fracture patterns mandating screening to rule out blunt cerebrovascular injury. Surgery 2007; 141:76–82.

16. Delgado-Almandoz JE, Schaefer PW, Kelly HR, et al. Multidetector CT angiography in the evaluation of acute head and neck trauma: a proposed acute craniocervical trauma scoring system. Radiology 2010; 254:236–44.

17. Bae KT. Intravenous contrast medium administration and scan timing at CT: considerations and approaches. Radiology 2010;256:32–61.

18. Anderson SW, Soto JA, Lucey BC, et al. Blunt trauma: feasibility and clinical utility of pelvic CT angiography performed with 64–detector row. Radiology 2008;246:410–9.

19. Borisch I, Boehme T, Butz B, et al. Screening for carotid injury in trauma patients: image quality of 16-detector-row computed tomography angiography. Acta Radiol 2007;48:798–805.

20. Sliker CW, Shanmuganathan K, Mirvis SE. Diagnosis of blunt cerebrovascular injuries with 16-MDCT: accuracy of whole-body MDCT compared with neck MDCT angiography. AJR Am J Roentgenol 2008;190:790–9.

21. Miller PR, Fabian TC, Croce MA, et al. Prospective screening for blunt cerebrovascular injuries analysis of diagnostic modalities and outcomes. Ann Surg 2002;236:386–95.

22. Eastman AL, Chason DP, Perez CL, et al. Computed tomographic angiography for the diagnosis of blunt cervical vascular injury: is it ready for primetime? J Trauma 2006;60:925–9.

23. Malhotra AK, Camacho M, Ivatury RR, et al. Computed tomographic angiography for the diagnosis of blunt carotid/vertebral artery injury: a note of caution. Ann Surg 2007;246:632–42.

24. Goodwin RB, Beery PR 2nd, Dorbish RJ, et al. Computed tomographic angiography versus conventional angiography for the diagnosis of blunt cerebrovascular injury in trauma patients. J Trauma 2009;67:1046–50.

25. DiCocco JM, Emmett KP, Fabian TC, et al. Blunt cerebrovascular injury screening with 32-channel

multidetector computed tomography: more slices still don't cut it. Ann Surg 2011;253:444–50.

26. Biffl WL, Moore EE, Offner PJ, et al. Blunt carotid arterial injuries: implications of a new grading scale. J Trauma 1999;47:845.

27. Biffl WL, Moore EE, Offner PJ, et al. Blunt carotid and vertebral arterial injuries. World J Surg 2001;25(8): 1036–43.

28. Munera F, Soto JA, Palacio D, et al. Diagnosis of arterial injuries caused by penetrating trauma to the neck: comparison of helical CT angiography and conventional angiography. Radiology 2000;216:356–62.

29. Nunez DB, Torres-Leon M, Munera F. Vascular injuries of the neck and thoracic inlet: helical CT-angiographic correlation. Radiographics 2004;24:1087–98.

30. Munera F, Soto JA, Palacio D, et al. Penetrating neck injuries: helical CT angiography for initial evaluation. Radiology 2002;224:366–72.

31. Inaba K, Munera F, McKenney M, et al. Prospective evaluation of screening multislice helical computed tomographic angiography in the initial evaluation of penetrating neck injuries. J Trauma 2006;61:144–9.

32. Munera F, Soto JA, Nunez D. Penetrating injuries of the neck and the increasing role of CTA. Emerg Radiol 2004;10:303–9.

33. Munera F, Danton G, Rivas LA, et al. Multidetector row computed tomography in the management of penetrating neck injuries. Semin Ultrasound CT MR 2009;30:195–204.

34. Sliker CW. Blunt cerebrovascular injuries: imaging with multidetector CT angiography. Radiographics 2008;28:1689–710.

35. Cogbill TH, Moore EE, Meissner M, et al. The spectrum of blunt injury to the carotid artery: a multicenter perspective. J Trauma 1994;37:473–9.

36. DiCocco JM, Fabian JC, Emmett KP, et al. Optimal outcomes for patients with blunt cerebrovascular injury (BCVI): tailoring treatment to the lesion. J Am Coll Surg 2011;212:549–57.

37. Stein DM, Boswell S, Sliker CW, et al. Blunt cerebro-vascular injuries: does treatment always matter? J Trauma 2009;66:132–44.

38. Eastman AL, Muraliraj V, Sperry JL, et al. CTA-based screening reduces time to diagnosis and stroke rate in blunt cervical vascular injury. J Trauma 2009;67: 551–6.

39. Deen HG, McGirr SJ. Vertebral artery injury associated with cervical spine fracture. Report of two cases. Spine 1992;17:230–4.

40. Schellinger PD, Schwab S, Krieger D, et al. Masking of vertebral artery dissection by severe trauma to the cervical spine. Spine 2001;26:314–9.

41. Cloud GC, Markus HS. Diagnosis and management of vertebral artery stenosis. QJM 2003;96:27–54.

42. Bromberg WJ, Collier BC, Diebel LN, et al. Blunt cere-brovascular injury practice management guidelines: the eastern association for the surgery of trauma. J Trauma 2010;68:471–7.

43. Biffl WL, Ray CE Jr, Moore EE, et al. Treatment-related outcomes from blunt cerebrovascular injuries: importance of routine follow-up arteriography. Ann Surg 2002;235:699–706 [discussion: 706–7].

44. Chokshi FH, Munera F, Rivas LA, et al. 64-MDCT angiography of blunt vascular injuries of the neck. AJR Am J Roentgenol 2011;196:W309–15.

45. Anaya C, Munera F, Bloomer CW, et al. Screening multidetector computed tomography angiography in the evaluation on blunt neck injuries: an evidence-based approach. Semin Ultrasound CT MR 2009;30:205–14.

Imaging of Acute Head and Neck Infections

Aldo Gonzalez-Beicos, MD, Diego Nunez, MD, MPH*

KEYWORDS

- Acute infection • Paranasal • Floor of the mouth
- Suprahyoid and infrahyoid neck

Facial and cervical infectious processes represent a common clinical problem in patients of all ages, in particular children and young adults. In the head and neck, symptoms and signs of infection are usually clinically evident and allow for a presumptive diagnosis. Imaging studies, in particular CT and, to a lesser extent MR imaging, are frequently requested in the emergency setting to confirm the diagnosis and, more importantly, to locate the infection and exclude the possibility of abscess formation. The contribution of diagnostic imaging becomes more relevant in patients with clinical suspicion of the deep neck infection where access to an adequate clinical exploration may be limited. This article reviews the role of imaging in the evaluation of patients with infectious diseases of the head and neck, recognizing knowing the anatomic cervical partitions and spaces for an optimal diagnosis. It also discusses the most common infections involving the head and neck, with attention to its complications.

SOURCES OF INFECTION AND IMAGING OPTIONS

Infections of the neck typically originate from a single source. Tonsillar infection is the most common cause in children and young adults whereas odontogenic infection is the most common cause in older population groups.[1,2] Other potential sources of neck infection include the salivary glands, nasal sinuses, middle ear and mastoids, cervical lymph nodes, and trauma.[3]

The exact incidence of neck infections is not currently known but the frequency is likely rising, given the increasing number of immunocompromised patients at risk for atypical infections and its complications. These patients often lack the typical signs and symptoms of infection; this can mask the severity of a rapidly progressive infectious condition. The possibility of underestimating the severity of a neck infection makes diagnostic imaging a first step in an emergency department in choosing the best therapeutic approach.

In an emergency setting, the use of radiography is usually limited to the initial screening of suspected retropharyngeal infection and other acute upper airway infections in children, such as epiglottitis and croup. Ultrasound is occasionally used in the evaluation of more superficial infections to exclude the possibility of the fluid collection. Unquestionably, CT and MR imaging have higher sensitivity for the recognition of deep infections, particularly for the identification of abscess formation as well as its precise location and extension of disease.

The immediate availability, the high quality of anatomic detail, and the ability to create multidimensional reformatted images make CT with intravenous contrast the optimal modality for imaging neck infections in an emergency department.

The characteristic findings of infection include the loss of definition between contiguous anatomic spaces of the neck. The muscles can be thickened with hazy contours secondary to edema, which can also extend to the superficial soft tissues, resulting in stranding of the subcutaneous fat planes. With the use of intravenous contrast, diffuse enhancement of the inflamed tissue is seen. The existence of an abscess can be recognized by the higher attenuation in the periphery and a central zone of lesser density. Areas of low attenuation, however, can be seen

The authors have nothing to disclose.
Department of Radiology, Hospital of Saint Raphael, Yale School of Medicine, 1450 Chapel Street, New Haven, CT 06511, USA
* Corresponding author.
E-mail address: dnunez@srhs.org

Radiol Clin N Am 50 (2012) 73–83
doi:10.1016/j.rcl.2011.08.004

within inflamed tissue, not necessarily representing liquefaction. When the infectious process progresses without prompt diagnosis and treatment, it is more likely to evolve into formation of an inflammatory cavity or abscess, which typically establishes within 1 or 2 weeks of the onset of the infection. The usual appearance of a cervical abscess on contrast-enhanced CT is that of a lesion with peripheral enhancement and central coalescent areas of lower density.[4–7] In the neck, this appearance can be confused occasionally with necrotic lymph nodes when they are affected by metastatic disease, particularly from squamous cell carcinoma. MR imaging provides exquisite anatomic detail and can be used as a secondary method to aid in the evaluation of the infectious processes, particularly when further characterization or differentiation is needed between abscess and adenopathy. Also, in infections arising behind the upper airway, MR imaging can be useful in excluding the possibility of diskitis or vertebral osteomyelitis.

ANATOMY

Despite the typically easy visual inspection and palpation of the mouth and superficial structures of the face, the presence of infection can significantly affect the mobility of the mandible, thus limiting adequate clinical assessment. That is why the evaluation can largely depend on imaging findings. Knowledge of the fascial reflections and spaces in the neck is essential to understanding the etiology, imaging findings, and routes of infectious spread. The superficial fascia completely surrounds the head and neck separating the deep layers of the neck from the skin. It contains fat, superficial lymph nodes, nerves and hair follicles as well as the platysma muscle and the external jugular vein. The deep cervical fascia forms the boundaries of the cervical spaces and creates the normal symmetry of the neck. It is composed of three layers: superficial, middle, and deep. The reflections of these layers form the masticator, parotid, vascular, and parapharyngeal spaces laterally as well as the mucosal, retropharyngeal, and perivertebral spaces deeper around the midline. These fibrous boundaries also determine the communicative pathways for infection spread in the neck. In addition, based on the centered midline position of the hyoid bone, the neck is topographically subdivided into two broad compartments with different anatomic and physiologic features: the suprahyoid and infrahyoid segments. The specific infectious entities are reviewed, based on three distinct areas: the anterior suprahyoid neck, including the nasal and oral cavities; the lateral and deep suprahyoid spaces; and the infrahyoid neck.

Anterior Facial and Suprahyoid Neck Infections

Paranasal sinuses

Infections of the paranasal sinuses are usually diagnosed on clinical grounds and imaging is often reserved for the exclusion of the orbital and intracranial complications of rhinosinusitis. The majority of sinus infections are uncomplicated and caused by viruses, whereas bacterial causes become more likely when the common symptoms of viral infection do not subside or worsen after several days. Sinus and ear pain, fever, and purulent secretions usually develop. Sinus infection may spread by direct extension or through the valveless communicating veins of the face, particularly to the orbit. The inflammatory process in the orbit produces edema and cellulitis, progressing to subperiosteal and intraorbital abscess (Fig. 1). In severe cases, the infectious process may be

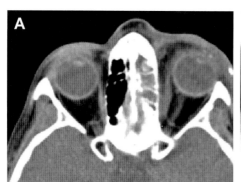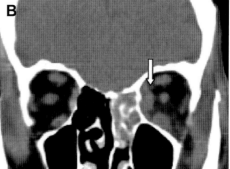

Fig. 1. Ethmoid sinusitis with subperiosteal orbital abscess. (*A*) Axial and (*B*) coronal CT images show left ethmoid sinus opacification and increased intraorbital soft tissues along the surface of the lamina papyracea, resulting in thickening and bulging of the medial rectus muscle (*arrow*).

complicated by ophthalmic vein thrombophlebitis and cavernous sinus thrombosis. Both CT and MR imaging play a critical role in the evaluation of these complications (**Fig. 2**). Similarly, an infection can permeate the osseous wall of the sinus and spread intracranially. Although rare, osteomyelitis, epidural and subdural empyema, meningitis, cerebritis, and brain abscess are all possible consequences of intracranial spread of sinus infections (**Fig. 3**). MR imaging best evaluates these complications of sinusitis because it can definitely show meningeal thickening and enhancement as well as adjacent signal abnormalities in the brain parenchyma. Of particular interest are the acute mycotic sinus infections that can rapidly progress and become necrotizing. Mucormycosis and aspergillosis can be aggressive infections that start usually in the nose and rapidly extend to the orbit and then intracranially by means of perivascular spread and bone destruction. The imaging diagnosis of mycotic sinus infections can be made using either CT or MR imaging, when the combination of bone destruction, nodular sinonasal mucosal thickening, and orbital or intracranial involvement is identified, typically in immunocompromised patients.

The oral cavity, sublingual, and submandibular spaces

The oral cavity should be differentiated from the oropharynx, which is actually part of the deep suprahyoid neck. These two spaces are separated by the ring-like plane that is formed by the soft palate, the tonsillar pillars, and the anterior line of the lingual tonsils, which separate the oral tongue from its own base or posterior third. This plane represents the posterior limit of the oral cavity. The dental arcades, as well as the hard palate superiorly and the mylohyoid muscle inferiorly, complete the boundaries of this space. It is particularly important to be familiar with the anatomy of the floor of the mouth. The mylohyoid muscle represents the anatomic floor of the mouth. It is shaped like a handheld fan forming a halved diaphragm that extends transversely from the medial aspect of the mandible to the midline. Above the mylohyoid muscle is the sublingual space, which is part of the oral cavity. Below the muscle is the submandibular space, which is part of the anterior suprahyoid neck. Posteriorly, the mylohyoid muscle has a free edge that extends approximately to the level of the second and third molar teeth, leaving no anatomic division between the sublingual and submandibular spaces. It is precisely at this free edge of the muscle that the submandibular gland straddles, with the duct coursing in the sublingual space. These anatomic features need to be taken into account when assessing infections that involve either of these compartments. Infections in these spaces generally occur as a result of a radicular dental lesion or a periodontogenic infection, most frequently of the second or third motor tooth. The roots of the more posterior molar teeth usually extend below the level of insertion of the mylohyoid muscle in the mandible. Therefore, infections originating in these teeth are more prone to extend into the submandibular space. When the infection is localized in the more anterior teeth, the extension occurs above the mylohyoid muscle and the infection tends to be confined to the sublingual space. Dental infections typically break through the

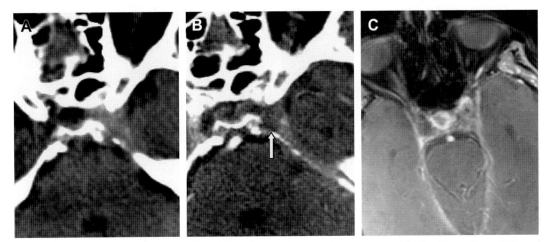

Fig. 2. Cavernous sinus thrombosis. (*A*) Axial CT image shows enlargement and high attenuation of the left cavernous sinus. (*B*) Contrast-enhanced axial CT image shows large filling defect within the medial aspect of the partially enhanced left cavernous sinus (*arrow*). (*C*) Axial T1-weighted image with fat suppression demonstrates heterogeneous enhancement of both cavernous sinuses, consistent with bilateral thrombosis.

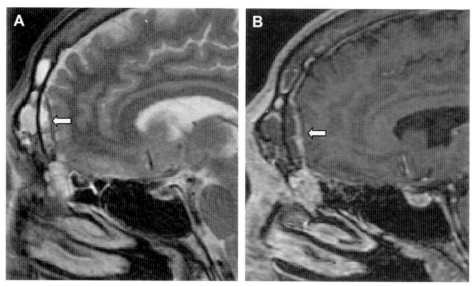

Fig. 3. Frontal sinusitis with epidural empyema. (*A*) Sagittal T2-weighted image shows hyperintense fluid within the frontal sinus and a small heterogenous epidural collection. Notice the low-signal posteriorly displaced dura (*arrow*). (*B*) Postcontrast sagittal T1-weighted image shows partial mucosal enhancement within the frontal sinus and enhancement of the posteriorly displaced thickened dura (*arrow*).

mandibular cortex more frequently on the medial or lingual aspect, which is anatomically thinner.[8] Other forms of infections in the submandibular and sublingual space originate in the submandibular gland (**Fig. 4**), more frequently complicating ductal obstruction by sialolithiasis.

An aggressive infection of the floor of the mouth with involvement across the midline and rapid extension to deeper cervical spaces, if untreated, is known as Ludwig angina. Usually odontogenic in origin, this infection typically presents as an advanced phlegmonous process without liquefaction (**Fig. 5**) and relative sparing of the salivary glands. Imaging assessment of posterior extension, tongue involvement, and potential airway compromise is paramount. Not commonly seen

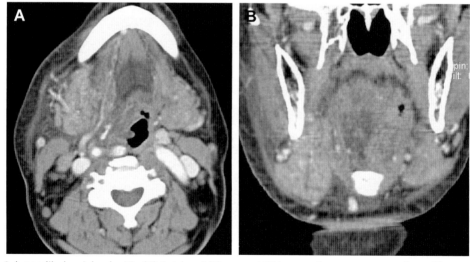

Fig. 4. Submandibular sialoadenitis. (*A*) Axial and (*B*) coronal CT images demonstrate an enlarged heterogenous right submandibular gland. Notice the soft tissue stranding superficial and deep to the thickened superficial layer of the deep cervical fascia.

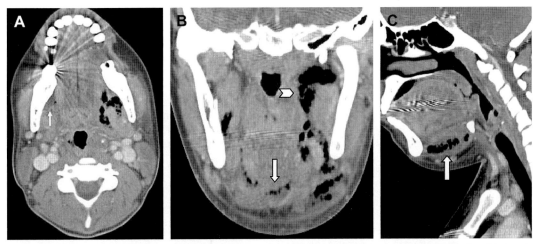

Fig. 5. Ludwig angina. A 22-year-old woman with facial swelling and pain, status post right inferior third molar extraction. (A) Enhanced axial CT image shows a small fluid collection along the medial border of the mandible on the right side (arrow) and air within the left masticator and submandibular spaces. (B) Coronal and (C) sagittal CT images show the extension of the gas-producing infection, also involving the left parapharyngeal space (arrowhead) and floor of the mouth. Note air within the substance of the mylohyoid muscle (arrows).

with the current antibiotic armamentarium is the described extension of Ludwig angina to the mediastinum.[9–11]

Lateral and Deep Suprahyoid Neck Spaces

Parotid space
The parotid space is enclosed by the superficial layer of the deep cervical fascia and contains the parotid gland, portions of the external carotid artery, facial nerve, retromandibular vein, and lymph nodes. The deep lobe of the gland reaches medially the parapharyngeal space and the parotid tail is adjacent to and communicates with the masticator and submandibular spaces. These relationships or communications serve as pathways for infectious spread.[12,13] Infection and abscess formation can arise in the parotid gland (Fig. 6). The cause of parotid infection is usually related to the presence of calculi that result in recurrent infections and chronic sialoadenitis. Acute parotitis of bacterial origin is uncommon

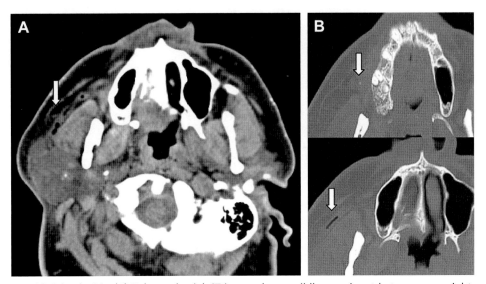

Fig. 6. Parotid sialoadenitis. (A) Enhanced axial CT image shows mildly prominent heterogenous right parotid gland and air within the salivary duct (arrow). (B) Axial CT images displayed in bone window settings show a small calcification (arrow, top) and confirm presence of air within duct (arrow, bottom).

but can present as a rapidly progressive purulent and necrotizing process leading to abscess formation. CT and MR imaging show glandular enlargement with heterogeneous density and signal and with abnormal nonhomogeneous enhancement. In severe cases, the masticator, submandibular, and parapharyngeal spaces are also involved by direct extension. A more typical form of bilateral parotitis occurs as a result of an acute viral infection, but this is not frequently an indication for imaging. Patients with immunologic compromise can also present parotid hypertrophy as a result of lymphoepithelial lesions and small cysts. These lesions should be included in the differential diagnosis of infections of the parotid space as well as Sjögren syndrome, an inflammatory autoimmune process that also affects the parotid glands, usually bilaterally. Appropriate clinical correlation is important in these cases.

Masticator space

The masticator space is located anterior to the parotid gland and anterolateral to the parapharyngeal space and is surrounded by the superficial layer of the deep cervical fascia. This space contains the medial and lateral pterygoid muscles, the masseter and temporalis muscles, the pterygoid venous plexus, and the ramus and posterior body of the mandible. Clinically, infections involving this space are characterized by trismus and pain along the mandibular ramus, secondary to the frequent involvement of the masseter and pterygoid muscles. Masticator space infections are classically odontogenic in origin and can lead to abscess formation and osteomyelitis of the mandible.[1,13] Infections frequently extend medially to the sublingual and submadibular spaces and there is potential for infectious spread into the parotid space and the parapharyngeal space. Aggressive infections can spread superiorly along the temporalis muscle into the temporal fossa as well (**Fig. 7**).

Carotid space

The carotid space is a potential compartment bounded by all three layers of the deep cervical fascia that spans from the skull base to the aortic arch. Within this space is the internal carotid artery, internal jugular vein, cranial nerves IX through XII superiorly, and the sympathetic plexus. Septic thrombophlebitis of the internal jugular vein is a frequent pathology and can occur as a primary event or, more commonly, as a complication from indwelling catheters. CT findings include reactive inflammatory changes in the perivascular space and the presence of a thrombus within the vessel lumen. Lemierre syndrome represents infectious thrombophlebitis complicated by septic pulmonary emboli (**Fig. 8**).[13–15] Other potential complications of infections in this space are cephalad extension of intraluminal clots causing cerebral venous sinuses thrombosis[16] and carotid

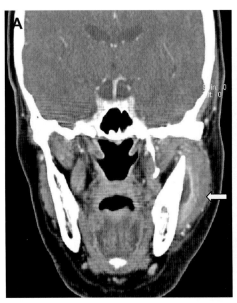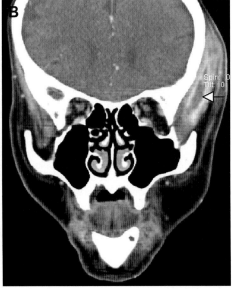

Fig. 7. Masticator space abscess. Coronal contrast-enhanced CT images show a rim-enhancing abscess (*A*) in the left masseter muscle (*arrow*) with thickening of the superficial layer of the deep cervical fascia. The infection has spread superiorly to the left temporal fossa, where there is another rim-enhancing abscess (*B*) in the left temporalis muscle (*arrowhead*). The patient presented 2 weeks after tooth extraction with left facial swelling and fever.

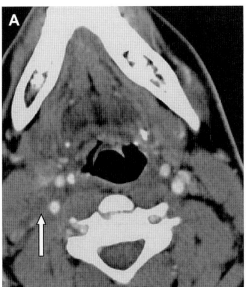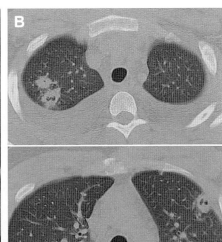

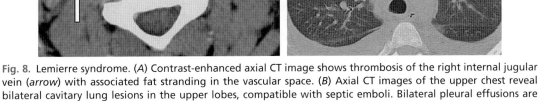

Fig. 8. Lemierre syndrome. (A) Contrast-enhanced axial CT image shows thrombosis of the right internal jugular vein (arrow) with associated fat stranding in the vascular space. (B) Axial CT images of the upper chest reveal bilateral cavitary lung lesions in the upper lobes, compatible with septic emboli. Bilateral pleural effusions are noted.

artery pseudoaneurym. Additional sources of carotid space infection include deep cervical lymphadenitis, spread of infection involving the parapharyngeal space, and traumatic infections from direct needle punctures in intravenous drug users.

Parapharyngeal space

The parapharyngeal space is created by the three deep cervical fascia reflections. The superficial layer is present laterally, the middle layer represents the medial boundary, and the deep reflection limits the space posteriorly. The parapharyngeal space spans from the skull base to the hyoid bone. It contains fat, branches of the trigeminal nerve, the ascending pharyngeal vessels, internal maxillary artery, and accessory salivary tissue. This space communicates inferiorly with the submandibular space and is limited by the masticator space anteriorly, the pharyngeal mucosal space medially, the parotid space laterally, and the vascular compartment posteriorly. Typically, an infection in the parapharyngeal space (**Fig. 9**) represents extension of disease originating from one of the bordering spaces (discussed previously).[17–19] The source of infection includes the pharynx, the tonsils, the parotid glands, the middle ear and mastoids, or can also be odontogenic.[13,20] Once deep neck infections reach the parapharyngeal space, they can subsequently spread to the submandibular or parotid glands and even to the skull base.

Pharyngeal mucosal space

The pharyngeal mucosal space is a common site of neck infection because it contains the adenoids and tonsils as well as the mucosa of the upper

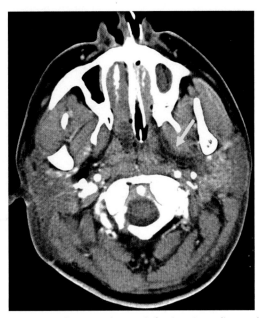

Fig. 9. Parapharyngeal space infection. Stranding and narrowing of the left parapharynegeal space (arrow) secondary to adjacent infection involving the left parotid gland. Note the normal fat density of the right parapharyngeal space.

aerodigestive tract.[2] A superficial mucosal pharyngitis in this space can progress to tonsillitis and even tonsillar abscess formation (**Fig. 10**). Contrast-enhanced CT is useful in establishing the extent of tonsillar infection and allows evaluation of potential deep extension and parapahryngeal abscesses formation. The primary lymphatic drainage of the tonsils is to the retropharyngeal chain, and lymphadenopathy within this space can be depicted on cross-sectional imaging. Asymmetric tonsils, pharyngeal mucosal wall thickening, and mass effect on the parapharyngeal space are expected findings in pharyngeal mucosal space infection.[21–23]

Retropharyngeal space

The retropharyngeal space extends from the skull base to the mediastinum. It is formed anteriorly by the visceral division of the middle cervical layer of the deep fascia with the posterior and lateral borders formed by the alar division of the deep layer. The retropharyngeal space normally contains only lymph nodes and fat.

Infection within the retropharyngeal space is most common among children, and abscess formation is usually the end result of a suppurative adenitis of the retropharyngeal lymph nodes (**Fig. 11**) but can also be secondary to penetrating trauma or iatrogenic injury from endoscopy or intubation.[13,24] Retropharyngeal infections typically localize off the midline, on either side, posterolateral to the pharyngeal mucosal space. Cervical spine infections can also serve as the nidus for eventual retropharyngeal space infection.[2,25,26] Because the retropharyngeal space extends to approximately the level of T3 in the mediastinum, a retropharyngeal abscess can result in mediastinitis.[27]

Prevertebral-paravertebral spaces

The prevertebral and paravertebral spaces are enclosed peripherally by the deep layer of the cervical fascia and both comprise the perivertebral space. The vertebral bodies are the deep boundary of the prevertebral space, which contains prevertebral muscles, the brachial plexus, the phrenic nerve, the vertebral arteries, and veins. The posterior vertebral elements are the deep boundary of the paravertebral space, which contains the paraspinal muscles. Infection in these spaces typically arises from cervical diskitis (pyogenic infection or tuberculosis) or as direct extension from the retropharyngeal space. Aggressive infections can lead to vertebral osteomyelitis or cervical instability and even spread into the epidural space.[13] In such cases, MR imaging has high sensitivity for the diagnosis and can better characterize epidural extension and possible compression or involvement of the spinal cord (**Fig. 12**). Longus colli tendinitis produced by deposition of crystals of hydroxyapatite in the prevertebral tendons can present with dysphagia of acute onset and clinically mimic acute infection. CT demonstrates longus colli tendon enlargement with calcifications, usually at the C1-C2 vertebral level.

Infrahyoid Neck

The visceral space is enclosed by the visceral division of the middle layer of the deep cervical fascia. It extends from the hyoid bone to the aortic arch

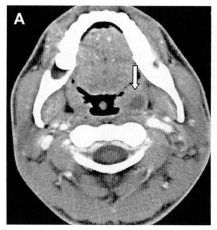
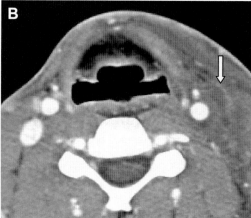

Fig. 10. Tonsillar abscess. (*A*) Contrast-enhanced axial CT image shows a left tonsillar abscess causing partial effacement of the left parapharyngeal space (*arrow*). (*B*) Magnified view of a contrast-enhanced axial CT image in the same patient shows extension of the infectious process into a left superficial facial vein causing septic thrombosis (*arrow*).

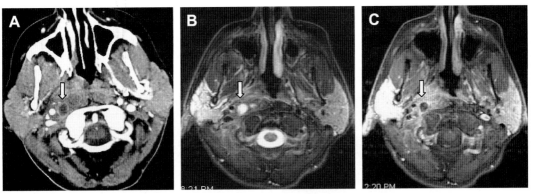

Fig. 11. Retropharyngeal abscess. A 58-year-old male patient who presented clinically with sore throat, fever, and dyspnea. (*A*) Contrast-enhanced axial CT image shows a small rim-enhancing abscess within the right aspect of the retropharyngeal space (*arrow*). (*B*) Axial T2-weighted and (*C*) postcontrast, fat-suppressed, T1-weighted images illustrate the fluid collection (*arrows*) and surrounding phlegmonous changes within the retropharyngeal space.

and contains the trachea, larynx, pharynx, esophagus, thyroid gland, parathyroid glands, and lymph nodes.[2] Infection in this space typically originates from traumatic anterior perforation of the trachea and can extend into the anterior mediastinum.

Less commonly, neck trauma or thyroiditis can also lead to visceral space infections.[13] Additionally, it is important to consider that the carotid, retropharyngeal and perivertebral spaces span the suprahyoid and infrahyoid neck regions.

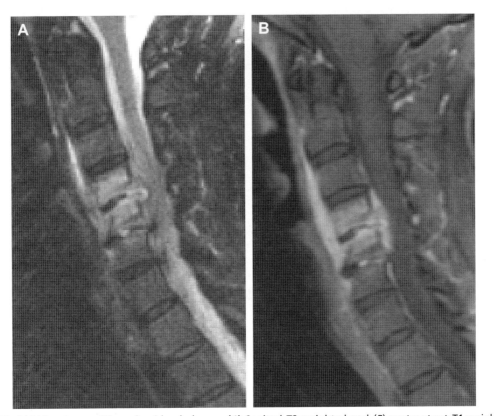

Fig. 12. Diskitis-osteomyelitis and epidural abscess. (*A*) Sagittal T2-weighted and (*B*) postcontrast T1-weighted images show increased signal and enhancement of the C4 and C5 vertebral bodies. There is associated enhancing prevertebral and epidural extension of the infectious process, with compression of the spinal cord.

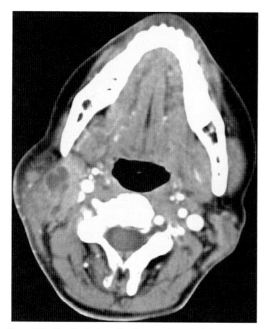

Fig. 13. Cervical lymphadenopathy. Axial contrast-enhanced CT image shows right cervical level II lymph node enlargement with central nodal necrosis in a patient with tuberculous lymphadenitis. Note the surrounding stranding and deformity of the subcutaneous tissue consistent with extracapsular spread of infection.

The posterior cervical space is located within the posterolateral aspect of the neck, extending from the skull base to the clavicle deep to the sternomastoid and trapezius muscles but superficial to the prevertebral space. The majority of the posterior cervical space is topographically within the infrahyoid neck. Together with the submandibular and retropharyngeal spaces, the posterior cervical space is a common area for development of infectious lymphadenitis. In adults, pharyngotonsillitis and odontogenic infections caused by *Streptococcus*, *Staphylococcus*, and *Bacteroides* species are common causes of cervical lymphadenitis. Viral causes of cervical lymphadenitis are common, particularly in the pediatric population. Involvement of the cervical lymph nodes is the most common presentation of tuberculous lymphadenitis. The appearance on cross-sectional imaging can vary from nonspecific enlarged enhancing lymph nodes to necrotic lymph nodes that can coalesce to form large multiloculated masses within the neck, with or without extranodal soft tissue involvement (**Fig. 13**).

SUMMARY

Understanding the anatomy of the cervical fascia as well as the relationships and communications between the various neck spaces is essential for radiologists to make an accurate diagnosis and help guide management of infectious processes.

The role of diagnostic imaging is to define the location of the infection and the possible presence of a drainable fluid collection and to search for extension of disease beyond the site of origin. A careful assessment of potential severe complications, such as vascular compromise, osteomyelitis, and airway narrowing, should be performed routinely. These goals can be achieved with the appropriate use of contrast-enhanced CT and MR imaging in selected cases.

REFERENCES

1. Chow AW, Roser SM, Brady FA. Orofacial odontogenic infections. Ann Intern Med 1978;88(3): 392–402.
2. Hurley MC, Heran MK. Imaging studies for head and neck infections. Infect Dis Clin North Am 2007;21(2): 305–53, v–vi.
3. Johnson RF, Stewart MG, Wright CC. An evidence-based review of the treatment of peritonsillar abscess. Otolaryngol Head Neck Surg 2003;128(3): 332–43.
4. Hudgins PA. Nodal and nonnodal inflammatory processes of the pediatric neck. Neuroimaging Clin N Am 2000;10(1):181–92, ix.
5. Lazor JB, Cunningham MJ, Eavey RD, et al. Comparison of computed tomography and surgical findings in deep neck infections. Otolaryngol Head Neck Surg 1994;111(6):746–50.
6. Nyberg DA, Jeffrey RB, Brant-Zawadzki M, et al. Computed tomography of cervical infections. J Comput Assist Tomogr 1985;9(2):288–96.
7. Weber AL, Siciliano A. CT and MR imaging evaluation of neck infections with clinical correlations. Radiol Clin North Am 2000;38(5):941–68, ix.
8. Barakate MS, Jensen MJ, Hemli JM, et al. Ludwig's angina: report of a case and review of management issues. Ann Otol Rhinol Laryngol 2001;110(5 Pt 1): 453–6.
9. Brondbo K, Rubin A, Chapnik JS, et al. Ludwig's angina following dental extraction as a cause of necrotizing mediastinitis. J Otolaryngol 1983;12(1): 50–2.
10. Furst IM, Ersil P, Caminiti M. A rare complication of tooth abscess—Ludwig's angina and mediastinitis. J Can Dent Assoc 2001;67(6):324–7.
11. Sofianou D, Peftoulidou M, Manolis EN, et al. A fatal case of Ludwig's angina and mediastinitis caused by an unusual microorganism, Gemella morbillorum. Scand J Infect Dis 2005;37(5):367–9.
12. Brook I. Acute bacterial suppurative parotitis: microbiology and management. J Craniofac Surg 2003; 14(1):37–40.

13. Vieira F, Allen SM, Stocks RM, et al. Deep neck infection. Otolaryngol Clin North Am 2008;41(3): 459–83, vii.

14. Gowan RT, Mehran RJ, Cardinal P, et al. Thoracic complications of Lemierre syndrome. Can Respir J 2000;7(6):481–5.

15. Patel S, Brennan J. Diagnosis of internal jugular vein thrombosis by computed tomography. J Comput Assist Tomogr 1981;5(2):197–200.

16. Chirinos JA, Lichtstein DM, Garcia J, et al. The evolution of Lemierre syndrome: report of 2 cases and review of the literature. Medicine (Baltimore) 2002;81(6):458–65.

17. Branstetter BF 4th, Weissman JL. Normal anatomy of the neck with CT and MR imaging correlation. Radiol Clin North Am 2000;38(5):925–40, ix.

18. Harnsberger HR, Osborn AG. Differential diagnosis of head and neck lesions based on their space of origin. 1. The suprahyoid part of the neck. AJR Am J Roentgenol 1991;157(1):147–54.

19. Paonessa DF, Goldstein JC. Anatomy and physiology of head and neck infections (with emphasis on the fascia of the face and neck). Otolaryngol Clin North Am 1976;9(3):561–80.

20. Tanner A, Stillman N. Oral and dental infections with anaerobic bacteria: clinical features, predominant pathogens, and treatment. Clin Infect Dis 1993; 16(Suppl 4):S304–9.

21. Johnson JT. Abscesses and deep space infections of the head and neck. Infect Dis Clin North Am 1992;6(3):705–17.

22. McRae D, Dilkes M, Jacob-Hood J, et al. Computerized tomography of acute, tender peritonsillar swellings. Clin Otolaryngol Allied Sci 1993;18(5): 350–4.

23. Sichel JY, Dano I, Hocwald E, et al. Nonsurgical management of parapharyngeal space infections: a prospective study. Laryngoscope 2002;112(5): 906–10.

24. Barratt GE, Koopmann CF Jr, Coulthard SW. Retropharyngeal abscess—a ten-year experience. Laryngoscope 1984;94(4):455–63.

25. Faidas A, Ferguson JV Jr, Nelson JE, et al. Cervical vertebral osteomyelitis presenting as a retropharyngeal abscess. Clin Infect Dis 1994;18(6):992–4.

26. Jang YJ, Rhee CK. Retropharyngeal abscess associated with vertebral osteomyelitis and spinal epidural abscess. Otolaryngol Head Neck Surg 1998;119(6):705–8.

27. Takao M, Ido M, Hamaguchi K, et al. Descending necrotizing mediastinitis secondary to a retropharyngeal abscess. Eur Respir J 1994;7(9):1716–8.

Imaging of Aortic and Branch Vessel Trauma

Martin L. Gunn, MBChB, FRANZCR

KEYWORDS

- Aortic injury • Multidetector-row computed tomography
- Trauma

Although infrequently encountered even in busy trauma centers, injuries to the aorta and branch vessels remain an important cause of trauma-related mortality.[1] Advances in the diagnosis and management of these injuries have led to more accurate and timely imaging, and improved patient outcomes.[2] Thoracic multidetector-row computed tomography (MDCT) has now supplanted catheter angiography as the reference standard for the diagnosis of thoracic aortic injury, and endovascular repair has reduced mortality. Delays in evaluating the aorta have been reduced with implementation of rapid multiregional computed tomography (CT) in the severely injured patient, and previously unrecognized minor aortic injuries are now increasingly apparent.[3–5]

Despite these advances, several challenges in evaluating the severely injured trauma patient remain. Although liberal use of MDCT will result in the diagnosis of nearly all blunt aortic injuries, effective clinical prediction rules to determine the exact indications for CT have not yet been developed.[6] This drawback is of particular concern, as radiation exposure from radiographs and CT is high in multitrauma patients and health care costs of imaging are rising.[7,8] Moreover, some findings on CT can be challenging to interpret, and in some cases require further imaging.[9] This review provides an overview of current concepts in the imaging of aortic and branch vessel injuries, and provides pointers to improve detection and interpretation of more challenging cases.

NORMAL AORTIC ANATOMY

The thoracic aorta can be divided into anatomic segments. The aortic root is a short segment of the aorta arising from the heart, and contains the aortic valve, aortic annulus, and coronary sinuses. The aortic root and proximal ascending aorta is surrounded by the superior aortic recess of the pericardium. This recess is a cranial extension of the transverse pericardial sinus and is composed of anterior, right lateral, and posterior portions. It can usually be seen on CT.[10] The ascending aorta extends from the root to the proximal edge of the brachiocephalic artery. The aortic arch continues from brachiocephalic artery to the attachment of the ligamentum arteriosum and gives rise to the brachiocephalic artery, left common carotid, and left subclavian arteries. The descending thoracic aorta is the segment between the ligamentum arteriosum and the aortic hiatus of the diaphragm. The portion of the descending aorta between left subclavian artery and the ligamentum arteriosum is termed the aortic isthmus.

Variants in arch anatomy are common. In 13% of patients there is a common origin of the brachiocephalic and left common carotid arteries; the so-called bovine-arch.[11] In 6% of cases, the left vertebral artery has an aortic origin.[12]

EPIDEMIOLOGY, OUTCOME, AND PATHOPHYSIOLOGY

Blunt thoracic aortic injury (BTAI) is a highly lethal injury. Although aortic injuries occur in less than 0.5% to 2% of nonlethal motor vehicle collisions (MVCs), it has been found in up to 34% of trauma fatalities at autopsy.[1,13,14] Up to 80% of patients die from aortic injury at the scene. The incidence of aortic injury associated with MVCs does not appear to be declining, although the patterns of vehicular intrusion have been changing from

Disclosures: No funding support provided for this project, or relevant disclosures.
Department of Radiology, University of Washington, 325 9th Avenue, Box 359728, Seattle, WA 98104, USA
E-mail address: marting@uw.edu

frontal impact to side (especially near-side) impact.[14–16] Other causes of aortic injury include motorcycle and aircraft crashes, pedestrian injuries, falls from height, and crush injuries.

BTAI has traditionally been considered a surgical emergency, based largely on the work of Parmley in the 1950s, when there was a 1% mortality rate per hour in the first 48 hours of hospitalization.[17] Following the widespread implementation of early blood pressure control for aortic injury, a different mortality pattern has emerged over the last several years. Patients arriving in the emergency department in extremis still have a very high probability of death, approaching 100%.[18] However, patients who arrive hemodynamically stable and are managed with β-blockade and definitive repair do considerably better, even with "delayed" repair. Between the first American Association for the Surgery of Trauma trial ($AAST_1$) in 1997 and the second trial in 2007 ($AAST_2$), there was a significant reduction in both mortality and morbidity from blunt aortic injury.[2,18] Over this period, the short-term mortality (excluding patients who arrive in extremis) improved from 22% to 13%, and the paraplegia rate fell from 8.7% to 1.6%. There are multiple reasons for this mortality reduction. Over this period, CT scanning virtually replaced catheter aortography and transesophageal echocardiography (TEE) as the primary diagnostic test. In addition, the time from admission to definitive repair increased, and the means of repair switched from exclusively open repair to predominantly endovascular repair. Although recent short and medium term outcome studies are very promising, outcome studies evaluating the long-term outcome of endovascular repair, especially in young patients, are awaited.

Despite several proposed pathophysiological mechanisms for blunt aortic injury, the exact mechanism has not been determined. In reality, a combination of mechanisms likely accounts for the spectrum of injuries that are encountered.

The deceleration shear force theory proposes that shearing forces are generated in the aorta at points of differential deceleration. During rapid deceleration, fixation of the aorta by the great vessels, heart, and ligamentum arteriosum cause shearing injuries where these points intersect with more mobile sections of the aorta. This theory accounts for the tendency of aortic injuries to occur adjacent to the aortic isthmus, and for the incidence of aortic injuries correlating with deceleration of more than 20 mph (32 km/h) and vehicular intrusion.[19,20] The "osseous pinch" theory hypothesizes that rupture of the aorta is due to entrapment of the aorta between the anterior thoracic bony structures (manubrium, clavicle, and first ribs) and the vertebral column, resulting in transverse lacerations at the aortic isthmus.[21] This mechanism may also explain concomitant injuries to some branch vessels.[13] The water-hammer theory proposes that sudden increased intravascular pressure from aortic occlusion at the diaphragm results in transmission of a significant pressure pulse to the aortic arch, resulting in transverse tears in the aortic arch at the level of the isthmus, which is the weakest point.[22,23]

In autopsy series, 58% to 90% of thoracic aortic injuries occur at the level of the aortic isthmus.[14,17,24,25] The next most common region, the aortic root and ascending aorta, comprises 5% to 10% of aortic injuries. Injury to the aortic root and ascending aorta is usually immediately fatal, and clinical presentation is extremely rare.[25] Between 3% and 8% of injuries occur in the distal descending thoracic aorta.[24] Five to seventeen percent of aortic injuries occur at branch vessel origins.[26,27] Aortic injuries are multifocal in 13% to 18% of patients.[14,24,25]

Blunt abdominal aortic injuries (BAAI) represent only about 5% of blunt aortic injuries.[28] BAAI are associated with high-speed MVCs, and have been linked to steering-wheel injury to the lower abdomen and the use of lap-belt restraints.[28] Like BTAI, the mechanism of injury is unclear, but theories include direct compression of the aorta against the spine, stretching of the aortic wall by elevation of the intraluminal pressure following sudden compression, differential shearing forces at the aortic bifurcation, and longitudinal aortic stretching accompanying distraction injuries of the lumbar spine.[29,30] As with BTAI, there has been a recent shift to endovascular repair of BAAI, with good short-term outcomes.[28–30] Endovascular repair avoids the potential for surgical graft infection from concurrent bowel injury. Surgical treatment is associated with an overall mortality of 27%.

Penetrating aortic injury represents 14% of aortic injuries at autopsy. These injuries are almost always attributable to knife and gunshot injuries.[25] Rare causes include misplacement of spinal fixation screws, and lacerations from spinal fractures.[31] Gunshot injuries to the thoracic aorta have a strong predilection for the ascending aorta. Stab wounds are strongly associated with branch vessel injuries.[25] Most patients who arrive alive at the hospital with penetrating aortic injuries will have injuries to the abdominal aorta rather than the thoracic aorta.[32] Patients often arrive at the hospital in hypovolemic shock. The outcome of penetrating aortic injuries is usually dismal, with thoracic aortic injuries faring worse than abdominal aortic injuries (92% vs 76% mortality).[32] Endovascular repair has been described.[33]

CLASSIFICATION OF AORTIC INJURY

Over the years, classification systems for BTAI have been developed based on time course, pathologic appearance, and imaging appearance.[34–36] For the radiologist and vascular surgeon, the best classification system to guide management may be one based on imaging appearances, proposed by Azizzadeh and colleagues[34] in 2009 (**Fig. 1**). This system is valuable because it includes minimal aortic injuries, which are increasingly identified with the use of screening CT.[4]

ASSOCIATED INJURIES

Associated injuries can provide clues to the presence of an aortic injury. Historically first rib fractures, which are associated with high-energy injury trauma, have been considered to be strongly associated with aortic and great vessel injuries. However, recent evidence suggests that angiography is not indicated solely by the presence of first-rib fractures in both children and adults. In a series by Hamilton and colleagues,[37] none of the 22 pediatric patients with a first-rib fracture and a normal mediastinum on plain radiography had a traumatic vascular injury on CT or clinical follow-up. Although there does appear to be an association between vascular injuries and fractures of the upper ribs, the conclusion of multiple series is that decision to perform angiography should not be based solely on the presence of a first-rib fracture, but on clinical signs of vascular injury and/or an abnormal mediastinum.[38] Commonly identified on chest CT, first-rib and second-rib fractures were present in almost half of the trauma CTs performed in one series. These investigators found similar rates of aortic and great vessel injury in patients with and without first-rib or second-rib fractures.[39]

In a recent autopsy study by Teixeria and colleagues,[14] the extent and distribution of associated injuries was well documented. These

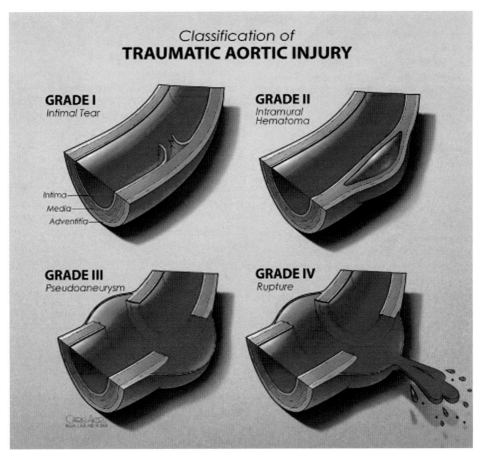

Fig. 1. Classification of traumatic aortic injury. Grades I and II are considered minimal aortic injuries, and are treated conservatively when small. Grade III injuries are the most common to present clinically. Survival from Grade IV injuries is rare. (*From* Azizzadeh A, Keyhani K, Miller CC III, et al. Blunt traumatic aortic injury: initial experience with endovascular repair. J Vasc Surg 2009;49(6):1403–8; with permission.)

investigators found extrathoracic injuries in 96% of patients with BTAI. Almost all these injuries are associated with a high energy mechanism of trauma. Patients with BTAI are significantly more likely than trauma patients without BTAI to have cardiac injury, diaphragmatic lacerations, hemothorax, rib fractures, pelvic fractures, and intra-abdominal injuries. Sternal fractures and head injuries were not associated with BTAI.[14] Posterior sternoclavicular dislocation has been associated with injuries to aortic branch vessels.

IMAGING TECHNIQUES
Plain Radiography

Chest radiography, specifically the supine chest radiograph, has long been used as the initial means of screening for thoracic aortic injury. However, the chest radiograph may be normal in 7% to 11% of cases of acute aortic injury (**Fig. 2**).[40–42] Although it has greater specificity,[43] an erect chest radiograph often cannot be obtained in unstable trauma patients and in the setting of potential spine injury. A "widened mediastinum" is the best known sign of aortic injury.[44] However, the definition of a widened mediastinum varies. Quantitatively, it refers to a mediastinal width of 8 cm at the level of the aortic arch on a supine (or erect) chest anteroposterior radiograph.[43] Due to variation in patient size, a mediastinum to chest-width ratio of (>0.25 [and >0.38]) has been suggested as a more accurate measure.[2,43,45] However, a subjective assessment of mediastinal width is usually used in practice.

Due to several potential causes of mediastinal widening on a supine radiograph (eg, mediastinal lipomatosis, vascular ectasia or engorgement, atelectasis), other signs of aortic contour abnormality are usually used to increase specificity (**Box 1**).

One technique to improve visualization of the aortic contour in supine patients is a coned mediastinal view with craniocaudal tilt, although routine use has not been systemically validated. This view has been termed the reverse Trendelenburg radiograph.[46] As a Trendelenburg position is usually impractical in the acutely ill patient, at the author's institution a coned view of the mediastinum is performed with higher tube potential and 15° of craniocaudal tilt whenever an aortic or mediastinal contour abnormality is suspected on a supine radiograph.

Due to the imperfect sensitivity and poor specificity of chest radiography, further imaging (almost always with CT) should be performed whenever an abnormality is suspected on chest radiography, or when the mechanism of injury is compatible with aortic injury.

Computed Tomography

Multidetector CT angiography (CTA) is the reference-standard imaging study for the diagnosis of blunt traumatic aortic injury.[2,47–50] Accordingly, it has almost completely replaced catheter aortography and TEE.[2] Indications for chest CTA include an abnormal aortic contour on plain radiography, clinical signs, and injury mechanism suggestive of aortic injury. Several series have shown that helical CTA has a sensitivity of 95% or more for the detection of BTAI.[50–53] In the early days of helical CT for aortic injury, reliance of mediastinal hematoma as an indirect sign led to a lower reported specificity for aortic injury, and reliance on catheter angiography as the reference standard. However, as is described later, the finding of isolated mediastinal hematoma does not warrant further investigation following a high-quality MDCT examination. Unfortunately, CT is not fail-safe. CT artifacts, variants in the aorta, and subtle aortic injuries can still be challenging even for the experienced radiologist.

At most trauma centers, CTA of the thorax in patients at risk of BTAI is not performed as a sole examination. Rather, it is usually integrated into a whole-body CT (the so-called trauma pan-scan), a technique that has been shown to improve survival and reduce imaging time.[3,5] There is now the potential to use electrocardiographic (ECG) cardiac gating for the assessment of aortic injury. Due to its higher temporal resolution, dual-source CT (DSCT) ECG-gated (or nongated) CTA can be performed without β-blockade in patients with regular heart rates, and can achieve acceptable motion suppression at radiation doses below 5 mSv.[20,54,55] Hence, it is now technically feasible to perform ECG-gated CTA as a screening tool for aortic injury. In cases of indeterminate nongated aortic CTAs, a follow-up gated CTA using single-source scanners and β-blockade also offers promise.

Transesophageal Echocardiography

TEE has sensitivity for the diagnosis of BTAI in the 56% to 99% range, with specificity in the 89% to 99% range.[56] With the increased use of screening helical CTA, it is now rarely used; only 1% of BTAI cases were diagnosed with TEE in the $AAST_2$ trial.[2] Potential reasons for this include lack of availability, the need for sedation, and concerns about potential suboptimal sensitivity. TEE does have a "blind spot" in the distal ascending aorta and proximal branch vessels. TEE can be useful as a diagnostic tool for the evaluation of equivocal CTA or catheter aortogram.[57]

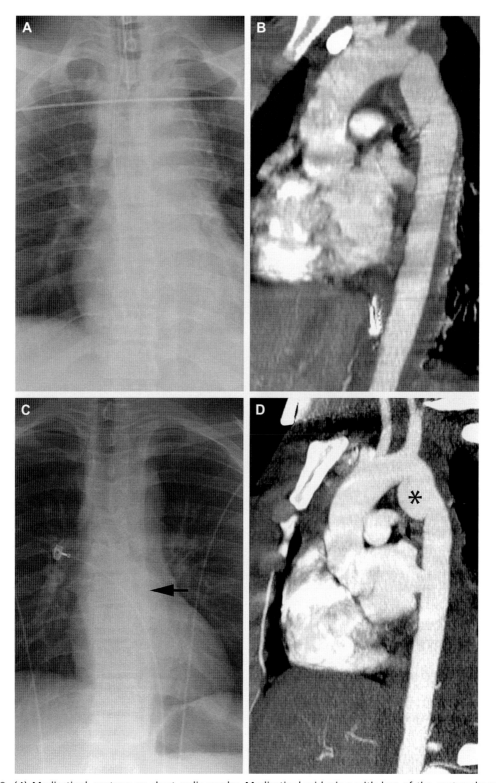

Fig. 2. (A) Mediastinal contour on chest radiography. Mediastinal widening with loss of the aortopulmonary window, right paratracheal stripe thickening, left apical pleural cap, loss of the descending aortic contour, and widening of the paravertebral stripe. (B) Thin-slab maximum-intensity projection from a chest CTA shows an aortic transection with a pseudoaneurysm at the level of the aortic isthmus. (C) Chest radiograph initially reported as negative for aortic injury. Although the mediastinum does not appear widened, there is thickening of the left paravertebral stripe (arrow) and a left pleural cap. (D) Chest CTA revealed a large pseudoaneurysm in the aortic isthmus (asterisk), which was successfully managed with endovascular repair.

Intravascular Ultrasonography

Intravascular ultrasonography (IVUS) is performed by introducing a high-frequency (approximately 10 MHz) miniature ultrasound transducer through a large arterial sheath (approximately 8F) and obtaining real-time 360° images of the aorta. Although limited by the absence of a reference-standard technique, a recent study found that IVUS performed better than catheter aortography in patients who had equivocal CTAs.[9] The high cost of the disposable transducers, invasive nature, and operating room time limit IVUS to a problem-solving tool at present.

Catheter Aortography

Catheter aortography was long considered to be the reference-standard examination for the diagnosis of aortic injury, with previously reported sensitivity, specificity, and accuracy all approaching 100%. However, studies were usually limited by the absence of another test. It does appear that false-positive catheter angiograms do occur, particularly in the setting of an atypical ductus arteriosus.[58] Moreover, there is significant interobserver variability in the interpretation of catheter angiograms in equivocal cases, greater than that of IVUS.[9,59] Furthermore, since CTA use became widespread, it has been recognized that minimal injuries such as intimal tears comprise up to 10% of BTAI, and most of these are occult on catheter aortography (**Fig. 3**).[4] The role of catheter aortography in the initial diagnosis of BTAI is now limited; it can be performed without significant delay or

risk of morbidity following pelvic angioembolization, but in most cases the assessment for aortic injury is better performed using CTA integrated with MDCT of other body regions. Moreover, catheter angiography may have a limited role as a problem-solving tool in the equivocal CTA, for which IVUS, or even follow-up gated CTA, are better options.[9]

Imaging Algorithm

A recent systematic review of 10 studies to evaluate predictors for blunt aortic injuries found that clinical and radiographic predictors of BTAI did not perform adequately enough to safely omit chest CT.[6] Consequently, the liberal use of CT was recommended; this corresponds with the author's clinical experience at a high-volume trauma center. The imaging algorithm performed at Harborview Medical Center for the assessment of BTAI is shown in **Fig. 4**. This algorithm has not been prospectively tested, although it was shown to be effective retrospectively.[60] Patients who undergo CTA of the chest for potential aortic injury usually visit the emergency CT scanner for other investigations, particularly CT of the head, cervical spine, and abdomen/pelvis. In these patients, CTA or CT of the chest is performed as part of a single helical acquisition, without significantly greater radiation dose or additional contrast exposure.

IMAGING APPEARANCES OF AORTIC INJURY
Blunt Thoracic Aortic Transection: Pseudoaneurysm and Rupture

Radiographic signs of BTAI are largely confined to the detection of mediastinal hematoma, and are discussed in some detail in earlier sections.

Historically, signs of blunt traumatic injury on CT of the chest have been classified as indirect and direct (**Box 2**). The principal indirect sign of aortic injury visible on CT of the chest is periaortic hematoma.[61] Periaortic hematoma usually does not arise directly from exsanguination of blood from the aorta, but from injury to small mediastinal vessels or fractures of the spine or thoracic cage. The importance of periaortic and perivascular mediastinal hematoma is that it is a marker of mediastinal injury, and it should prompt an extremely careful evaluation for direct signs of aortic injury. Periaortic hemorrhage identified at the level of the diaphragm visible on abdominal CT in a trauma patient should prompt CTA of the chest (**Fig. 5**).[62] Mediastinal hematoma without direct signs of aortic injury was previously believed to be an indication for aortography. However, evidence now suggests that it is unnecessary when mediastinal hematoma is encountered in

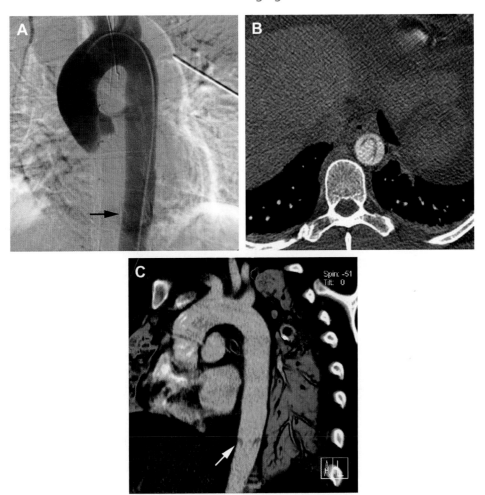

Fig. 3. Aortic intimal tears not identified on catheter angiography. High-speed motor vehicle collision in a young woman. (*A*) Catheter aortogram immediately following pelvic angioembolization was reported as negative for aortic injury, but in retrospect a subtle intimal tear is visible (*arrow*). (*B*) Axial and (*C*) oblique sagittal volume rendered images from a CT performed immediately after angiography reveal a circumferential intimal tear (*arrow*) of the descending aorta. This tear is likely to be a stretch-type injury. The patient was treated with an endovascular stent graft.

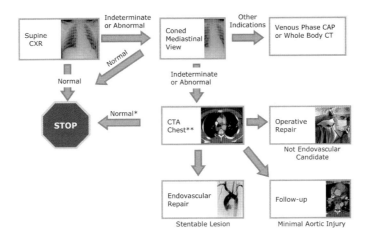

* Includes isolated periaortic hematoma
** Usually combined with other examinations.

Fig. 4. Harborview Medical Center Screening algorithm for blunt thoracic aortic injury.

Box 2
CT signs of aortic injury

Periaortic hematoma (indirect)

End-organ arterial infarcts (indirect)

Aortic pseudoaneurysm

Active vascular extravasation

Intimal flap

Small intraluminal filling defects

Narrow aortic caliber

Periaortic hematoma at the diaphragm

Coarctation

Intramural hematoma

the absence of direct signs, especially if it can be explained by the presence of other adjacent injuries.[49,63,64] End-organ infarcts, another indirect sign, are occasionally seen (**Fig. 6**).

An aortic pseudoaneurysm is the most commonly identified injury on CT. It is thought to be caused by near complete transection of the aortic wall, with sparing of the adventitia, or tamponade due to hematoma.[17] In most patients who present to hospital the injury is at the level of the aortic isthmus. Pseudoaneurysms frequently occupy the inferomedial surface but they can also be circumferential (**Fig. 7**). On axial images, the pseudoaneurysm may resemble a beret sitting on top of the aorta, which forms the face (**Fig. 8**). Pseudoaneurysms typically

have acute angles with the adjacent aortic lumen, a feature that helps to distinguish them from ductus diverticula. Active vascular extravasation (**Fig. 9**) is rarely identified, and is thought to indicate a poor outcome.[49]

Traumatic coarctation typically refers to a small descending aorta distal to a large pseudoaneurysm. The mechanism for this has not been determined, but compression by a proximally located pseudoaneurysm has been suggested.[51]

Minimal Aortic Injury

Minimal aortic injuries comprise small (<10 mm) intimal tears (grade I) and intramural hematomas (grade II).[4,34,65] These injuries have been increasingly recognized as the use of CT screening has increased. In an early helical CT series, they were estimated to represent 10% of aortic injuries.[4] These injuries are likely to have been underdiagnosed when catheter angiography was the primary diagnostic test. Conservative management of minimal aortic injuries has been examined in a few small series and is probably effective and safe. Imaging surveillance is necessary, especially for intimal tears greater than 10 mm.[66,67]

Minimal aortic injuries commonly appear as small luminal filling defects, intimal flaps, and intramural hematomas (**Figs. 10** and **11**). Serial imaging may reveal resolution of the injury. There should be no associated pseudoaneurysm, and mediastinal hematoma is uncommonly encountered.[4]

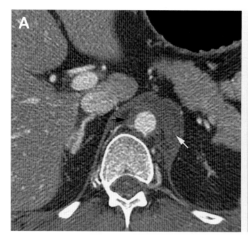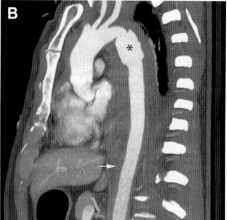

Fig. 5. Retrocrural periaortic hematoma on an upper abdominal CT image. (*A*) CT at the level of the diaphragm reveals retrocrural blood (*white arrow*) and subadventitial blood around the descending thoracic aorta. (*B*) Oblique sagittal thick-slab maximum-intensity projection shows the blood (*white arrow*) tracking around the aorta and a large pseudoaneurysm at the level of the aortic isthmus (*asterisk*). The finding of unexplained retrocrural blood on the upper cuts of a CT of the abdomen in the setting of trauma should prompt CTA of the chest.

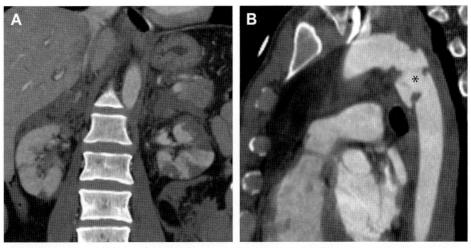

Fig. 6. Indirect signs of aortic injury. (*A*) Wedge-shaped bilateral renal infarcts (in addition to renal lacerations) are present. No renal vascular injuries were noted on CTA. Note the perinephric hemorrhage. (*B*) Transection of the isthmus of the aorta (*asterisk*) with unusually thick intimomedial flaps (likely with adherent thrombus) in the same patient. Note the periaortic blood extending inferiorly around the aorta.

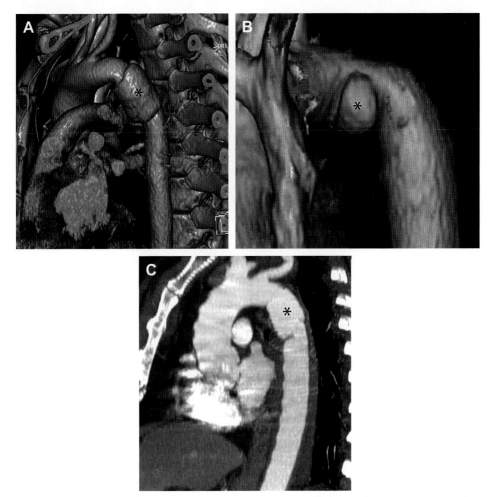

Fig. 7. Common appearances of traumatic pseudoaneurysms. (*A*) Volume-rendered projection (VR) of a CTA showing a circumferential transection centered in aortic the isthmus (*asterisk*). (*B*) VR from a CT in another patient showing a more localized pseudoaneurysm (*asterisk*). Note the acute angles on both the upper and lower edges, a finding (along with periaortic hematoma) that helps differentiate from a ductus diverticulum. (*C*) Oblique sagittal thin-slab maximum-intensity projection revealing a transection with large intimomedial tears extending into the aortic lumen (*asterisk*).

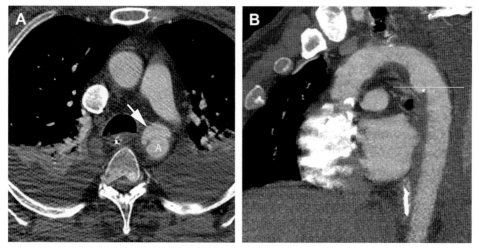

Fig. 8. Beret sign on axial CT. (*A*) Contrast-enhanced CT of the chest shows a pseudoaneurysm resembling a beret cap (*arrow*) sitting on the head, formed by the aortic lumen (A). (*B*) Oblique sagittal reformat shows the level of the corresponding axial slice (*white line*). The axial appearance has also been likened to a mushroom.

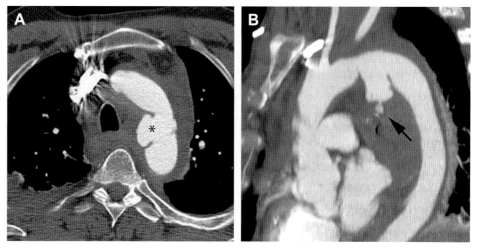

Fig. 9. Active vascular extravasation. (*A*) Axial CTA at the level of the aortic arch shows a large aortic traumatic pseudoaneurysm (*asterisk*) surrounded by a large quantity of mediastinal blood. In addition, there was a right hemothorax. (*B*) Oblique sagittal thin-slab maximum-intensity projection demonstrates active bleeding (*arrow*). Unfortunately, the patient died soon after leaving the CT scanner.

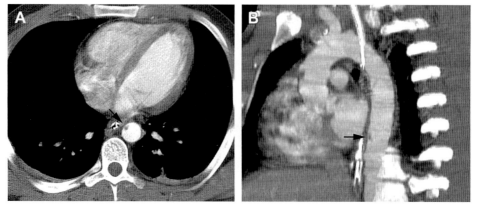

Fig. 10. Minimal aortic injury. (*A*) Axial and (*B*) oblique sagittal images from a CTA showing a small filling defect in the descending aorta (*black arrow*) resembling an intimal tear with adherent thrombus. The patient was treated with β-blockers. A follow-up CTA 5 days later (not shown) revealed resolution of the filling defect.

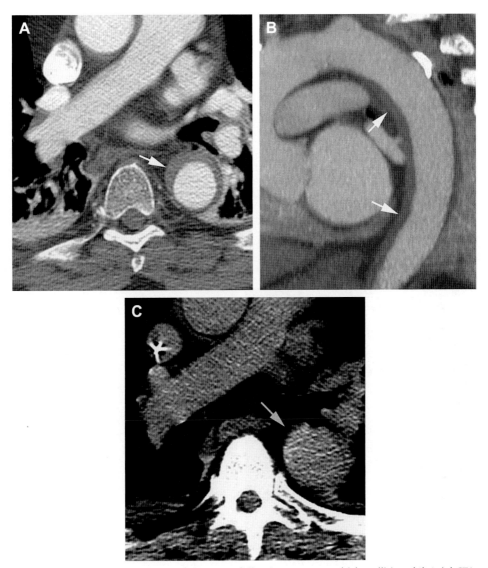

Fig. 11. Traumatic intramural hematoma of the aorta following a motor vehicle collision. (*A*) Axial CTA and (*B*) oblique sagittal maximum-intensity projection reveal mural thickening of the descending aorta (*white arrows*). (*C*) A noncontrast phase is not routinely performed to evaluate for aortic injury. However, in this patient the lower slices of a noncontrast cervical spine CT revealed a hyperdense crescent of blood (*gray arrow*) correlating with the mural thickening, confirming an intramural hematoma. The patient was treated conservatively.

Branch Vessel Injury

Although uncommon, injury to the aortic branch vessels can be subtle, and should be specifically sought when there are fractures of the adjacent thoracic cage or posterior sternoclavicular dislocation. No large series has evaluated the accuracy of CTA for the diagnosis of branch vessel injury. As the branch vessels pass perpendicular to the plane of axial images, subtle changes in vessel caliber due to pseudoaneurysms may be difficult to detect (**Fig. 12**). Multiplanar reformats,

particularly in the coronal and "candy-cane" planes, are invaluable for the diagnosis of these injuries. Intimal flaps are also seen. Perivenous artifacts from concentrated intravenous contrast in the subclavian and brachiocephalic veins may obscure these injuries, so a right upper extremity injection is preferred.[68]

Blunt Abdominal Aortic Injury

BAAI almost always occurs inferior to the renal arteries, usually at the levels of the

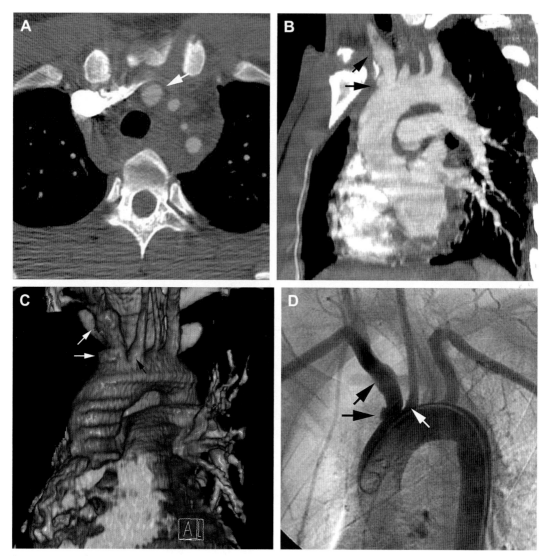

Fig. 12. Value of multiplanar imaging. (*A*) Axial CT in a patient with posterior right sternoclavicular fracture-dislocation reveals perivascular blood surrounding the great vessels. The unusually large size of the brachioce-phalic artery (BCA) (*white arrow*) is difficult to appreciate. (*B*) Oblique sagittal maximum-intensity projection reveals 2 pseudoaneurysms of the BCA (*black arrows*). (*C*) On volume-rendered views a small pseudoaneurysm of the origin of the right internal carotid artery (ICA) was identified (*black arrow*) in addition to the BCA pseudoaneurysms (*white arrows*). (*D*) Catheter angiogram reveals all 3 pseudoaneurysms (*arrows*).

inferior mesenteric artery or aortic bifurcation.[30] It is typically limited in length.[28] Intimal disruption, which may be circumferential, is the most commonly encountered finding on imaging studies (**Fig. 13**). The distal intimal flaps may be dissected or inverted by the blood flow or may be a nidus for thrombus formation, leading to arterial insufficiency.[30] Pseudoaneurysms, true rupture, and thrombosis may also occur.

Penetrating Aortic Injury

Preoperative imaging is not commonly performed for patients with penetrating aortic and branch vessel injury, as these patients usually undergo immediate surgery. When imaging is performed, the findings include pseudoaneurysm, vascular occlusion, active contrast extravasation, and intimal flaps (**Fig. 14**).[69] In cases of gunshot injury, the patient should always be surveyed for the presence of an exit wound as well as vascular embolization of projectiles (**Fig. 15**).

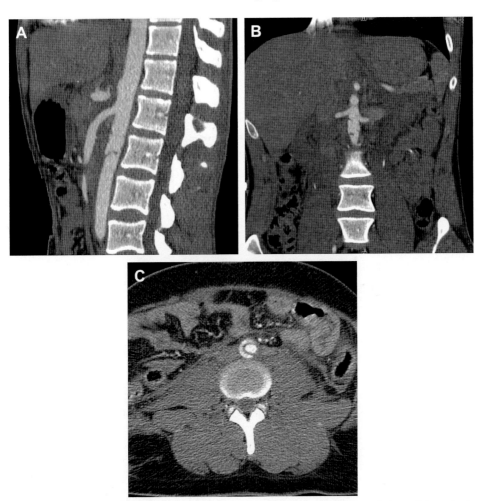

Fig. 13. Blunt abdominal aortic injuries (BAAI) from high-speed motor vehicle collisions. (*A*) Sagittal and (*B*) coronal images from a CTA of the abdomen reveal a stretch-type injury to the infrarenal abdominal aorta. The proximal and distal intimal flaps are visible, and there is a small intervening aortic pseudoaneurysm. (*C*) Axial CTA in a different patient reveals a circumferential intimal tear just above the bifurcation, not an unusual finding in BAAI.

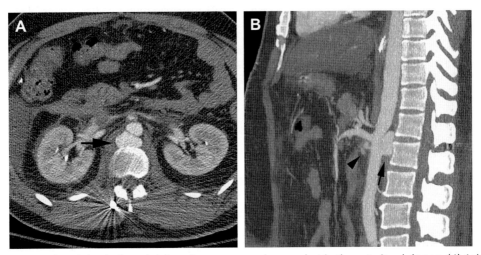

Fig. 14. Penetrating abdominal aortic injury. A young man who was shot in the anterior abdomen. (*A*) Axial and (*B*) sagittal images from a CTA following laparotomy for repair of injuries to the bowel and mesentery reveal pseudoaneurysms arising from the posterior (*arrows*) and anterior (*arrowhead*) surfaces of the abdominal aorta. The bullet is in the paraspinal muscles. Following open repair of the pseudoaneurysm, the man made a good recovery.

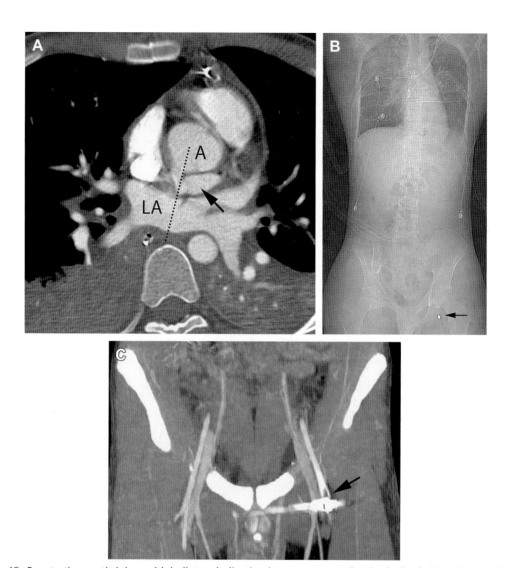

Fig. 15. Penetrating aortic injury with bullet embolization in a young man shot in the back. No exit wound was found. (A) Axial CTA following emergent thoracotomy reveals the bullet course (*dotted line*) through the left atrium (LA) and noncoronary sinus of the aorta [shown as (A)]. A pseudoaneurysm is visible between the aorta and coronary sinus (*arrow*). The bullet entered at a lower level (not shown) and traveled cranially, hence the injured vertebral body injury is not shown. (B) A CT scout image reveals a metallic body in the left groin (*arrow*). (C) CTA of the pelvis performed in combination with the chest CTA demonstrates the bullet lodged in the common femoral artery bifurcation (*arrow*) with adherent thrombus. The patient received aortic and groin surgery and survived.

PITFALLS IN THE INTERPRETATION OF AORTIC INJURY ON MDCT
Aortic Arch Variants: Ductus Diverticulum, Aortic Spindle, Branch Infundibula, and Physiologic Shape Variation

Ductus diverticulum (DD) is a common developmental outpouching of the thoracic aorta, present in 33% of newborns and between 9% and 26% of normal adults.[58,70] The DD is usually located on the anteromedial aspect of the aortic isthmus at the site of the ligamentum arteriosum, the remnant of the fetal ductus arteriosum. Some propose that, it might be a remnant of the right dorsal aortic root.[71] Unfortunately, this is also by far the most common site of BTAI. Although a DD typically has smooth obtuse angles at its junction with the normal aortic wall, in a minority of cases a DD may form an acute angle at its superior margin. If the obtuse angles are not present, the best means of excluding injury are noting the absence of peri-aortic hematoma adjacent to the DD (**Fig. 16**A). Penetrating atherosclerotic ulcers, which may also occur in a similar location, can also simulate a traumatic pseudoaneurysm.

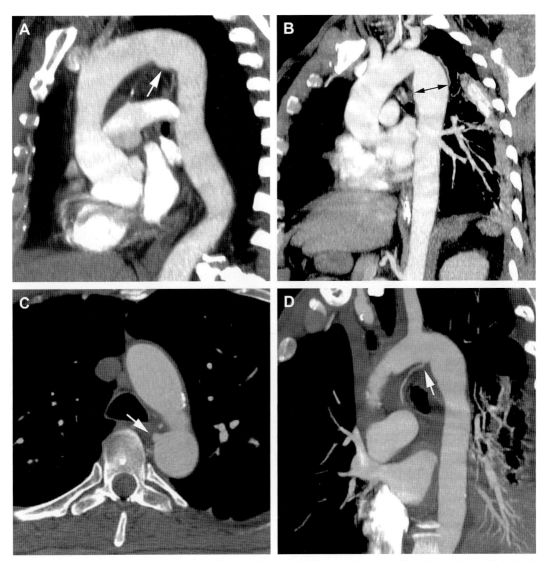

Fig. 16. (*A*) Thin-slab maximum-intensity projection demonstrating a small ductus diverticulum (*arrow*). Note the gentle angles with the aortic arch and the slightly more acute angle at the superior margin, a common finding. (*B*) Aortic spindle deformity with widening of the aorta immediately beyond the isthmus (*double-headed arrow*). (*C*) Bronchial artery infundibulum. Axial CTA shows a small outpouching of the aorta in the region of the isthmus (*arrow*), which on thin-slab sagittal maximum-intensity projection (*D*) is shown to connect to a bronchial artery (*arrow*).

The aortic spindle is a fusiform dilation of the aorta immediately beyond the aortic isthmus that is present in the fetal aorta. This spindle may persist into adulthood and mimic a circumferential aortic pseudoaneurysm (**Fig. 16**B).[72]

Branch vessel infundibula are occasionally seen at the origin of bronchial and intercostal arteries, and may simulate small pseudoaneurysms as they project beyond the expected contour of the aortic lumen. Close inspection of the infundibulum will reveal smooth margins, and a vessel originating from the apex (**Fig. 16**C, D).

Recent work has demonstrated considerable physiologic variation in the diameter, shape, and length of the normal thoracic aorta during the cardiac cycle, especially in younger patients who have more elastic vessel walls.[73,74] In one series, a change in maximum aortic diameter of 12% to 17% was observed in the aorta distal to the left subclavian artery.[75] During nongated aortic CTA, these changes in aortic contour and size can mimic aortic injury. Smooth variation in the shape of the thoracic aorta in young patients should not be misinterpreted as a sign of aortic injury.

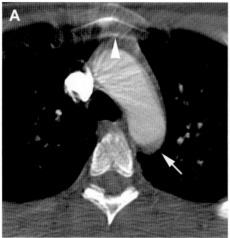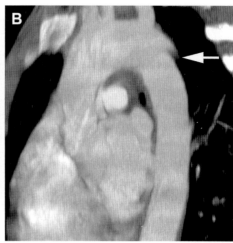

Fig. 17. Pulsation artifact. (*A*) Axial and (*B*) sagittal images from a chest CT in a patient stabbed in the chest reveal a double contour to the aortic arch (*white arrows*). A double contour to the sternum (*arrowhead*) is also visible, indicating motion artifact. Motion artifact can arise from voluntary movement, breathing, vascular pulsation, or cardiac motion. Adjacent vessels (eg, the pulmonary artery), bones, and tubes should always be examined for similar artifacts to confidently exclude an aortic injury.

Pulsation Artifact

Pulsation artifacts most commonly occur in the ascending aorta and aortic root, although they can be identified throughout the length of the thoracic aorta. Ninety-two percent of aortic motion artifacts are simultaneously seen in the left anterior and right posterior quadrants of the aorta. In 93% of cases, motion artifact can also be demonstrated in the superior vena cava (SVC), with a "pseudointimal" flap.[73,76] An important discriminatory clue to the presence of a motion artifact is the observation of similar artifacts in adjacent structures. Whenever a motion artifact is suspected, the SVC, pulmonary artery, adjacent tubes and lines, and bones should be inspected for concurrent artifacts at the same level (**Fig. 17**). Concurrent traumatic injuries to the pulmonary artery and SVC at the same level almost never occur.

SUMMARY

Liberal use of multidetector-row CTA will allow for the accurate diagnosis of aortic and branch vessel injury in almost all cases, and provides a baseline for endovascular repair and surgical planning. Greater integration of rapid CT into the evaluation of the severely injured patients, and the evolving use of DSCT and ECG-gated CTA for the evaluation of more subtle and challenging injuries, provide opportunities for further improvement in the evaluation of aortic injuries.

REFERENCES

1. Neschis DG, Scalea TM, Flinn WR, et al. Blunt aortic injury. N Engl J Med 2008;359(16):1708–16.
2. Demetriades D, Velmahos GC, Scalea TM, et al. Diagnosis and treatment of blunt thoracic aortic injuries: changing perspectives. J Trauma 2008; 64(6):1415–8 [discussion: 1418–9].
3. Huber-Wagner S, Lefering R, Qvick LM, et al. Effect of whole-body CT during trauma resuscitation on survival: a retrospective, multicentre study. Lancet 2009;373(9673):1455–61.
4. Malhotra AK, Fabian TC, Croce MA, et al. Minimal aortic injury: a lesion associated with advancing diagnostic techniques. J Trauma 2001;51(6): 1042–8.
5. Nguyen D, Platon A, Shanmuganathan K, et al. Evaluation of a single-pass continuous whole-body 16-MDCT protocol for patients with polytrauma. AJR Am J Roentgenol 2009;192(1):3–10.
6. Brink M, Kool DR, Dekker HM, et al. Predictors of abnormal chest CT after blunt trauma: a critical appraisal of the literature. Clin Radiol 2009;64(3): 272–83.
7. Inaba K, Branco BC, Lim G, et al. The increasing burden of radiation exposure in the management of trauma patients. J Trauma 2011;70(6):1366–70.
8. Blackmore CC. Evidence-based imaging in trauma radiology: where we are and how to move forward. Acta Radiol 2009;50(5):482–9.
9. Azizzadeh A, Valdes J, Miller CC 3rd, et al. The utility of intravascular ultrasound compared to angiography in the diagnosis of blunt traumatic aortic injury. J Vasc Surg 2011;53(3):608–14.

10. Groell R, Schaffler GJ, Rienmueller R. Pericardial sinuses and recesses: findings at electrocardiographically triggered electron-beam CT. Radiology 1999;212(1):69–73.

11. Layton KF, Kallmes DF, Cloft HJ, et al. Bovine aortic arch variant in humans: clarification of a common misnomer. AJNR Am J Neuroradiol 2006;27(7): 1541–2.

12. Cloud GC, Markus HS. Diagnosis and management of vertebral artery stenosis. QJM 2003;96(1):27–54.

13. Steenburg SD, Ravenel JG, Ikonomidis JS, et al. Acute traumatic aortic injury: imaging evaluation and management. Radiology 2008;248(3):748–62.

14. Teixeira PG, Inaba K, Barmparas G, et al. Blunt thoracic aortic injuries: an autopsy study. J Trauma 2011;70(1):197–202.

15. Schulman CI, Carvajal D, Lopez PP, et al. Incidence and crash mechanisms of aortic injury during the past decade. J Trauma 2007;62(3):664–7.

16. Fitzharris M, Franklyn M, Frampton R, et al. Thoracic aortic injury in motor vehicle crashes: the effect of impact direction, side of body struck, and seat belt use. J Trauma 2004;57(3):582–90.

17. Parmley LF, Mattingly TW, Manion WC, et al. Nonpenetrating traumatic injury of the aorta. Circulation 1958;17(6):1086–101.

18. Fabian TC, Richardson JD, Croce MA, et al. Prospective study of blunt aortic injury: multicenter trial of the American Association for the Surgery of Trauma. J Trauma 1997;42(3):374–80 [discussion: 380–3].

19. Richens D, Field M, Neale M, et al. The mechanism of injury in blunt traumatic rupture of the aorta. Eur J Cardiothorac Surg 2002;21(2):288–93.

20. Horton TG, Cohn SM, Heid MP, et al. Identification of trauma patients at risk of thoracic aortic tear by mechanism of injury. J Trauma 2000;48(6):1008–13 [discussion: 1013–4].

21. Crass JR, Cohen AM, Motta AO, et al. A proposed new mechanism of traumatic aortic rupture: the osseous pinch. Radiology 1990;176(3):645–9.

22. Lundervall J. The mechanism of traumatic rupture of the aorta. Acta Pathol Microbiol Scand 1964;62: 34–46.

23. Nzewi O, Slight RD, Zamvar V. Management of blunt thoracic aortic injury. Eur J Vasc Endovasc Surg 2006;31(1):18–27.

24. Burkhart HM, Gomez GA, Jacobson LE, et al. Fatal blunt aortic injuries: a review of 242 autopsy cases. J Trauma 2001;50(1):113–5.

25. Dosios TJ, Salemis N, Angouras D, et al. Blunt and penetrating trauma of the thoracic aorta and aortic arch branches: an autopsy study. J Trauma 2000; 49(4):696–703.

26. Ahrar K, Smith DC, Bansal RC, et al. Angiography in blunt thoracic aortic injury. J Trauma 1997;42(4): 665–9.

27. Chen MY, Regan JD, D'Amore MJ, et al. Role of angiography in the detection of aortic branch vessel injury after blunt thoracic trauma. J Trauma 2001; 51(6):1166–71 [discussion: 1172].

28. Gunn M, Campbell M, Hoffer EK. Traumatic abdominal aortic injury treated by endovascular stent placement. Emerg Radiol 2007;13(6):329–31.

29. Inaba K, Kirkpatrick AW, Finkelstein J, et al. Blunt abdominal aortic trauma in association with thoracolumbar spine fractures. Injury 2001; 32(3):201–7.

30. Roth SM, Wheeler JR, Gregory RT, et al. Blunt injury of the abdominal aorta: a review. J Trauma 1997; 42(4):748–55.

31. Lopera JE, Restrepo CS, Gonzales A, et al. Aortoiliac vascular injuries after misplacement of fixation screws. J Trauma 2010;69(4):870–5.

32. Demetriades D, Theodorou D, Murray J, et al. Mortality and prognostic factors in penetrating injuries of the aorta. J Trauma 1996;40(5):761–3.

33. Ding X, Jiang J, Su Q, et al. Endovascular stent graft repair of a penetrating aortic injury. Ann Thorac Surg 2010;90(2):632–4.

34. Azizzadeh A, Keyhani K, Miller CC III, et al. Blunt traumatic aortic injury: initial experience with endovascular repair. J Vasc Surg 2009;49(6):1403–8.

35. Duhaylongsod FG, Glower DD, Wolfe WG. Acute traumatic aortic aneurysm: the Duke experience from 1970 to 1990. J Vasc Surg 1992;15(2):331–42 [discussion: 342–3].

36. Prijon T, Ermenc B. Classification of blunt aortic injuries a new systematic overview of aortic trauma. Forensic Sci Int 2010;195(1–3):6–9.

37. Hamilton NA, Bucher BT, Keller MS. The significance of first rib fractures in children. J Pediatr Surg 2011; 46(1):169–72.

38. Gupta A, Jamshidi M, Rubin JR. Traumatic first rib fracture: is angiography necessary? A review of 730 cases. Cardiovasc Surg 1997;5(1):48–53.

39. Khosla A, Ocel J, Rad AE, et al. Correlating first- and second-rib fractures noted on spine computed tomography with major vessel injury. Emerg Radiol 2010;17(6):461–4.

40. Ekeh AP, Peterson W, Woods RJ, et al. Is chest x-ray an adequate screening tool for the diagnosis of blunt thoracic aortic injury? J Trauma 2008;65(5): 1088–92.

41. Woodring JH. The normal mediastinum in blunt traumatic rupture of the thoracic aorta and brachiocephalic arteries. J Emerg Med 1990;8(4):467–76.

42. Benjamin ER, Tillou A, Hiatt JR, et al. Blunt thoracic aortic injury. Am Surg 2008;74(10):1033–7.

43. Mirvis SE, Bidwell JK, Buddemeyer EU, et al. Value of chest radiography in excluding traumatic aortic rupture. Radiology 1987;163(2):487–93.

44. Nagy K, Fabian T, Rodman G, et al. Guidelines for the diagnosis and management of blunt aortic

injury: an EAST Practice Management Guidelines Work Group. J Trauma 2000;48(6):1128–43.

45. Woodring JH, King JG. Determination of normal transverse mediastinal width and mediastinal-width to chest-width (M/C) ratio in control subjects: implications for subjects with aortic or brachiocephalic arterial injury. J Trauma 1989;29(9):1268–72.

46. Barker DE, Crabtree JD Jr, White JE, et al. Mediastinal evaluation utilizing the reverse Trendelenburg radiograph. Am Surg 1999;65(5):484–9.

47. Dyer DS, Moore EE, Ilke DN, et al. Thoracic aortic injury: how predictive is mechanism and is chest computed tomography a reliable screening tool? A prospective study of 1,561 patients. J Trauma 2000;48(4):673–82 [discussion: 682–3].

48. Fabian TC, Davis KA, Gavant ML, et al. Prospective study of blunt aortic injury: helical CT is diagnostic and antihypertensive therapy reduces rupture. Ann Surg 1998;227(5):666–76 [discussion: 676–7].

49. Mirvis SE, Shanmuganathan K. Diagnosis of blunt traumatic aortic injury 2007: still a nemesis. Eur J Radiol 2007;64(1):27–40.

50. Steenburg SD, Ravenel JG. Acute traumatic thoracic aortic injuries: experience with 64-MDCT. AJR Am J Roentgenol 2008;191(5):1564–9.

51. Mirvis SE, Shanmuganathan K, Miller BH, et al. Traumatic aortic injury: diagnosis with contrast-enhanced thoracic CT–five-year experience at a major trauma center. Radiology 1996;200(2):413–22.

52. Dyer DS, Moore EE, Mestek MF, et al. Can chest CT be used to exclude aortic injury? Radiology 1999; 213(1):195–202.

53. Bruckner BA, DiBardino DJ, Cumbie TC, et al. Critical evaluation of chest computed tomography scans for blunt descending thoracic aortic injury. Ann Thorac Surg 2006;81(4):1339–46.

54. Karlo C, Leschka S, Goetti RP, et al. High-pitch dual-source CT angiography of the aortic valve-aortic root complex without ECG-synchronization. Eur Radiol 2011;21(1):205–12.

55. Donnino R, Jacobs JE, Doshi JV, et al. Dual-source versus single-source cardiac CT angiography: comparison of diagnostic image quality. AJR Am J Roentgenol 2009;192(4):1051–6.

56. Cinnella G, Dambrosio M, Brienza N, et al. Transesophageal echocardiography for diagnosis of traumatic aortic injury: an appraisal of the evidence. J Trauma 2004;57(6):1246–55.

57. Patel NH, Hahn D, Comess KA. Blunt chest trauma victims: role of intravascular ultrasound and transesophageal echocardiography in cases of abnormal thoracic aortogram. J Trauma 2003; 55(2):330–7.

58. Morse SS, Glickman MG, Greenwood LH, et al. Traumatic aortic rupture: false-positive aortographic diagnosis due to atypical ductus diverticulum. AJR Am J Roentgenol 1988;150(4):793–6.

59. Lee DE, Arslan B, Queiroz R, et al. Assessment of inter- and intraobserver agreement between intravascular US and aortic angiography of thoracic aortic injury. Radiology 2003;227(2):434–9.

60. Kirkham JR, Blackmore CC. Screening for aortic injury with chest radiography and clinical factors. Emerg Radiol 2007;14(4):211–7.

61. Fishman JE, Nunez D Jr, Kane A, et al. Direct versus indirect signs of traumatic aortic injury revealed by helical CT: performance characteristics and interobserver agreement. AJR Am J Roentgenol 1999; 172(4):1027–31.

62. Wong H, Gotway MB, Sasson AD, et al. Periaortic hematoma at diaphragmatic crura at helical CT: sign of blunt aortic injury in patients with mediastinal hematoma. Radiology 2004;231(1): 185–9.

63. Sammer M, Wang E, Blackmore CC, et al. Indeterminate CT angiography in blunt thoracic trauma: is CT angiography enough? AJR Am J Roentgenol 2007; 189(3):603–8.

64. Scaglione M, Pinto A, Pinto F, et al. Role of contrast-enhanced helical CT in the evaluation of acute thoracic aortic injuries after blunt chest trauma. Eur Radiol 2001;11(12):2444–8.

65. Steenburg SD, Ravenel JG. Multi-detector computed tomography findings of atypical blunt traumatic aortic injuries: a pictorial review. Emerg Radiol 2007;14(3):143–50.

66. Mosquera VX, Marini M, Lopez-Perez JM, et al. Role of conservative management in traumatic aortic injury: comparison of long-term results of conservative, surgical, and endovascular treatment. J Thorac Cardiovasc Surg 2011;142(3):614–21.

67. Caffarelli AD, Mallidi HR, Maggio PM, et al. Early outcomes of deliberate nonoperative management for blunt thoracic aortic injury in trauma. J Thorac Cardiovasc Surg 2010;140(3):598–605.

68. You SY, Yoon DY, Choi CS, et al. Effects of right-versus left-arm injections of contrast material on computed tomography of the head and neck. J Comput Assist Tomogr 2007;31(5):677–81.

69. Fisher RG, Ben-Menachem Y. Penetrating injuries of the thoracic aorta and brachiocephalic arteries: angiographic findings in 18 cases. AJR Am J Roentgenol 1987;149(3):607–11.

70. Fisher RG, Sanchez-Torres M, Whigham CJ, et al. "Lumps" and "bumps" that mimic acute aortic and brachiocephalic vessel injury. Radiographics 1997; 17(4):825–34.

71. Agarwal PP, Chughtai A, Matzinger FR, et al. Multi-detector CT of thoracic aortic aneurysms. Radiographics 2009;29(2):537–52.

72. Gray H, Lewis WH. Anatomy of the human body. 23rd edition. Philadelphia: Lea & Febiger; 1936.

73. Morrison TM, Choi G, Zarins CK, et al. Circumferential and longitudinal cyclic strain of the human

thoracic aorta: age-related changes. J Vasc Surg 2009;49(4):1029–36.

74. Ganten M, Krautter U, Hosch W, et al. Age related changes of human aortic distensibility: evaluation with ECG-gated CT. Eur Radiol 2007;17(3):701–8.

75. Muhs BE, Vincken KL, van Prehn J, et al. Dynamic cine-CT angiography for the evaluation of the thoracic aorta; insight in dynamic changes with implications for thoracic endograft treatment. Eur J Vasc Endovasc Surg 2006;32(5):532–6.

76. Ko SF, Hsieh MJ, Chen MC, et al. Effects of heart rate on motion artifacts of the aorta on non-ECG-assisted 0.5-sec thoracic MDCT. AJR Am J Roentgenol 2005;184(4):1225–30.

Splenic Trauma: What is New?

Alexis Boscak, MD*,
Kathirkamanthan Shanmuganathan, MD

KEYWORDS

- Trauma • Spleen • Ultrasound • Computed tomography
- Angiography • Embolization

The spleen remains the most frequently injured abdominal organ after blunt trauma. The diagnosis of splenic injury and the identification of features salient to prognosis and management are major goals of imaging assessment after trauma. Computed tomography (CT) has become the predominant modality for definitive trauma imaging in most trauma centers in the United States; it permits rapid and accurate assessment for life-threatening injuries throughout the body and is reliable for determining the presence and severity of splenic injury. CT imaging plays an increasing role in identification and characterization of splenic vascular lesions, guiding the selection of patients for catheter angiography with splenic artery embolization as an adjunct to nonoperative management. This article reviews current trends and controversies in imaging splenic trauma, with an emphasis on CT assessment and indications for catheter angiography and embolization.

ANATOMY AND TRAUMATOLOGY

The spleen is a highly vascular organ, receiving up to 5% of cardiac output (200 mL/min) and containing approximately 500 mL of blood.[1] Its intraperitoneal position creates the potential for uncontained hemorrhage resulting in fatal exsanguination after trauma. Constrained by a thin fibrous capsule on a minimally mobile vascular pedicle, the spleen is relatively fragile, subject to delayed and acute rupture. Although usually at least partially protected by the ribcage,

inspiratory excursion may inferiorly displace the spleen to a more exposed subcostal position; when fractured, the ribs may lacerate the spleen, while the retroperitoneum and even the diaphragm provide inflexible surfaces against which the spleen may be compressed. Splenomegaly of any cause (portal hypertension, infection, hematologic disorders) increases the risk of injury and rupture. Blunt splenic trauma is associated with injury of other abdominal organs in approximately 36.5% of cases, and approximately 80% of patients with blunt splenic injury also have extra-abdominal injury.[2] Optimal imaging assessment must provide accurate diagnosis of splenic injury while also screening for other major abdominopelvic as well as thoracic, cervical, and head injuries. In some cases, other injuries may mandate operative intervention regardless of splenic status; if the spleen is the solely or most significantly injured structure, then specific imaging features will play a role in determining management, in concert with clinical indications.

MANAGEMENT OF SPLENIC INJURY

The management of splenic injury continues to evolve toward conservative strategies maximizing splenic salvage. Before the integration of imaging modalities, including ultrasound (US) and CT, into routine trauma work-up protocols, the diagnosis of splenic injury was based on physical examination and diagnostic peritoneal lavage, with all patients suspected to have intra-abdominal injury

The authors have nothing to disclose.
Trauma/Emergency Section, Department of Radiology, University of Maryland Medical Center, University of Maryland, 22 South Greene Street, Baltimore, MD 21201, USA
* Corresponding author.
E-mail address: aboscak@umm.edu

Radiol Clin N Am 50 (2012) 105–122
doi:10.1016/j.rcl.2011.08.008

directed toward laparotomy, frequently resulting in splenectomy. Pioneered in the pediatric population,[3] splenic salvage is now an important goal in the management of both children and adults with splenic injury. Avoiding splenectomy not only spares patients immediate operative morbidity and lifelong risk of postsplenectomy sepsis (2%, with mortality exceeding 50%) but contributes to decreased duration of hospitalization and may reduce cost.[4] With increased awareness of splenic function and the morbidities associated with the postsplenectomy state, operative strategy has trended toward splenic conservation by subtotal resection and splenorrhaphy when possible. In addition, nonsurgical management has become a key goal in trauma care. Both operative and nonoperative splenic conservation leads to decreased early infection rates.[5] Higher rates of nonoperative management are associated with decreased risk-adjusted mortality.[6]

Most patients with splenic injury are now managed nonoperatively, with overall success rates around 90%, depending on selection criteria; splenic salvage rates can exceed 80% even in high-grade splenic injury, with adjunctive embolotherapy.[7,8] Prediction of failure of nonoperative management, defined as worsening imaging or clinical parameters necessitating delayed intervention, has become an integral component of initial trauma assessment and a key goal of trauma CT. CT findings impacting the success of nonoperative management include injury grade, amount of hemoperitoneum, evidence of ongoing hemorrhage, and presence of splenic vascular lesions. Injuries corresponding to the American Association for the Surgery of Trauma (AAST) grade III or higher and large-volume hemoperitoneum (defined as blood extending from the splenic fossa into the pelvis) increase the risk of failure of nonoperative therapy.[9–11] CT identification of active bleeding or contained intrasplenic vascular injury (pseudoaneurysm or arteriovenous fistula) increases the risk of failing nonoperative management by 40% to 67%.[12] Transfusion requirement in excess of 1 unit in the first 24 hours may also predict failure in patients with high-grade spleen injuries ($\geq$ AAST III), although this is dependent on the source of blood loss in polytrauma patients.[13] Management of older patients remains controversial because of conflicting published outcomes; the early proposal of age older than 55 years as a contraindication for nonoperative management was met by several studies describing acceptably low failure rates in that population[14,15] versus others affirming age older than 55 years as an independent predictor of failure.[8,10]

Although these various parameters provide relative indications for surgical intervention and should impact decision making, none are absolute contraindications to attempting nonoperative management; as diagnostic and therapeutic modalities have evolved, the one remaining absolute indication for surgery after splenic injury is intractable hypotension referable to the spleen. At the University of Maryland Shock Trauma Center (UMSTC), any hemodynamically stable patient with any grade of splenic injury who has no other injuries requiring surgery is considered for nonoperative management (**Fig. 1**).

TRIAGE OF ABDOMINAL TRAUMA

Many patients at risk of blunt splenic injury have suffered multisystem trauma. The spleen may not be the only or the most severely injured organ. Initial triage of patients after blunt trauma depends on physical examination, hemodynamic status, staff clinical expertise, and available diagnostic modalities. Physical examination alone may be insufficient to exclude intra-abdominal injury when traumatized patients have suffered severe distracting injury, have altered mental status because of intoxication or head injury, or altered sensation because of spinal cord injury.[16]

Hemodynamically unstable patients can be most readily assessed for intra-abdominal blood by sonography or diagnostic peritoneal lavage (DPL), either of which can be performed in the resuscitation area. A grossly positive DPL or large-volume intraperitoneal blood on sonography in unstable patients are indications for urgent laparotomy.[9,17] For hemodynamically stable patients able to tolerate further investigation and transfer, CT is the imaging modality of choice for definitive assessment.

ULTRASOUND IN SPLENIC TRAUMA

US can provide rapid noninvasive assessment of the injured abdomen and can be accomplished at the bedside with minimal disruption of resuscitation efforts. Focused assessment with sonography for trauma (FAST) exploits these features, delineating a streamlined protocol tailored to optimize the detection of hemoperitoneum with acquisition of 4 standard abdominal views (subxiphoid, suprapubic, and bilateral upper quadrants) in less than 5 minutes.[18]

Reported sensitivity of US for detection of free intraperitoneal fluid varies, ranging from 62% to 99%, with negative predictive values of 89% to 99%.[19,20] FAST is readily integrated into the resuscitation assessment and can be performed by

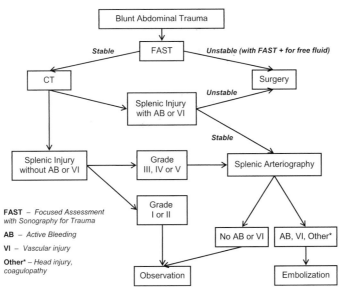

Fig. 1. UMSTC splenic injury management algorithm.

a radiologist or a nonradiologist provider. In many institutions, FAST imaging has replaced DPL for the identification of hemoperitoneum in unstable patients who can then be directed to laparotomy without additional imaging.[21] For hemodynamically stable patients, CT scan may be indicated regardless of the FAST result to allow direct assessment of viscera and vasculature not evaluated by FAST protocol. Although DPL typically results in iatrogenic pneumoperitoneum and by definition introduces intraperitoneal fluid, US does not alter the abdomen and, therefore, adds no artifactual complexity to subsequent CT assessment.

While sonography supplants diagnostic peritoneal lavage for identification of hemoperitoneum, it must be borne in mind that up to 27% to 29% of patients with CT-proven splenic injury may have no detectable hemoperitoneum[19,22]; this number may be as high as 40% in children.[23] Many of these injuries may be minor and amenable to expectant management but as many as 40% are high grade (AAST III–V). Although ultrasound could be used to assess for solid organ injury, such an examination would be more time consuming and more disruptive to resuscitation than FAST; furthermore, reported sensitivities vary widely and seem more operator dependent than the highly standardized FAST examination.[24] Thorough sonographic examinations of the abdomen performed by experienced technologists were 84% sensitive and 96% specific for fluid

or organ disruption in a large study but required 10 minutes of imaging time.[25] A smaller study demonstrated US sensitivity of 72% overall and only 41% for organ injury despite scan performance by trained radiology residents or fellows.[26] Contrast-enhanced US examination seems to provide increased sensitivity for solid organ injury (**Fig. 2**) and can even demonstrate active bleeding and vascular lesions,[27–29] but US contrast agents are not commonly used for trauma in the United States.

CT OF SPLENIC TRAUMA

Widespread availability of multi-detector CT (MDCT) at most trauma centers in the United States allows CT to play the principal role in the detection and characterization of splenic injury. Evolving CT technology allows acquisition of isotropic data with generation of high-quality multiplanar reformatted images and rapid scan repetition after intravascular contrast-agent administration providing multiphase data sets. Acquisition of images in the arterial phase for CT angiography can provide similar diagnostic information to catheter angiography, with good, if not perfect, accuracy.[11]

CT Protocol

Although noncontrast CT can demonstrate some sequelae of trauma, including hemoperitoneum and major splenic disruption, intravascular

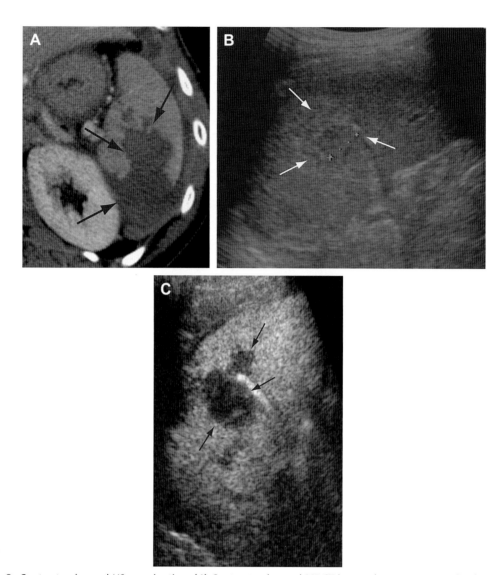

Fig. 2. Contrast-enhanced US examination. (*A*) Contrast-enhanced MDCT image demonstrates a mixed attenuation grade III splenic contusion/hematoma (*arrows*). (*B*) Noncontrast US image shows a vague area of mixed echogenicity (*arrows*) within the spleen. (*C*) Postcontrast US images more clearly demonstrate a hypoechoic lesion (*arrows*) corresponding to the splenic injury seen by CT. (*Courtesy of* Poletti PA, et al, University Hospital of Geneva, Switzerland.)

contrast-enhanced CT is required for optimal depiction of parenchymal and vascular injury. In the authors' experience of using 40- and 64-slice MDCT in evaluating patients with blunt splenic trauma at the UMSTC, arterial phase images optimally demonstrate the main splenic and intrasplenic arteries and are required for the identification of small vascular injuries (**Fig. 3**) but are suboptimal for the evaluation of splenic parenchymal injury because of the typically heterogeneous pattern of early splenic enhancement (**Fig. 4**A). In the portal venous phase, normal splenic parenchyma enhances homogeneously (see **Fig. 4**B), providing the best demonstration of the various parenchymal injuries. Delayed (eg, excretory/urographic) phase imaging is suboptimal for the direct assessment of either vasculature or parenchyma; however, dual-phase imaging of the spleen is useful in differentiating between active bleeding and vascular injuries, including pseudoaneurysm and traumatic arteriovenous fistulae.[30]

Most patients admitted to the UMSTC have suffered multisystem injury, so the abdomen is assessed as part of a total-body CT in which scans are obtained from the circle of Willis through the symphysis pubis in the arterial phase after the injection of intravenous contrast material, followed

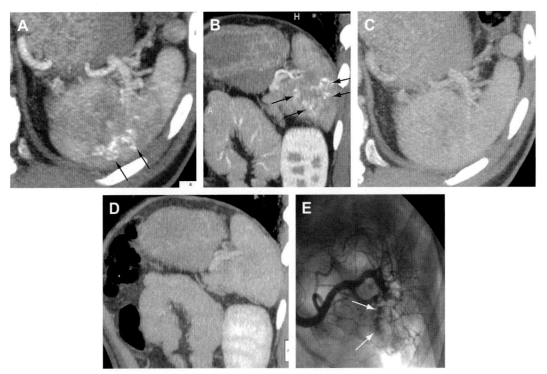

Fig. 3. Splenic vascular injury only visualized on arterial phase images. (A) Axial and (B) sagittal reformatted arterial phase CT images demonstrate multiple, rounded, high-attenuation areas (arrows) within the splenic parenchyma. (C) Axial and (D) sagittal reformatted portal venous phase CT images show washout of these vascular injuries, which now seem isoattenuating with the splenic parenchyma. (E) Splenic arteriogram shows multiple PA (arrows). Main splenic artery embolization was performed (not shown).

by a repeat scan through the abdomen in the portal venous phase (Table 1). For patients younger than 50 years of age and without known cardiac disease, this protocol is performed with scan initiation 18 seconds after contrast injection.

CT Appearances of Splenic Injury

MDCT is highly accurate (98%) in diagnosing splenic injury.[11] Possible CT findings in splenic injury are perisplenic, intrasplenic, and subcapsular hematoma; laceration; infarction; active bleeding; and contained vascular injuries, including pseudoaneurysm and arteriovenous fistula.

Hematoma

Perisplenic hematoma, consisting of blood collection around the spleen, may reflect splenic bleeding (implying capsule violation or rupture) or

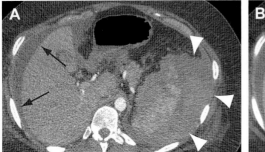
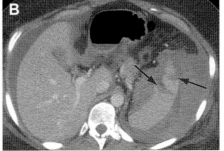

Fig. 4. Heterogeneous enhancement of splenic parenchyma during arterial phase. (A) Axial arterial phase CT image shows perihepatic hemoperitoneum (arrows) and perisplenic clot (arrowheads). Heterogeneous parenchymal enhancement pattern makes it difficult to determine the extent of splenic injury. (B) Axial portal venous phase CT image obtained at the same anatomic level better defines 2 lacerations in the anterior spleen (arrows).

| Table 1 | | | | | | | | |
| MDCT protocol for blunt abdominal trauma | | | | | | | | |
MDCT	IV Contrast Volume	I₂ mg/mL	Injection Rate	Scan Delay	Detector Width	Pitch	Rotation Time	Location of Bolus Pro
40 or 64 slice <50 y	100 mL	350 mg/mL Normal saline	50 mL @ 6 mL/s 50 mL @ 4 mL/s 50 mL @ 5 mL/s	18 s	0.625 mm	0.976	0.5 s	n/a
40 or 64 slice >50 y	100 mL	350 mg/mL Normal saline	50 mL @ 6 mL/s 50 mL @ 4 mL/s 50 mL @ 5 mL/s	Bolus pro 90 HU	0.625 mm	0.976	0.5 s	Ascending aorta

Abbreviation: IV, intravenous; n/a, not applicable.

represent blood from a distant injury. Highest-attenuation sentinel clot around the spleen is more specific for splenic origin of hemorrhage (**Fig. 5**).[31] Intrasplenic hematomas may be intra-parenchymal or subcapsular. Intraparenchymal hematomas are rounded, ovoid, or irregular collections of nonenhancing blood-attenuation fluid within the spleen (**Fig. 6**). Subcapsular hematomas are crescentic peripheral collections just deep to the splenic capsular surface. A subcapsular hematoma is constrained by the splenic capsule, so its mass effect compresses underlying splenic parenchyma; this finding aids discrimination between subcapsular (**Fig. 7**) and perisplenic hematomas, which can coexist. The diameter of an intrasplenic hematoma and the percentage of splenic surface area involved by subcapsular hematoma are considerations in injury grading (AAST scale).

Hematomas decrease in attenuation over time, reflecting clot liquefaction before reabsorption. Increase in the size of intrasplenic or subcapsular hematoma indicates further splenic hemorrhage and may warrant surgery, angiography, or close clinical surveillance with follow-up CT.

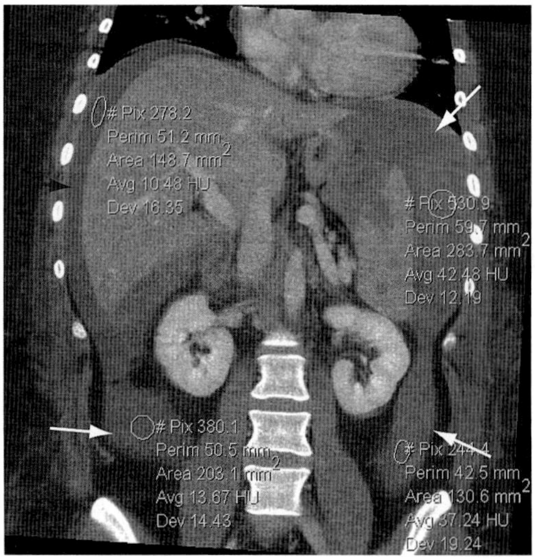

Laceration

On contrast-enhanced CT, acute splenic lacerations appear as irregular, linear, branching, or stellate nonenhancing low-attenuation areas within the parenchyma (**Fig. 8**). Lacerations may extend to the splenic capsule, which may be intact or torn. Nontraumatic splenic clefts or lobulations appear as splenic contour defects that can be confused with lacerations but have more clearly defined, smooth, or rounded margins and always extend to the splenic surface; identification of fat within clefts may allow the correct diagnosis. Artifact arising from adjacent ribs, streak artifact from electrocardiogram leads or other metal devices, motion artifact, and heterogeneous splenic perfusion during early phase imaging can also mimic splenic laceration. Laceration depth and extension to/through splenic trabecular, segmental, or hilar

Fig. 5. Sentinel clot sign. Multiplanar reformatted CT image demonstrates a grade III splenic injury with multiple contusions. Hemoperitoneum is seen in multiple anatomic locations (*arrows*). The highest-attenuation blood is adjacent to injured spleen.

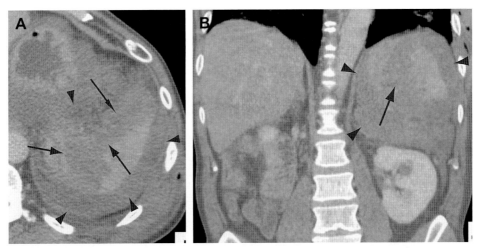

Fig. 6. Splenic hematoma in a 55-year-old man admitted following a fall. (*A*) Axial and (*B*) coronal reformatted CT images show an ill-defined area of intermediate attenuation (*arrows*) within the spleen, a grade III splenic hematoma, with similar attenuation perisplenic clot (*arrowheads*).

vessels are considerations in injury grading (AAST scale).

Over time, lacerations become less well defined, decreasing in size and number. Although such maturational changes may begin within days, resolution may take weeks to months, depending on the size and extent of the original injury. Increase in number or size of lacerations on

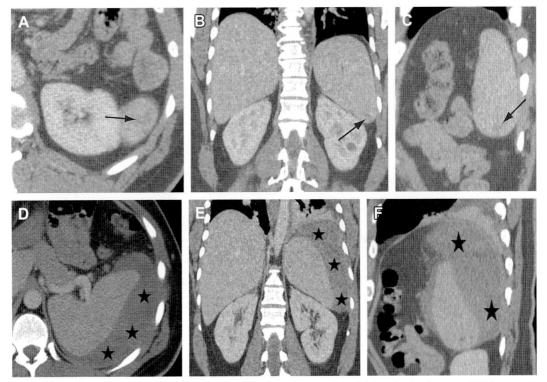

Fig. 7. Delayed onset of subcapsular hematoma. (*A*) Axial, (*B*) coronal, and (*C*) sagittal reformatted CT images obtained at admission demonstrate a subtle low-attenuation grade I contusion (*arrows*) in the lower aspect of the spleen. (*D*) Axial, (*E*) coronal, and (*F*) sagittal reformatted CT images obtained 8 days later, for new-onset abdominal pain, show a mixed-attenuation grade III subcapsular splenic hematoma (*asterisks*) causing mass effect on the underlying parenchyma.

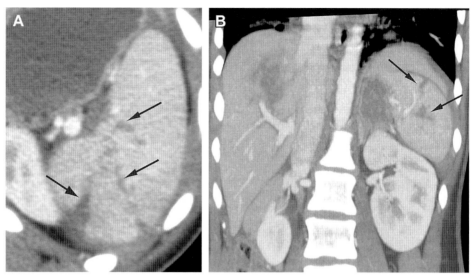

Fig. 8. Splenic lacerations. (*A*) Axial and (*B*) coronal maximum intensity CT images show multiple irregular linear low-attenuation splenic lacerations (*arrows*). Low-attenuation area within liver also represents injury.

follow-up CT indicates progression of injury and may warrant surgery, angiography, or close clinical surveillance with follow-up CT.

Splenic infarction

Traumatic splenic infarction is a rare entity seen in 1.4% of patients with blunt splenic injury.[32] Splenic segmental infarction appears on contrast-enhanced CT as a well-defined wedge-shaped area of nonenhancing hypoattenuation, typically involving 25% to 50% of the spleen (**Fig. 9**). Although the exact mechanism of splenic infarction after blunt trauma is not known, angiographic findings suggest arterial thrombosis after intimal tear resulting from mechanical stretching of intrasplenic arteries. Infarct size may reflect both the injured artery territory and the presence of collateral perfusion. Significant splenic devascularization resulting in greater than 25% infarction is relevant to injury grading (AAST scale).

Most splenic infarcts heal without complication, decreasing in size over time. Rare complications include delayed appearance of new areas of infarction, abscess formation, and splenic rupture.[32]

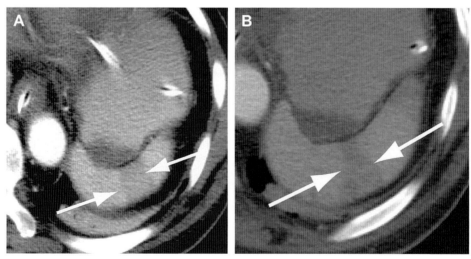

Fig. 9. Splenic segmental infarction in a 72-year-old man admitted following a fall. (*A, B*) Axial CT images show a well-defined wedge-shaped area of low attenuation (*arrows*) representing a splenic infarct.

Active bleeding

Active bleeding during contrast-enhanced CT appears as extravasation of contrast-enhanced blood from the splenic artery and its branches, resulting in collection of high-attenuation (up to 300–400 HU) material that is similar in attenuation to contrast material within the adjacent vessels, conspicuously different from clotted blood (40–70 HU; mean = 50 HU).[33] CT is potentially as sensitive as first-order selective digital subtraction angiography for the detection of active bleeding, with a threshold rate of 0.35 mL/min in an in-vitro model,[34] although studies suggest decreased sensitivity in vivo.[11] Active splenic bleeding on CT is often arterial, resulting in irregular or linear highest-attenuation areas (**Fig. 10**). On delayed imaging, the area of active extravasation typically remains high in attenuation and characteristically increases in size, reflecting ongoing bleeding (see **Fig. 10**). With multidetector CT, active bleeding may be found in as many as 18% to 19% of patients with splenic injury.[35]

Numerous studies have concluded that the presence of active arterial bleeding on CT indicates the need for surgical management,[11,36–38] although some reports have questioned the predictive strength of contrast extravasation, cautioning against its consideration as an absolute indication for either surgical or angiographic intervention.[39,40] A few studies suggest that splenic contrast extravasation in children may be less predictive for failure of conservative management than in adults.[41,42] Active bleeding confined to the spleen and active bleeding into the peritoneal cavity may portend different prognoses. In a recent study of initially stable patients with splenic injury on CT, 88% of those with active bleeding from the spleen into the peritoneum on CT experienced clinical deterioration during preparation for angiography, resulting in emergent

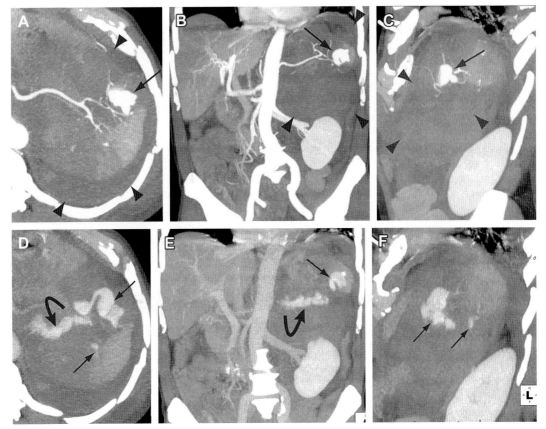

Fig. 10. Splenic active bleeding in a 55-year-old man admitted following blunt force trauma. (*A*) Axial, (*B*) coronal, and (*C*) sagittal maximum-intensity projection arterial phase CT images show an irregular area of active bleeding (*arrows*) from the spleen. Large-volume perisplenic intraperitoneal blood (*arrowheads*) is also seen. (*D*) Axial, (*E*) coronal, and (*F*) sagittal maximum-intensity projection portal venous phase CT images show increase in the amount of prior-visualized active bleeding (*arrows*) and new areas of intraperitoneal active bleeding (*curved arrows*). Splenectomy was performed to control hemorrhage.

laparotomy, whereas only 23% of patients with limited intrasplenic active bleeding suffered such early failure.[43] At UMSTC, the presence of active contrast material extravasation on MDCT is an indication for immediate angiography in patients who are hemodynamically stable and for splenic surgery in patients who are hemodynamically unstable.

Vascular injuries

Posttraumatic splenic vascular injuries include intrasplenic pseudoaneurysms (PA) and arteriovenous fistulae (AVF) (**Fig. 11**). PA and AVF appear as well-circumscribed foci of contrast material with attenuation similar to adjacent contrast-enhanced arteries (see **Figs. 3**A, B and **11**A). These nonbleeding vascular injuries may be

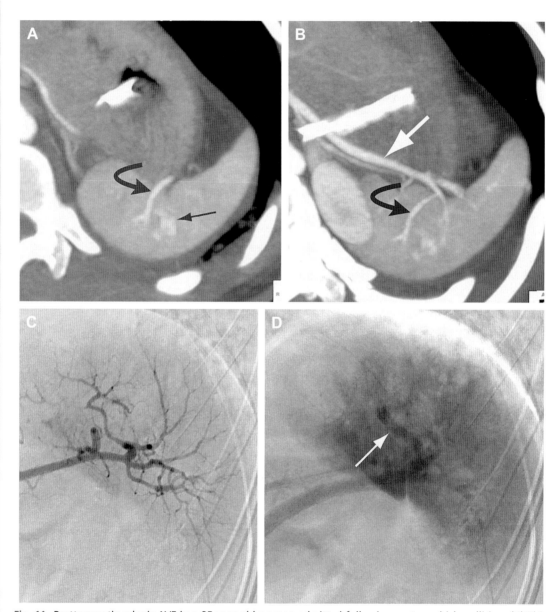

Fig. 11. Posttraumatic splenic AVF in a 25-year-old woman admitted following motor vehicle collision. (*A*) Thin and (*B*) thick axial maximum-intensity projection late arterial phase CT images demonstrate a splenic vascular injury (*black arrow*) and early opacification of an intrasplenic venous branch (*curved arrows*) draining into the main splenic vein (*white arrow*). (*C*) Early arterial phase image from splenic arteriogram shows no PA. (*D*) Delayed image from splenic arteriogram shows an abnormal draining vein (*arrow*) within the spleen. The AVF was embolized (not shown).

surrounded by low-attenuation parenchyma or hematoma. On delayed imaging, vascular lesions typically decrease in attenuation from washout of contrast material and become similar to or slightly higher in attenuation than adjacent normal parenchyma (see **Figs. 3**C and **11**B). The attenuation values of these lesions are typically within 10 HU of the adjacent contrast-enhanced artery on all phases. On contrast-enhanced CT, these two lesions have the same imaging characteristics and can be differentiated only on splenic angiography.

A posttraumatic splenic PA is formed by an injury to the arterial wall, typically involving the media, allowing a small amount of blood to track into the injured vessel wall and distend the adventitia; the inability to maintain normal integrity of the vessel wall results in the formation of a PA. AVF may develop in the immediate posttraumatic period as a result of injury to both the artery and adjacent vein.

Although the natural history of these lesions is not fully understood, the major potential complication of visceral PA is rupture, with rates reported to be 3% to 46%.[44] Their presence represents a predictor for failure of nonsurgical management, independent of other factors contributing to injury grade. Schurr and colleagues[36] reported the presence of vascular blush in a significantly higher number of patients who failed nonoperative management than in patients successfully managed nonoperatively (67% and 6%, respectively), whereas Gavant and colleagues[45] noted well-defined intrasplenic vascular injury on helical CT in 82% of 11 patients failing nonsurgical management of their blunt splenic injuries. These contained vascular injuries seem to warrant intervention in many, if not all, cases and are more likely to be successfully managed by angiographic embolization than are cases of active bleeding,[11,43] indicating the need to accurately distinguish these entities during initial imaging assessment of the victim of blunt splenic trauma.

REPORTING AND GRADING SPLENIC INJURY

The radiologist's report for patients with splenic injury must accurately convey the nature and extent of splenic disruption and describe the presence or absence of the specific findings most relevant to immediate management: large-volume hemoperitoneum, active arterial bleeding, and contained vascular injury. The term "contrast blush" has been used in the surgical literature to describe any localized extravasation of contrast from vasculature, which may represent either active bleeding or contained vascular injury.

Confident discrimination of these lesions is possible in many cases, particularly if multiphase acquisition is performed, and can help guide optimal clinical decision making. The radiology report should, therefore, provide an explicit description of active bleeding (and name the suspected source), specifically diagnose vascular injury (PA or AVF) when findings allow confident discrimination, or clearly communicate when the nature of a contrast blush is indeterminate.

Because data from diagnostic imaging has become integral to trauma management protocols, rapid availability of accurate CT interpretation is necessary to optimize patient care. It has been demonstrated that mortality increases 1% for every 3-minute delay in laparotomy,[46] and a recent study found a 47% increased risk of mortality per hour delay to interventional radiologic occlusion of active bleeding after trauma.[47] At the high-volume, high-acuity UMSTC, CT scan interpretation is provided by in-house attending trauma radiologists staffed around the clock. Delegation of off-hours scan interpretation to a trainee or even nonradiology personnel is common, but the increasing complexity of information available from CT requires expertise and experience to maximize its contribution to patient care.

Grading systems in clinical medicine improve clarity and efficiency of communication, structuring the description of the individual patient to aid standardization of assessment, reporting, and management. Availability of a common grading scale also facilitates research, allowing data to be shared and compared with different institutions. Application of a comprehensive grading scale to splenic trauma would be of particular value if grades of injury could predict success of specific nonoperative strategies, including observation or angiographic embolization, and accurately identify patients likely to fail conservative management who should proceed to surgical therapy. The AAST splenic injury grading scale, devised in 1987 and revised in 1994, is the most commonly used classification system in trauma centers in the United States (**Table 2**).[48] Although injuries identified at CT can often be matched to AAST categories, the scale is developed from and reflective of findings at laparotomy; salient findings depicted by CT, including active contrast extravasation and contained vascular lesions, are not represented within the AAST system. Furthermore, the AAST scale has demonstrated limited correlation with patient outcome. Although patients with high-grade (AAST grade III to V) injuries have worse prognosis and are most likely to require surgical therapy, patients with low-grade (AAST I to II) injuries may also fail

Table 2	
AAST: splenic injury scale (1994 revision)	
Grade	**Description of Injury**
I	Subcapsular hematoma <10% surface area Laceration <1 cm parenchymal depth
II	Subcapsular hematoma 10%–50% surface area Intraparenchymal hematoma <5 cm in diameter Laceration 1–3 cm parenchymal depth, which does not involve trabecular vessels
III	Subcapsular hematoma, >50% surface area or expanding Ruptured subcapsular or intraparenchymal hematoma Laceration >3 cm parenchymal depth or involving trabecular vessels
IV	Laceration involving segmental or hilar vessels producing major devascularization (>25% of spleen)
V	Shattered spleen Hilar vascular injury that devascularizes spleen

Table 3	
MDCT-based splenic injury grading system	
Grade	**Description of Injury**
I	Subcapsular hematoma <1 cm thick Laceration <1 cm parenchymal depth Parenchymal hematoma <1 cm diameter
II	Subcapsular hematoma 1–3 cm thick Laceration 1–3 cm parenchymal depth Parenchymal hematoma 1–3 cm diameter
III	Splenic capsular disruption Subcapsular hematoma >3 cm thick Laceration >3 cm parenchymal depth Parenchymal hematoma >3 cm diameter
IVA	Active intraparenchymal or subcapsular splenic bleeding Splenic vascular injury (PA or AVF) Shattered spleen
IVB	Active intraperitoneal bleeding

Data from Marmery H, Shanmuganathan K, Alexander M, et al. Optimization of selection for nonoperative management of blunt splenic injury: comparison of MDCT grading systems. AJR Am J Roentgenol 2007;189:1421–7.

nonoperative management and many could benefit from angiography.[9,49] Although an early CT-based grading system (deviating minimally from the AAST scale) demonstrated limited correlation with patient outcome,[50] an updated version, including identification of contained vascular injury and intraparenchymal versus intraperitoneal active bleeding as grading criteria, has been shown to provide improved accuracy of prediction of the need for angiography or surgery compared to the AAST scale (**Table 3**).[51] Other CT-based scoring systems have been proposed, incorporating additional relevant scan information, such as volume of hemoperitoneum; however, dissimilarity to the AAST system may limit familiarity and acceptability to trauma clinicians.[49,52–55]

SPLENIC ARTERIOGRAPHY AND EMBOLIZATION

Splenic arteriography with embolization can achieve effective hemostasis in cases of active bleeding after splenic injury and demonstrates utility as a prophylactic measure to reduce the incidence of delayed splenic hemorrhage.[56–61] The use of angioembolization decreases the operative intervention rate, resulting in decreased incidence of abdominal complications and blood use compared with surgery.[62] The addition of angioembolization to management protocols has increased the percentage of patients in whom nonoperative management is attempted, increased the nonoperative success rate, and increased overall splenic salvage.[63,64]

The two main methods of splenic embolization are selective distal embolization and proximal main splenic artery embolization; in some cases a combination of these techniques may be necessary.[56,59,60] While selective distal embolization attempts targeted occlusion of a bleeding or injured artery, proximal main splenic artery embolization reduces perfusion to the entire spleen, allowing hemostasis and healing, while patent collateral arterial supply contributes to the preservation of splenic function.[65–67] Segmental splenic infarction is nearly universal after selective distal embolization; infarction also occurs in more than half of patients after proximal main splenic artery embolization, but those lesions tend to be smaller and more peripheral.[68] Scintigraphic examination with ^{99m}Tc-sulfur colloid performed after main splenic artery embolization in 12 patients demonstrated preservation of splenic function in all of the patients examined.[69]

No conclusive difference in outcomes has been established between proximal versus distal embolization. In some patients, unusually robust collateral flow, as may result from preexisting celiac stenosis, may reduce the effectiveness of proximal embolization.[70] A few investigators have suggested that selective distal embolization may impart an increased risk of subsequent bleeding from latent lesions not identified at early angiography.[59,71] The routine use of main splenic artery embolization in all patients with severe (AAST grade III to V) splenic injury, with or without CT depiction of active bleeding or contained vascular injury, seems to reduce the failure rate of nonoperative management in this higher-risk setting; in one study, the splenectomy rate was reduced to 2.7% compared with 10.0% for the patients managed nonoperatively without embolization, despite the higher severity of injury in the former group.[66]

No uniformly accepted indications guide the use of splenic angiography and embolization. Indications for splenic angiography reported in the literature include CT evidence of active bleeding, vascular injury, high-grade injury (AAST grades III to V), and large-volume hemoperitoneum.[11,60,61] At the authors' institution, angiography is considered for any patient with splenic vascular injury or active bleeding on CT. All patients with high-grade (AAST grades III to V) injuries for whom nonoperative management is attempted also undergo splenic angiography. Pursuing this aggressive policy has helped to successfully and nonoperatively manage more than 80% of grade IV and V injuries.[61]

Postembolization Findings and Complications

Complications after splenic artery embolization include iatrogenic vascular injury; hemorrhage; infection, including abscess formation; and coil migration. Although reported complication rates vary, a large multi-institutional trial conducted by the Western Trauma Association including patients having undergone proximal main, selective distal, or combined embolizations, found iatrogenic vascular injury in 1%, hemorrhage in 10% (half requiring splenectomy), infection in 4% (3% proven abscesses), and coil migration in 2%.[60] One recent study suggests that patient age older than 65 years may be an independent risk factor for the development of complications after embolization, although age is not generally considered a contraindication to nonoperative management.[72]

As previously described, infarctions occur in almost all selective distal splenic embolizations and in 63% of proximal splenic embolizations, manifest on contrast-enhanced CT as roughly wedge-shaped areas of nonenhancement extending to the splenic periphery.[68] Patients with splenic infarcts may have a low-grade fever and left-upper-quadrant pain requiring analgesics. If followed by imaging, most infarcts decrease in size or remain unchanged and resolve without further complication.[68]

CT depiction of nonprogressive intrasplenic gas in the first few days after embolization can be within normal postprocedural limits (**Fig. 12**). Increasing or delayed intrasplenic gas accumulation, perisplenic pneumoperitoneum, and, in particular, intrasplenic gas-fluid level are suspicious findings, suggesting splenic necrosis or infection with abscess formation, which may require percutaneous aspiration for diagnostic confirmation.

Splenic vascular lesions identified by follow-up CT after embolization (**Fig. 13**) may have different implications than similar lesions identified on initial evaluation of the injured spleen. A study assessing the significance of splenic pseudoaneurysms detected after main splenic artery embolization demonstrated no significant change in splenic salvage rate (94%) in 32 patients with new or persistent PA after main splenic artery embolization; 29 of these patients did not require any additional therapy, whereas 3 underwent operation for clinical deterioration.[73]

IMAGING FOLLOW-UP AFTER SPLENIC INJURY

Controversy exists regarding appropriate follow-up imaging strategies during nonoperative management of splenic injury. Although failure of nonoperative management, defined as deterioration requiring surgery, is minimized by careful selection of candidates and use of angiography for prophylaxis and salvage, a small number of patients will remain at risk. A recent large study demonstrated a 1.4% risk of readmission for splenectomy in the 180 days after blunt splenic trauma; most occurred within 8 days.[74] Patients arriving in stable condition with mild (AAST grade I to II) splenic injury and no evidence of significant

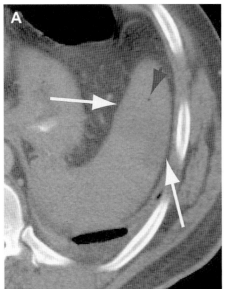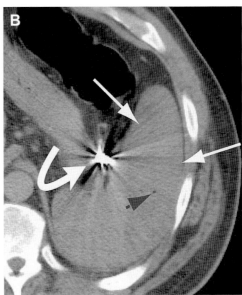

Fig. 12. Postembolization intrasplenic gas. (*A, B*) Axial CT images show a postembolization splenic infarct (*white arrows*) in the anterior aspect of the spleen. A few tiny bubbles of gas (*black arrowheads*) are seen in the infarcted parenchyma. Embolization coil (*curved arrow*) is seen in the main splenic artery at the hilum.

hemorrhage (no large hematoma or hemoperitoneum and no active extravasation or PA) are unlikely to deteriorate, and such patients are commonly managed conservatively without routine

Fig. 13. Persistent PA following main splenic artery embolization. A large PA (*arrow*) is seen following main splenic artery embolization with coils (*curved arrow*).

imaging follow-up. Although any patients suffering significant clinical deterioration warrant attention, which may include repeat imaging, early identification of failure while conservatively managed patients remain asymptomatic is the optimal situation, avoiding the worst-case scenario of catastrophic delayed hemorrhage requiring emergent splenectomy. At the same time, considerations of cost, radiation dose, and potential contrast agent nephrotoxicity mandate that CT surveillance not be overutilized with low yield.[75]

Numerous studies suggest that routine follow-up CT is not likely to reveal significant delayed complications in asymptomatic patients.[76–80] Contradictory results of other studies keep this issue in question; one recent retrospective review found worsening of injury on follow-up CT in slightly more than 9% of outpatients, most of whom were asymptomatic, although these did not require intervention.[81] The finding of delayed PA formation had been previously reported by Norotsky and colleagues[82] in a study that also emphasized the importance of obtaining follow-up CT scans in patients managed nonoperatively. Growth and rupture of intrasplenic PA is thought to be a major cause of delayed hemorrhage after blunt splenic injury. Although identification of delayed PA is more common in higher-grade injuries, as many as 24% of latent PA occur in patients with AAST grade I to II injuries.[83] Although restriction of follow-up CT to patients with high-grade injuries may result in nonidentification of some PA, the clinical significance of such lesions is unclear. Although there is no definite consensus as to utility of routine follow-up CT, generally accepted case-specific indications for repeat CT after trauma include clinical deterioration (hemodynamic instability or new/increasing abdominal pain or peritoneal signs); suspicion for extrasplenic injuries not confirmed by initial imaging (particularly bowel/mesenteric injury); and, in rare cases, to assess healing before the release of patients to resume high-risk activity (eg, contact sports).[80,84]

SUMMARY

Although hemodynamically unstable patients with abdominal injury suspected based on clinical assessment or hemoperitoneum identified by DPL or FAST still generally require laparotomy, stable patients may be considered for nonoperative management. CT contributes to this secondary triage, allowing direct noninvasive depiction of solid organ injury while providing increased sensitivity for hemoperitoneum. Evolving CT technology has progressively improved visualization and assessment of vasculature and vessel injury; improved detection and characterization of injury facilitates risk assessment, allowing the application of nonoperative management to an increasing percentage of patients with splenic injury. Specific CT findings may mandate laparotomy, predict success versus failure of nonoperative management, or prompt angiography. The increasing diagnostic capacity of CT requires refinement of radiologists' descriptive terminology to ensure optimal extraction and communication of imaging information. Catheter angiography remains the gold standard for depiction of vascular injuries, whereas angiographic embolization provides alternative primary therapy for the injured spleen and contributes to the success of nonoperative management. Controversies persist regarding the predictive value of specific imaging findings, usefulness of grading systems, indications for and utility of angiography, and strategies for imaging follow-up after splenic trauma. Ongoing research will continue to elucidate the evolving roles of imaging and imaging-guided intervention after splenic injury.

REFERENCES

1. Esposito TJ, Gamelli RL. Injury to the spleen. In: Mattox KL, Feliciano DV, Moore EE, editors. Trauma. 4th edition. New York: McGraw-Hill; 2000. p. 683–711.
2. Traub AC, Perry JF Jr. Injuries associated with splenic trauma. J Trauma 1981;21(10):840–7.
3. Hansen K, Singer DB. Asplenic-hyposplenic overwhelming sepsis: postsplenectomy sepsis revisited. Pediatr Dev Pathol 2001;4(2):105–21.
4. Izu BS, Ryan M, Markert RJ, et al. Impact of splenic injury guidelines on hospital stay and charges in patients with isolated splenic injury. Surgery 2009; 146:787–93.
5. Gauer J, Gerber-Paulet S, Seiler C, et al. Twenty years of splenic preservation in trauma: lower early infection rate than in splenectomy. World J Surg 2008;32:2730–5.
6. Shafi S, Parks J, Ahn C, et al. More operations, more deaths? Relationship between operative intervention rates and risk-adjusted mortality at trauma centers. J Trauma 2010;69(1):70–7.
7. Raikhlin A, Baerlocher MO, Asch MR, et al. Imaging and transcatheter arterial embolization for traumatic splenic injuries: review of the literature. Can J Surg 2008;51(6):464–72.
8. Renzulli P, Gross T, Schnuriger B, et al. Management of blunt injuries to the spleen. Br J Surg 2010;97: 1696–703.
9. Peitzman AB, Heil B, Rivera L, et al. Blunt splenic injury in adults: multi-institutional study of the Eastern Association for the Surgery of Trauma. J Trauma 2000;49(2):177–89.
10. Bee TK, Croce MA, Miller PR, et al. Failures of splenic nonoperative management: is the glass half empty or half full? J Trauma 2001;50(2):230–6.
11. Marmery H, Shanmuganathan K, Mirvis SE, et al. Correlation of multidetector CT findings with splenic arteriography and surgery: prospective study in 392 patients. J Am Coll Surg 2008;206: 685–93.
12. Saladyga A, Benjamin R. An evidence-based approach to spleen trauma: management and outcomes. Chapter 21. In: Cohn SM, editor. Acute care surgery and trauma: evidence based practice. London: Informa; 2009. p. 131–7.
13. Velmahos GC, Chan LS, Kamel E, et al. Nonoperative management of splenic injuries: have we gone too far? Arch Surg 2000;135:674–81.
14. Myers JG, Dent DL, Stewart RM, et al. Blunt splenic injuries: dedicated trauma surgeons can achieve a high rate of nonoperative success in patients of all ages. J Trauma 2000;48(5):801–6.
15. Nix JA, Costanza M, Daley BJ, et al. Outcome of the current management of splenic injuries. J Trauma 2001;50:835–42.
16. Swann IJ, Allister CA, Lewis HJ, et al. The value of peritoneal lavage in the assessment of patients with stab wounds of the abdomen and lower chest. J R Coll Surg Edinb 1986;31(1):40–3.
17. Peitzman AB, Harbrecht BG, Rivera L, et al. Failure of observation of blunt splenic injury in adults: variability in practice and adverse consequences. J Am Coll Surg 2005;201(2):179–87.

18. Korner M, Krotz MM, Degenhart C, et al. Current role of emergency US in patients with major trauma. Radiographics 2008;28:225–42.

19. Shanmuganathan K, Mirvis SE, Sherbourne CD, et al. Hemoperitoneum as the sole indicator of abdominal visceral injuries: a potential limitation of screening abdominal US for trauma. Radiology 1999;212:423–30.

20. Gaarder C, Kroepelien F, Loekke R, et al. Ultrasound performed by radiologists – confirming the truth about FAST in trauma. J Trauma 2009;67:323–9.

21. Lee BC, Ormsby EL, McGahan JP, et al. The utility of sonography for the triage of blunt abdominal trauma patients to exploratory laparotomy. AJR Am J Roentgenol 2007;188:415–21.

22. Chiu WC, Cushing BM, Rodriguez A, et al. Abdominal injuries without hemoperitoneum: a potential limitation of focused abdominal sonography for trauma. J Trauma 1997;42:617–25.

23. Taylor GA, Sivit CJ. Posttraumatic peritoneal fluid: is it a reliable indicator of intra-abdominal injury in children? J Pediatr Surg 1995;30:1644–8.

24. Sato M, Yoshii H. Reevaluation of ultrasonography for solid-organ injury in blunt abdominal trauma. J Ultrasound Med 2004;23:1583–96.

25. Brown MA, Casola G, Sirlin CB, et al. Blunt abdominal trauma: screening US in 2693 patients. Radiology 2001;218:352–8.

26. Poletti PA, Kinkel K, Vermeulen B, et al. Blunt abdominal trauma: should US be used to detect both free fluid and organ injuries? Radiology 2003;227:95–103.

27. Poletti P, Platon A, Becker D, et al. Blunt abdominal trauma: does the use of a second-generation sonographic contrast agent help to detect solid organ injuries? AJR Am J Roentgenol 2004;183:1293–301.

28. McGahan JP, Horton S, Gerscovich EO, et al. Appearance of solid organ injury with contrast-enhanced sonography in blunt abdominal trauma: preliminary experience. AJR Am J Roentgenol 2006;187:658–66.

29. Valentino M, Ansaloni L, Catena F, et al. Contrast-enhanced ultrasonography in blunt abdominal trauma: considerations after 5 years of experience. Radiol Med 2009;114(7):1080–93.

30. Anderson SW, Varghese JC, Lucey BC. Blunt splenic trauma: delayed-phase CT for differentiation of active hemorrhage from contained vascular injury in patients. Radiology 2007;243:88–95.

31. Orwig D, Federle MP. Localized clotted blood as evidence of visceral trauma on CT: the sentinel clot sign. AJR Am J Roentgenol 1989;153:747–9.

32. Miller LA, Mirvis SE, Shanmuganathan K, et al. CT diagnosis of splenic infarction in blunt splenic trauma: imaging features, clinical significance and complications. Clin Radiol 2004;59:342–8.

33. Shanmuganathan K, Mirvis SE, Sover ER. Value of contrast-enhanced CT in detecting active hemorrhage in patients with blunt abdominal or pelvic trauma. AJR Am J Roentgenol 1993;161(1):65–9.

34. Roy-Choudhury SH, Gallacher DJ, Pilmer J, et al. Relative threshold of detection of active arterial bleeding: in-vitro comparison of MDCT and digital subtraction angiography. AJR Am J Roentgenol 2007;189:W238–46.

35. Yao DC, Jeffrey RB Jr, Mirvis SE, et al. Using contrast-enhanced helical CT to visualize arterial extravasation after blunt abdominal trauma: incidence and organ distribution. AJR Am J Roentgenol 2002;178(1):17–20.

36. Schurr MJ, Fabian TC, Gavant M, et al. Management of blunt splenic trauma: computed tomographic contrast blush predicts failure of nonoperative management. J Trauma 1995;39(3):507–12.

37. Federle MP, Courcoulas AP, Powell M, et al. Blunt splenic injury in adults: clinical and CT criteria for management, with emphasis on active extravasation. Radiology 1998;206(1):137–42.

38. Nwomeh BC, Nadler EP, Meza MP, et al. Contrast extravasation predicts the need for operative intervention in children with blunt splenic trauma. J Trauma 2004;56(3):537–41.

39. Rhodes CA, Dinan D, Jafri SZ, et al. Clinical outcome of active extravasation in splenic trauma. Emerg Radiol 2005;11:348–52.

40. Diamond IR, Hamilton PA, Garber AB, et al. Extravasation of intravenous computed tomography scan contrast in blunt abdominal and pelvic trauma. J Trauma 2009;66:1102–7.

41. Cloutier DR, Baird TB, Gormley P, et al. Pediatric splenic injuries with a contrast blush: successful nonoperative management without angiography and embolization. J Pediatr Surg 2004;39(6):969–71.

42. Davies DA, Ein SH, Pearl R, et al. What is the significance of contrast "blush" in pediatric blunt splenic trauma? J Pediatr Surg 2010;45:916–20.

43. Fu CY, Wu SC, Chen RJ, et al. Evaluation of need for operative intervention in blunt splenic injury: intraperitoneal contrast extravasation has an increased probability of requiring operative intervention. World J Surg 2010;34:2745–51.

44. Smith JA, Macleish DG, Collier NA. Aneurysms of the visceral arteries. Aust N Z J Surg 1989;59:329–44.

45. Gavant ML, Schurr M, Flick PA, et al. Predicting clinical outcome of nonsurgical management of blunt splenic injury: using CT to reveal abnormalities of splenic vasculature. AJR Am J Roentgenol 1997;168:207–12.

46. Clarke JR, Trooskin SZ, Doshi PJ, et al. Time to laparotomy for intra-abdominal bleeding from trauma does affect survival for delays up to 90 minutes. J Trauma 2002;52:420–5.

47. Howell GM, Peitzman AB, Nirula R. Delay to therapeutic interventional radiology postinjury: time is of the essence. J Trauma 2010;68(6):1296–300.

48. Moore EE, Cogbill TH, Jurkovich GJ, et al. Organ injury scaling: spleen and liver (1994 revision). J Trauma 1995;38(3):323–4.

49. Becker CD, Spring P, Glattli A, et al. Blunt splenic trauma in adults: can CT findings be used to determine the need for surgery? AJR Am J Roentgenol 1994;162(2):343–7.

50. Mirvis SE, Whitley NO, Gens DR. Blunt splenic trauma in adults: CT-based classification and correlation with prognosis and treatment. Radiology 1989; 171:33–9.

51. Marmery H, Shanmuganathan K, Alexander M, et al. Optimization of selection for nonoperative management of blunt splenic injury: comparison of MDCT grading systems. AJR Am J Roentgenol 2007;189: 1421–7.

52. Resciniti A, Fink MP, Raptopoulos V, et al. Nonoperative treatment of adult splenic trauma: development of a computed tomographic scoring system that detects appropriate candidates for expectant management. J Trauma 1988;28(6):828–31.

53. Scatamacchia SA, Raptopoulos V, Fink MP. Splenic trauma in adults: impact of CT grading on management. Radiology 1989;171:725–9.

54. Williams RA, Black JJ, Sinow RM, et al. Computed tomography-assisted management of splenic trauma. Am J Surg 1997;174:276–9.

55. Thompson BT, Munera F, Cohn S, et al. Novel computed tomography scan scoring system predicts the need for intervention after splenic injury. J Trauma 2006;60(5):1083–6.

56. Sclafani SJ. The use of angiographic hemostasis in salvage of the injured spleen. Radiology 1981;141:645.

57. Sclafani SJ, Weisberg A, Scalea TM, et al. Blunt splenic injuries: nonsurgical treatment with CT, arteriography, and transcatheter arterial embolization of the splenic artery. Radiology 1991;181:189–96.

58. Sclafani SJ, Shaftan GW, Scalea TM, et al. Non-operative salvage of computed tomography-diagnosed splenic injuries: utilization of angiography for triage and embolisation for hemostasis. J Trauma 1995; 39(5):818–27.

59. Haan JM, Scott J, Boyd-Kranis RL, et al. Admission angiography for blunt splenic injury: advantages and pitfalls. J Trauma 2001;51(6):1161–5.

60. Haan JM, Biffl WB, Knudson MM, et al. Splenic embolization revisited: a multicenter review. J Trauma 2004;56(3):542–7.

61. Haan JM, Bochicchio GV, Kramer N, et al. Nonoperative management of blunt splenic injury: a 5-year experience. J Trauma 2005;58:492–9.

62. Wei B, Hemmila MR, Arbabi S, et al. Angioembolization reduces operative intervention for blunt splenic injury. J Trauma 2008;64:1472–7.

63. Gaarder C, Dormagen JB, Eken T, et al. Nonoperative management of splenic injuries: improved results with angioembolization. J Trauma 2006;61:192–8.

64. Sabe AA, Claridge JA, Rosenblum DI, et al. The effects of splenic artery embolization on nonoperative management of blunt splenic injury: a 16-year experience. J Trauma 2009;67:565–72.

65. Bessoud B, Denys A. Main splenic artery embolization using coils in blunt splenic injuries: effects on the intrasplenic blood pressure. Eur Radiol 2004; 14:1718–9.

66. Bessoud B, Denys A, Calmes JM. Nonoperative management of traumatic splenic injuries: is there a role for proximal splenic artery embolization? AJR Am J Roentgenol 2006;186:779–85.

67. Bessoud B, Duchosal MA, Siegrist CA, et al. Proximal splenic artery embolization for blunt splenic injury: clinical, immunologic and ultrasound-Doppler follow-up. J Trauma 2007;62:1481–6.

68. Killeen KL, Shanmuganathan K, Boyd-Kranis R, et al. CT findings after embolization for blunt splenic trauma. J Vasc Interv Radiol 2001;12:209–14.

69. Hagiwara A, Yukioka T, Ohta S, et al. Nonsurgical management of patients with blunt splenic injury: efficacy of transcatheter arterial embolization. AJR Am J Roentgenol 1996;167:159–66.

70. Requarth JA. Distal splenic artery hemodynamic changes during transient proximal splenic artery occlusion in blunt splenic injury patients: a mechanism of delayed splenic hemorrhage. J Trauma 2010;69(6): 1423–6. DOI:10.1097/TA.0b013e3181dbbd32 POST AUTHOR CORRECTIONS, 21 June 2010.

71. Smith HE, Biffl WL, Majercik SD, et al. Splenic artery embolization: have we gone too far? J Trauma 2006; 61(3):541–6.

72. Wu SC, Fu CY, Chen RJ, et al. Higher incidence of major complications after splenic embolization for blunt splenic injuries in elderly patients. Am J Emerg Med 2011;29(2):135–40.

73. Haan JM, Marmery H, Shanmuganathan K, et al. Experience with splenic main coil embolization and significance of new or persistent pseudoaneurysm: reembolize, operate or observe. J Trauma 2007;63: 615–9.

74. Zarzauer B, Vashi S, Magnotti L, et al. The real risk of splenectomy after discharge home following nonoperative management of blunt splenic injury. J Trauma 2009;66:1531–8.

75. Sinha S, Rajav SV, Lewis MH. Recent changes in the management of blunt splenic injury: effect on splenic trauma patients and hospital implications. Ann R Coll Surg Engl 2008;90:109–12.

76. Lawson DE, Jacobson JA, Spizarny DL, et al. Splenic trauma: value of follow-up CT. Radiology 1995;194(1):97–100.

77. Thaemert BC, Cogbill TH, Lambert PJ. Nonoperative management of splenic injury: are follow up

computed tomographic scans of any value? J Trauma 1997;43(5):748–51.

78. Shapiro MJ, Krausz C, Durham RM, et al. Overuse of splenic scoring and computed tomographic scans. J Trauma 1999;47(4):651–8.

79. Uecker J, Pickette C, Dunn E. The role of follow-up radiographic studies in nonoperative management of spleen trauma. Am Surg 2001;67(1): 22–5.

80. Sharma OP, Oswanski MF, Singer D. Role of repeat computerized tomography in nonoperative management of solid organ trauma. Am Surg 2005;71(3): 244–9.

81. Savage SA, Zarzauer BL, Magnotti LJ, et al. The evolution of blunt splenic injury: resolution and progression. J Trauma 2008;64:1085–92.

82. Norotsky MC, Roger FB, Shackford SR. Delayed presentation of splenic artery pseudoaneurysms following blunt abdominal trauma: case reports. J Trauma 1995;38:444–7.

83. Weinberg JA, Magnotti LJ, Croce MA, et al. The utility of serial computed tomography imaging of blunt splenic injury: still worth a second look? J Trauma 2007;62:1143–8.

84. Federle MP. Splenic trauma: is follow-up CT of value? Radiology 1995;194:23–4.

CT Imaging of Blunt Traumatic Bowel and Mesenteric Injuries

Christina A. LeBedis, MD, Stephan W. Anderson, MD,
Jorge A. Soto, MD*

KEYWORDS

• CT imaging • Blunt trauma • Bowel • Mesentery

Abdominal injuries are frequently the main cause of concern in patients who experience multiple traumas, especially from high-speed motor vehicle accidents. Clinical examination is challenging. After the initial evaluation and resuscitation in the trauma room, the decision to perform immediate laparotomy hinges on the hemodynamic status of the patient. Evidence of severe ongoing intra-abdominal hemorrhage with a compromised hemodynamic status, despite aggressive administration of blood products and fluids, is usually an indication for emergent laparotomy. A FAST (focused abdominal with sonography for trauma) ultrasonography examination that shows abundant free fluid (blood) in the abdomen often precedes the decision to transfer the patient to the operating room. Patients who do not require immediate laparotomy undergo further diagnostic evaluation. With the marked decrease in the use of peritoneal lavage, diagnosis usually relies on adequately performed and interpreted imaging studies, especially CT. Because conservative nonoperative therapy is preferred for all but the most severe injuries affecting the solid viscera, trauma surgeons and radiologists usually focus on detecting significant injuries to the hollow viscera and mesentery,[1–4] which often require operative repair. CT is superior to clinical evaluation and peritoneal lavage for diagnosing surgically important injuries to the bowel and mesentery.

GENERAL CONCEPTS AND PATHOPHYSIOLOGY

Although injuries to the hollow viscera and mesentery are rare, occurring in approximately 5% of patients who experience severe blunt abdominal trauma and require laparotomy,[1–5] one of the most essential tasks for a radiologist interpreting CT examinations of patients who experienced blunt trauma is to recognize the often subtle signs of bowel trauma. A delayed diagnosis of an injury to the bowel wall or mesentery that results in hollow viscus perforation leads to significant morbidity and mortality from hemorrhage, peritonitis, or abdominal sepsis. Delays in diagnosis as short as 8 to 12 hours after injury cause this increased morbidity and mortality.[6,7] Thus, early recognition with imaging is critical.

Three basic mechanisms have been proposed as the cause of bowel and mesenteric injuries in blunt abdominal trauma: shearing injuries caused by deceleration, crush injuries from direct impacts, and burst injuries from sudden increases in intraluminal pressure.[8] At least one-half of hollow visceral injuries involve the small bowel, with colonic, duodenal, and gastric injuries occurring in decreasing order of frequency.[1,9] The proximal jejunum (distal to the ligament of Treitz) and distal ileum (proximal to the ileocecal valve) are particularly susceptible to injuries from blunt traumatic forces. The points of fixation at these two sites allow shearing forces to injure the more mobile loops.[10]

The clinical diagnosis of bowel trauma is difficult. Spillage of blood and intestinal contents into the abdominal cavity causes peritonitis and subsequent complications. Abdominal pain and guarding from peritoneal irritation are the main early clinical manifestations of bowel and mesenteric injuries. In alert and noncomatose patients, the presence of these clinical findings should raise

Department of Radiology, Boston University School of Medicine, 820 Harrison Avenue, Boston, MA 02118, USA
* Corresponding author.
E-mail address: Jorge.Soto@bmc.org

Radiol Clin N Am 50 (2012) 123–136
doi:10.1016/j.rcl.2011.08.003
0033-8389/12/$ – see front matter © 2012 Elsevier Inc. All rights reserved.

the suspicion of a significant intra-abdominal injury. However, these are not specific and may not be present during the initial assessment after admission to the emergency room. Clear clinical signs of peritonitis may not appear for hours. In addition, these patients often have significant neurologic injuries to the head and spinal cord or receive medications that can mask pain and guarding, making physical examination of the abdomen difficult or unreliable. As a result, using clinical assessment alone as the indication for laparotomy to treat bowel or mesenteric injuries is associated with a negative laparotomy rate that may be as high as 40%.[11,12] Thus, diagnosing bowel and mesenteric injuries from blunt trauma requires the use of various diagnostic tests, especially CT. At most institutions, diagnostic peritoneal lavage has been abandoned as a diagnostic examination. In some practices, ultrasonography is used to triage patients with blunt trauma. Positive findings, such as free intraperitoneal fluid, may trigger the request for a CT examination.

CT TECHNIQUE

The efficacy of CT for diagnosing bowel and mesenteric injuries has been well established in the literature since the first reports from the early 1980s.[13,14] Numerous studies and reviews have been published detailing the performance of conventional, helical, and, more recently, multidetector CT in detecting bowel and mesenteric injury. Although all of the earlier studies were based on CT scanning performed with oral contrast media,[15–18] the need for oral contrast in this setting has been questioned by trauma surgeons, emergency medicine physicians, and radiologists.[19–21] The main reasons are safety issues (risk of aspiration and subsequent complications), potential delay in diagnosis, and lack of proven substantial added diagnostic information for detecting significant bowel and mesenteric injuries. Extraluminal oral contrast is seen on CT in approximately 10% to 15% of patients with surgically proven significant bowel or mesenteric injuries.[14–18] In addition to its low sensitivity, it is exceedingly rare for extraluminal oral contrast to be the only confirmatory sign of bowel or mesenteric trauma on CT. Almost 100% of the patients have additional highly suspicious CT findings that should alert the radiologist to the presence of a significant injury.

At the authors' institution, all emergent CT examinations for blunt trauma are currently performed with a 64-row multidetector scanner and without oral contrast material, using 1.25-mm thick images and a 1.25-mm reconstruction interval. The authors reserve the use of oral contrast material for follow-up CT in patients in whom possible bowel injury is suggested by the results of clinical examination or findings of the initial CT. Orthogonal (coronal and sagittal) reformations are generated for all patients for all series acquired, both with 2.5-mm thickness and a 2.5-mm reconstruction interval. Intravenous contrast (100–120 mL) is administered to all patients, and a 70-second delay is used for the portal venous phase acquisition. In addition, 5- to 7-minute delayed images of the abdomen and pelvis are obtained selectively in patients with injuries identified or suspected on the portal venous phase images.[22] These delayed-phase images are acquired with a low radiation dose technique, reducing the tube current by 50% to 70% of that used for the portal venous phase series.

SMALL BOWEL INJURIES

The timely diagnosis of significant bowel and mesenteric injuries (ie, those requiring operative repair) depends almost exclusively on their early recognition by the radiologist on the CT examination. Clinical signs and symptoms caused directly by the bowel injury are not specific and late to develop. Abdominal tenderness, rebound to palpation, and decreased peristalsis occurs in only one-third of the patients. Diagnosis with CT is also difficult and relies on careful inspection of the images for the presence of direct and indirect signs of injury. The significance of each individual finding varies. However, the presence of a combination of these findings increases the likelihood of a significant injury. Most patients with bowel and mesenteric injuries have associated injuries in other intra-abdominal organs, such as the liver and spleen. Therefore, all loops of bowel must be carefully scrutinized in patients with any abdominal injury identified on CT. In addition, patients with Chance vertebral fractures and those with abdominal wall hematomas also have a higher likelihood of having a significant injury in the bowel or mesentery.

The following are considered specific signs of bowel injury: transection of the wall with focal discontinuity, extraluminal oral contrast (in the rare occasions in which it is administered), pneumoperitoneum, and pneumoretroperitoneum. Specific signs of mesenteric trauma include mesenteric hematoma, intraperitoneal extravasation of intravenous contrast, and abrupt termination or unequivocal irregularity of the wall of mesenteric vessels. Other less-specific (but more sensitive) CT signs of bowel trauma include focal wall thickening, abnormal bowel wall enhancement, ill-defined increased attenuation ("stranding") of the mesentery, and free intraperitoneal fluid. Studies that used a different generation of scanners and relied on the multiple signs detailed in this article report a sensitivity between 70% and 95% and a specificity between 92% and 100% for the diagnosis of bowel and mesenteric injuries.[23–29]

The most severe bowel injuries are seen directly on CT as frank perforations with a focal interruption in the continuity of the bowel wall, and can be classified as bowel lacerations. Although this sign is almost 100% specific, its sensitivity is low, because only approximately 7% of injuries present with this finding.[30] More often, traumatic bowel perforations are small and cannot be directly identified on CT. Diagnosis of small bowel perforations demands careful attention from the radiologist to detect subtle signs.

Extraluminal gas is a highly suggestive but not a pathognomonic sign of bowel perforation. Pneumoperitoneum is found on CT in 20% to 75% of patients with proven bowel perforations.[21–30] The amount of free intraperitoneal gas varies widely and can be massive, filling all peritoneal compartments, or very small, with only a few bubbles noted outside of the bowel lumen (**Figs. 1** and **2**). In all patients with blunt trauma who have any CT finding that could potentially be associated with a hollow viscus injury, images should be reviewed with lung or bone window settings, in addition to the routine soft tissue settings. This approach facilitates the detection of small extraluminal gas collections. In addition, it is important to look for pneumoperitoneum in both the portal venous phase and delayed phase images, because occasionally the pneumoperitoneum may appear only on the second acquisition. Many patients with surgically proven perforations do not have

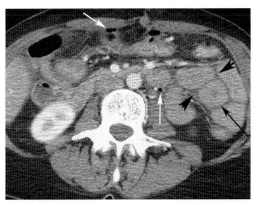

Fig. 2. CT of a 46-year-old woman who experienced significant blunt abdominal trauma and complained of abdominal pain at admission to the emergency room. The axial CT image shows wall thickening in a segment of jejunum (*black arrow*), associated fluid and stranding in the mesentery (*black arrowheads*), and small extraluminal gas collections (*white arrows*). The patient underwent surgical exploration and a focal perforation of the jejunum was repaired.

any evidence of pneumoperitoneum on CT. This circumstance may occur for various reasons: the perforation may be contained or may partially seal spontaneously, developing ileus prevents passage of gas into the abdominal cavity, or small gas collections may rapidly be reabsorbed through the peritoneal lining. A few potential causes of a false-positive finding of pneumoperitoneum should also be considered and ruled out before bowel perforation is diagnosed based on free intraperitoneal gas alone. Causes of pneumoperitoneum without bowel trauma include intraperitoneal rupture of the urinary bladder with an indwelling Foley catheter, massive pneumothorax (especially if a diaphragmatic rupture coexists), barotrauma, benign pneumoperitoneum (eg, as observed in some patients with systemic sclerosis), and the occasional diagnostic peritoneal lavage. Pseudopneumoperitoneum is another potential cause of a false-positive diagnosis of free intraperitoneal gas and bowel rupture. Pseudopneumoperitoneum, caused by air confined between the inner layer of the abdominal wall and the parietal peritoneum, may be found in patients who experience injuries to the extraperitoneal segments of the rectum, rib fractures, pneumothorax, or pneumomediastinum, with collections of extraluminal gas accumulating between the deep layers of the abdominal wall and the parietal peritoneum.[29] On CT, the appearance may closely resemble true pneumoperitoneum (**Figs. 3** and **4**). However, most patients with true pneumoperitoneum have collections of gas located deeper in the abdomen, often adjacent to the

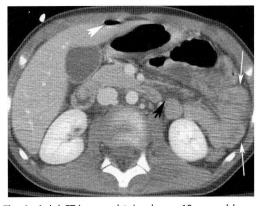

Fig. 1. Axial CT image obtained on a 19-year-old man who was a passenger in a high speed motor vehicle accident. A focal segment of thickened jejunum (*white arrows*) is shown, with associated pneumoperitoneum in the anterior peritoneal cavity (*white arrowhead*) and associated stranding of the small bowel mesentery (*black arrowhead*). Jejunal perforation was found at laparotomy.

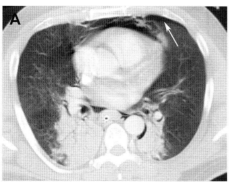
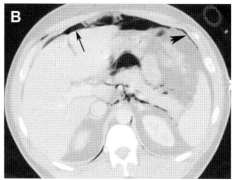

Fig. 3. Pneumoperitoneum and pseudopneumoperitoneum in a patient with thoracic trauma but no bowel injury. (*A*) Axial CT image of the lower chest, presented in lung window settings, shows a pneumomediastinum (air within the epicardial fat and surrounding the descending aorta and pulmonary arteries) and a left pneumothorax (*white arrow*). (*B*) Axial CT image of the upper abdomen, also presented in lung window settings, shows true pneumoperitoneum anterior to the surface of the liver (*black arrow*), and air within the extraperitoneal space of the abdominal wall (pseudopneumoperitoneum, *black arrowhead*). Although no additional CT findings suggested bowel injury, a laparotomy was performed; no bowel injury was found.

ruptured viscus, at the porta hepatis or outlining the falciform ligament. If in doubt, delayed images or a decubitus series may help make this distinction.

Unequivocal localized thickening of a small bowel loop or segment in the context of blunt trauma is usually an indication of a significant (surgically important) injury, such as a contusion, hematoma, ischemia secondary to mesenteric vascular trauma, or perforation (see **Figs. 1** and **2**; **Fig. 5**). Unequivocal focal abnormal enhancement (decreased or increased) of a segment of bowel is also a highly suspicious finding often

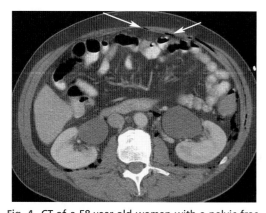

Fig. 4. CT of a 58-year-old woman with a pelvic fracture and a rectal wall tear, allowing leakage of gas into the extraperitoneal space of the pelvis. The axial CT image shows gas in the retroperitoneum (surrounding the kidneys and descending colon) and in the extraperitoneal space of the anterior abdominal wall (pseudopneumoperitoneum, *white arrows*). The patient underwent repair of the rectal tear but no laparotomy was performed.

associated with a significant injury (**Fig. 6**). The likelihood of focal wall thickening or focal abnormal enhancement representing a bowel injury that requires surgical intervention increases when found in association with pockets of fluid in the adjacent mesentery or free fluid in the peritoneal cavity.[31] Coronal and sagittal reformations are particularly useful for assessing the loops of small bowel and the associated mesentery for focal abnormalities. Focal full-thickness small bowel tears can be repaired with suture closure (enterorrhaphy); however, if multiple small bowel perforations are present, the affected loops of small bowel are typically resected and primary anastomosis is performed.[32]

Diffuse bowel wall thickening is usually not a result of direct trauma. Instead, the underlying pathophysiology is more likely edema secondary to volume overload or, in severely traumatized individuals with continued bleeding, to profound hypotension with hypoperfusion complex ("shock bowel") in which diffusely increased bowel wall enhancement.[33] Potential causes of increased bowel wall enhancement are leakage of contrast material from increased vascular permeability during hypoperfusion,[34] preferential shift of blood flow to the mucosa, or slowing of transit time of blood through the mucosa during hypotension. Other findings characteristic of shock and hypoperfusion complex on CT include a flat inferior vena cava, increased enhancement of the adrenal glands, and bowel and pancreatic and retroperitoneal edema (**Fig. 7**). Diffuse bowel wall thickening and edema can also be caused by overhydration and fluid overload. In this situation, the liver may show a heterogeneous pattern of enhancement

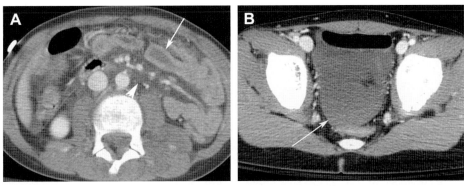

Fig. 5. CT of a 16-year-old man involved in a bicycle accident with abdominal pain and tenderness at presentation. The axial CT image of the mid-abdomen (*A*) shows a segment of thickened jejunum (*white arrow*), with fluid and stranding in the associated mesentery (*white arrowhead*). Axial CT image of the pelvis (*B*) shows a large amount of free fluid (*white arrow*). The mean attenuation of the fluid is 38 HU, consistent with hemoperitoneum. The air-fluid level is located inside the urinary bladder and does not represent pneumoperitoneum. At laparotomy, a jejunal wall hematoma and focal perforation were found.

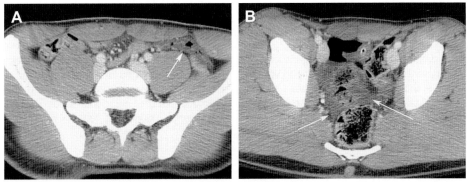

Fig. 6. Two axial CT images of the pelvis obtained in a 20-year-old man who was struck by a car while walking. A segment of thickened and poorly enhancing small bowel is seen in the left lower quadrant (*A, white arrow*), with associated free fluid in the pelvis (*B, white arrows*). A devascularized loop of proximal ileum, with an associated mural hematoma, was found at surgical exploration.

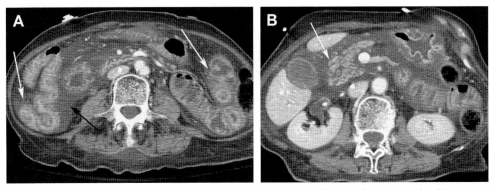

Fig. 7. Characteristic findings of hypoperfusion complex in a 64-year-old man who was involved in a motorcycle accident and experienced multiple extremity fractures with profuse bleeding. Diffuse thickening and hyperenhancement of the loops of small bowel is seen (*A, white arrows*), as are edema and free fluid in the mesentery (*A, black arrow*) and pancreatic and peripancreatic fat edema (*B, white arrow*). Aggressive resuscitation with intravenous fluids in polytraumatized patients is thought to be the cause of the abnormal accumulation of fluid in the peritoneal and retroperitoneal spaces.

("nutmeg" appearance) and a concentric halo of low attenuation around the portal veins (periportal edema), whereas the other abdominal organs and vessels have a normal appearance.

DUODENAL INJURIES

Duodenal injuries are uncommon and result from penetrating or, less frequently, blunt trauma.[35] Blunt duodenal injury is difficult to detect both clinically and radiologically, and may occur in isolation or with associated injuries of the pancreas, liver, or spleen. Blunt injuries of the duodenum most commonly occur from a crushing injury of the duodenum against the spine from an external force along the abdominal wall, such as a steering wheel or bicycle handlebars, and may be associated with a flexion/distraction fracture of L1–L2 (Chance fracture).[36] Rapid deceleration represents another mechanism of blunt duodenal injury causing tearing at the junction of the intraperitoneal (free) and retroperitoneal (fixed) portions of the duodenum, such as between the third and fourth portions.[36]

Clinically, patients with duodenal injuries most commonly present with epigastric pain and vomiting; however, in the emergent setting these symptoms may be masked by additional injuries, mental status changes, or medication. Additional symptoms frequently reported by these patients include diffuse abdominal pain, abdominal distention, and back pain.[35]

A high level of suspicion for duodenal injury should be maintained in patients who have sustained abdominal trauma given its high association with significant morbidity and mortality.[35] In addition, the clinical findings are nonspecific and laboratory values, such as serum amylase levels, lack sensitivity.[36] A delay in diagnosis longer than 24 hours has been reported to increase mortality from 11% to 40%.[37] Development of a duodenal fistula may cause serious fluid and electrolyte imbalances, and the extravasation of enzymes into the retroperitoneum can cause life-threatening peritonitis and sepsis.[36]

Imaging with CT has proven to be a valuable tool in the detection of often-subtle signs of duodenal injury. CT findings can include a duodenal hematoma manifesting as wall thickening; discontinuity of the duodenal wall possibly with intravenous or oral contrast extravasation from duodenal laceration; fluid adjacent to the duodenum, pancreatic head, and retroperitoneum; or retroperitoneal free air.[35] Physical examination findings, laboratory data, or imaging findings that suggest trauma to the duodenum warrant operative evaluation. Exploratory laparotomy with mobilization of the entire duodenum remains the gold standard for diagnosing duodenal injuries, because subtle injuries may be missed.[36]

Duodenal hematoma develops in the submucosal or subserosal layers of the intact duodenal wall (Fig. 8). Complications of duodenal hematomas include gastric outlet obstruction typically within 48 hours of injury. The management of a duodenal hematoma, when isolated, is conservative.[36,38]

Operative management of duodenal lacerations hinges on the extent and severity of the duodenal injury and the involvement of the adjacent vasculature, biliary tree, and pancreas.[39] Uncomplicated duodenal lacerations are repaired through primary surgical closure, known as *duodenorrhaphy*. More severe injuries of the duodenum such as duodenal lacerations with associated retroperitoneal infections, may require pyloric exclusion in addition to simple suture duodenal repair.[36,38,40] Pancreatico-duodenectomy is reserved for patients with severe combined duodenal and pancreatic head injuries, injury to the second portion of the duodenum involving the biliary tree, or devascularization of the duodenum.[36,38] Complex reconstructive procedures may not be possible initially if other abdominal injuries or signs of shock are present. In this setting, staged procedures are often pursued.[36] Complications of duodenal repair include suture dehiscence, duodenal fistula, pancreatitis, and sepsis.[35,36,38,40]

COLONIC INJURIES

Colonic and anorectal injuries represent a minority of traumatic bowel injuries, and are seen in up to

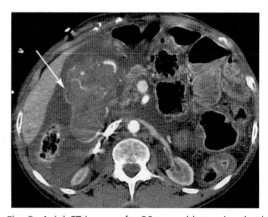

Fig. 8. Axial CT image of a 26-year-old man involved in a high-speed motor vehicle accident. The duodenum shows marked bowel wall thickening (*white arrow*) and extensive hemoperitoneum. CT examination showed multiple additional neurologic and thoracic injuries. The patient died as he was being transported to the operating room.

5% of patients with blunt abdominal trauma.[41] However, the colon is frequently affected in penetrating abdominal trauma from firearms and bladed weapons.[42]

Similar to those of the small bowel, the direct CT findings of blunt traumatic colonic perforation are free abdominal air, focal wall discontinuity, and extravasation of oral contrast. Free abdominal air is a highly specific (up to 95%) imaging finding for hollow viscus injury in blunt trauma; however, it has a low sensitivity (25%).[7,17] In the setting of colonic trauma, intraperitoneal air is most commonly identified. Retroperitoneal air may also be seen given the retroperitoneal course of both the ascending and descending colon; however, a duodenal source should also be considered. When retroperitoneal air is identified, it is most commonly seen in conjunction with intraperitoneal air rather than as an isolated finding. Alternative sources of retroperitoneal air should be considered, such as pneumothoraces and pneumomediastinum, because air may dissect into the retroperitoneum from the normal communications between these spaces. Conversely, air in the mediastinum may have its origin in the retroperitoneal space, such as in the setting of retroperitoneal bowel perforation. Multiplanar reconstructions and the use of lung or bone window settings can help identify air dissecting along the fascial planes of the torso and aid in the detection of subtle foci of air. Direct visualization of focal wall discontinuity is a highly specific finding for perforation, but is insensitive when the perforation is small.[43]

Given the relative insensitivity of direct signs of bowel injury, secondary signs of blunt colonic injury are crucial in detection. The indirect signs of colon injury are abnormal or focal bowel wall thickening or enhancement, stranding/infiltration of the adjacent mesentery or mesocolon, and free intraperitoneal fluid (**Figs. 9** and **10**).[30]

The bowel wall enhancement pattern and distribution are useful in suggesting the origin of injury. Patchy or irregular increases in bowel wall enhancement after the administration of intravenous contrast material are suggestive but not diagnostic of full-thickness injury.[31] However, areas of decreased or absent contrast enhancement are indicative of ischemic bowel.

As in small bowel injuries, adjacent fat stranding and infiltration are helpful CT findings in diagnosing colonic injury; however, these findings have a fairly low specificity because they may be caused by an isolated mesenteric injury. In the absence of solid visceral organ injury, free intraperitoneal fluid may be a secondary sign of blunt bowel injury. This finding is sensitive in diagnosing bowel injury, although it has been shown to lack specificity. For example in one series of 90 patients with isolated free fluid, only 7 had a bowel injury.[44] Despite the low specificity of these findings, suspicion of a bowel injury should be raised given the often-subtle imaging findings.

ANORECTAL INJURY

Given the propensity for concomitant injury of pelvic structures, such as the urinary bladder, urethra, and pelvic vasculature, blunt anorectal trauma is associated with high morbidity and mortality.[45] The mortality in these patients with blunt anorectal trauma has been shown to be nearly three times as high as in those with blunt colonic injury, with one series reporting mortality

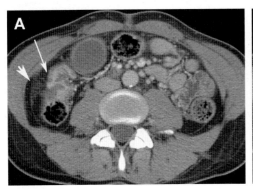
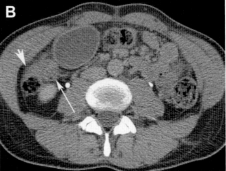

Fig. 9. CT of a 35-year-old woman who was struck by a moving vehicle. Axial CT image in the portal venous phase (A) shows focal segment of ascending colonic wall thickening and mucosal hyperenhancement (*white arrow*). Adjacent pericolonic fat stranding is seen (*white arrowhead*). On delayed phase axial CT (B), these imaging findings are more conspicuous, with persistent ascending colonic wall thickening (*white arrow*) and worsened pericolonic fat stranding with new free fluid (*white arrowhead*). At laparotomy, a hematoma in the wall of the ascending colon was found and a right hemicolectomy performed.

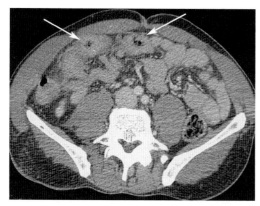

Fig. 10. Axial CT image of a 52-year-old woman who experienced blunt abdominal trauma. Marked transverse colonic wall thickening (*arrows*) with adjacent fat stranding is seen. Findings were confirmed at laparotomy.

from blunt rectal trauma to be up to 50%.[46] The frequency of rectal injuries was reported to be slightly higher than 2% of cases in a large series of patients with pelvic fractures secondary to blunt trauma (**Fig. 11**).[47] Specific pelvic fracture patterns

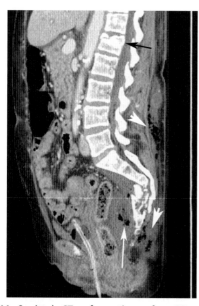

Fig. 11. Sagittal CT reformation of a 22-year-old woman who was a passenger in a motorcycle accident. Extensive extraluminal air is seen in the presacral space (*white arrow*) and tracking along the soft tissues posterior to the sacrum and lower lumbar spine (*white arrowheads*). Comminuted, displaced fractures of the lower sacrum and an anterior wedge compression fracture of L1 (*black arrow*) are also visualized. At surgery, this patient was found to have a rectal tear requiring repair and temporary diverting colostomy.

from blunt trauma have been shown to be associated with increased risks of rectal injury, such as widening of the pubic symphysis, which was noted to be an independent risk factor for rectal injury and anteroposterior compression type injury, which was seen in 75% of patients with rectal injury.[47]

Distinction between injuries to the intraperitoneal and extraperitoneal segments of the rectum is an important consideration in patients with rectal injury given differences in their subsequent management.[41,45] The anterior and lateral sidewalls of the upper two-thirds of the rectum are covered with peritoneum, and injuries to these segments are considered intraperitoneal. The distal one-third of the rectum circumferentially and the upper two-thirds of the rectum posteriorly are not covered with peritoneum and are considered extraperitoneal.

Primary CT findings of blunt anorectal injury that have the highest specificity include extraluminal air, direct evidence of a transmural injury, active hemorrhage related to a mural injury (an uncommon imaging presentation), and active extravasation of intravenously administered contrast into the bowel lumen (when no oral contrast is administered). The delayed phase of image acquisition is expected to show a change in the size or position of the intraluminal collection of contrast-enhanced blood in the setting of active extravasation.

As with the remainder of bowel injuries, these more-specific findings of blunt anorectal trauma are fairly insensitive. The indirect signs of blunt anorectal injury are similar to those previously described for the small bowel and colon, and include wall thickening, mesenteric stranding/infiltration, and free intraperitoneal fluid in the setting of injury to the intraperitoneal segment of the rectum when no solid visceral organ injury is identified. Rectal mesenteric and perianal fat stranding and infiltration have a fairly low specificity and may simply be related to an isolated mesenteric or perianal fat injury. However, the suspicion of an anorectal injury must be raised and, if the patient is to be conservatively managed, close clinical follow-up should be provided.

Patients with blunt trauma involving the intraperitoneal rectum are typically managed with primary repair, often with fecal diversion.[41] Low, extraperitoneal injuries from blunt trauma are repaired when accessible or when the injury is severely destructive. Alternatively, presacral drainage can be used to manage low, blunt rectal injury. Perineal injuries may disrupt the anal sphincter. Treatment of concomitant injuries, such as external fixation of unstable pelvic fractures and control of associated bleeding, is also necessary. Fecal diversion is typically used in patients unable to undergo immediate repair given their clinical status. Minimizing the risks of subsequent infection is crucial in blunt injury and typically requires extensive debridement, irrigation, and use of antibiotics.

INJURIES TO THE MESENTERY AND MESENTERIC VESSELS

Patients with evidence of bowel trauma on CT often have findings indicating presence of associated injuries to the mesentery. Mesenteric injuries can also be an isolated finding on CT. Specific findings of mesenteric trauma include intraperitoneal active extravasation of contrast-enhanced blood, mesenteric hematoma (**Figs. 12** and **13**), infiltration of the mesentery (**Fig. 14**), mesenteric rent with internal hernia (**Fig. 15**), and beading or abrupt termination of the mesenteric vessels.[30]

Active extravasation into the peritoneal cavity is uncommon, but the finding is almost 100% specific for presence of a significant injury that requires operative repair or, occasionally, endovascular therapy with coil embolization.[30] Nonoperative therapy with endovascular approaches can be attempted in patients with injuries to smaller vessels. The risk of inducing bowel ischemia must always be considered, and therefore these patients should be observed carefully in the postprocedure period with clinical examination and liberal use of follow-up CT. A hematoma is a well-defined collection of blood within the

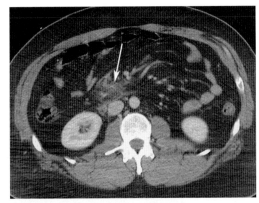

Fig. 13. Axial CT image obtained on a 30 year-old man involved in an automobile accident. A small focal hematoma in the root of the mesentery is seen (*arrow*). This patient was treated conservatively, with observation alone, and recovered without the need for laparotomy.

mesentery of the small bowel, mesocolon, or omentum. Small isolated mesenteric hematomas are not always an indication for immediate surgery and can be treated with observation alone (see **Fig. 12**). Larger hematomas occur in injuries to major mesenteric vessels, and therapeutic laparotomy is usually required to avoid the risk of delayed bowel ischemia (see **Fig. 13**). The finding of a mesenteric hematoma on portal venous-phase CT images should be further evaluated with delayed-phase images. Enlargement or increased attenuation of the hematoma on the delayed-phase is a sign of associated active bleeding that requires immediate action. Isolated mesenteric injuries can also manifest on CT as focal, poorly defined, haziness, and fat stranding of the mesentery (see **Fig. 14**). Abrupt termination, focal dilatation, and irregular beading of the mesenteric arterial or venous branches in the setting of trauma are signs of significant vascular injury. Mesenteric vascular injuries are uncommon but are significant because they are associated with the risk of subsequent bowel ischemia. Therefore, operative repair is usually indicated. Mesenteric tears are difficult to detect on CT and may only become apparent when a segment of bowel migrates through the defect causing an internal hernia (see **Fig. 15**). Closed loop bowel obstruction, volvulus, and strangulation can occur as complications of a traumatic internal hernia.

FREE INTRAPERITONEAL FLUID

Free intraperitoneal fluid is often found in patients with injuries to the bowel or mesentery. In fact, most studies cite free intraperitoneal fluid as the

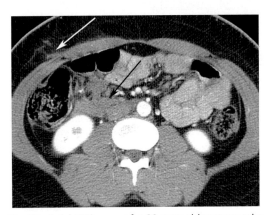

Fig. 12. Axial CT image of a 28-year-old woman who was the victim of an assault. A large focal collection of high attenuation fluid is seen in the root of the mesentery of the small bowel (*black arrow*). Note also a hematoma in the anterior abdominal wall (*white arrow*). The patient was complaining of abdominal pain at admission. Given the size of the hematoma, the decision was made to operate. At laparotomy, a laceration of a branch of the ileocolic artery was found, which required resection of a segment of ileum.

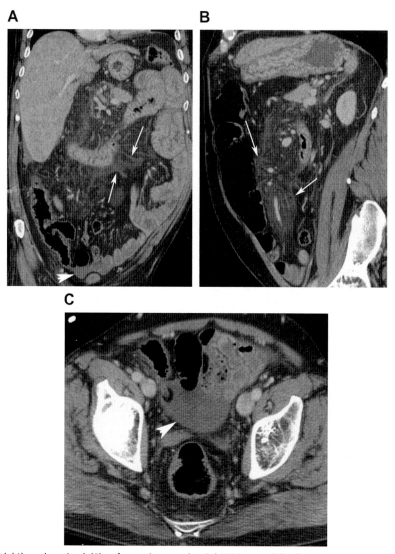

Fig. 14. Coronal (*A*) and sagittal (*B*) reformations and axial CT image (*C*) of a 43-year-old man who fell from a ladder and experienced a direct trauma to his abdomen. Ill-defined increased attenuation (stranding) and infiltration of the leaves of the mesentery of the small bowel (*A* and *B, arrows*) are seen, caused by mesenteric bleeding. Note also evidence of hemoperitoneum in the lower abdomen and pelvis (*A* and *C, arrowheads*). The patient was taken to the operating room and a lacerated jejunal branch of the superior mesenteric artery was found.

most common finding on CT (most sensitive sign).[22–31] In a retrospective study, Atri and colleagues[27] showed that the absence of free intraperitoneal fluid practically excludes the presence of a surgically important bowel or mesenteric injury in patients with blunt abdominal trauma. In most patients with significant (surgically important) bowel injuries, the finding of free peritoneal fluid is associated with other direct signs of trauma described previously (ie, focal wall thickening, wall perforation, abnormal wall enhancement, or pneumoperitoneum). Most patients with injuries to the intraperitoneal solid organs (ie, liver or

spleen) have variable amounts of associated hemoperitoneum. The attenuation is highest in the vicinity of the injured organ or organs; this is the "sentinel clot" sign. Thus, the finding of free intraperitoneal fluid in a trauma patient should trigger a careful evaluation of the solid organs and hollow viscera by the radiologist to detect the potential source (**Fig. 16**). The location of the fluid is important. Hemoperitoneum arising from the solid organs tends to accumulate in the paracolic gutters, Morrison's pouch, subphrenic spaces, and pelvis. Localized pockets of fluid, described as the "triangle sign" (fluid trapped between the

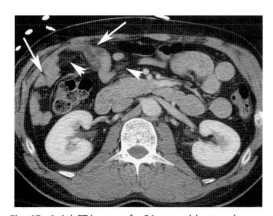

Fig. 15. Axial CT image of a 21-year-old man who was an unrestrained driver involved in an automobile accident. A cluster of abnormally positioned loops of small bowel is seen in the right hemiabdomen (*white arrows*), with associated subtle stranding of the corresponding mesentery (*white arrowheads*). These findings are characteristic of a traumatic internal hernia. At laparotomy, a rent in the mesentery with migrated loops of ileum was found and repaired.

leaves of the root of the mesentery), are unusual with injuries to the solid organs and are more specific for bowel or mesenteric injuries.[15,48]

In patients who have experienced blunt trauma, the finding on CT of free intraperitoneal fluid with absence of an identifiable injury makes interpretation difficult for radiologists and trauma surgeons, particularly in male patients. In women of reproductive age, ruptured ovarian follicular cysts can explain isolated free fluid in the pelvis. In men, the clinical importance of this finding is often questioned; that is, should management change because of the presence of free fluid alone. In the late 1990s, research suggested that the finding of free intraperitoneal fluid in the setting of blunt

trauma, in the absence of identifiable injury to explain the finding, necessitated exploratory laparotomy.[49,50] More recent work has led to a more conservative approach, with some of these patients being admitted for observation without immediate surgical intervention.[44,51–54] With advances in CT technology, the sensitivity for detecting small amounts of free intraperitoneal fluid has improved, and the radiologist must use all of the tools available to help guide further management.

Unexplained hemoperitoneum raises the likelihood of an underlying small bowel or mesenteric injury.[30] The attenuation of free blood in the peritoneal cavity is high (>30 to 40 Hounsfield units [HU]). In a study performed at the authors' institution, they showed that measuring the attenuation of the pockets of free fluid may help the radiologist and surgeon determine the significance of the isolated free fluid in men. In their study, isolated free fluid with low attenuation was found in 2.8% of men who experienced blunt trauma, and none was found to have a surgically important bowel or mesenteric injury.[55] The mean attenuation of the pockets of fluid on the portal venous-phase images was 13.1 HU (**Fig. 17**), considerably lower than the mean attenuation of free fluid in the patients who had an identifiable injury to explain the finding on CT (mean attenuation, 45.6 HU) (see **Fig. 16**). Yu and colleagues[56] reported similar results, with the only finding on CT being a small amount of free fluid in the pelvis in 4.8% of men who experienced blunt trauma. In this setting, the radiologist must carefully evaluate the CT images for findings that could explain the presence of low-attenuation fluid, such as intraperitoneal bladder rupture (urine) or biliary tract injury (bile). A trend for increased incidence of isolated free fluid can be seen in patients who receive

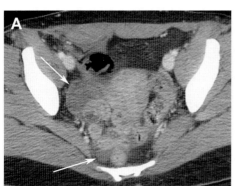
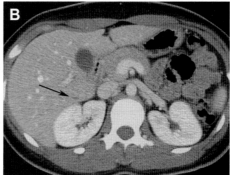

Fig. 16. Axial CT images obtained in a 31-year-old woman who was involved in an automobile accident. A moderate amount of free fluid is seen, consistent with hemoperitoneum (mean attenuation, 39 HU), in the pelvis (*A*, *arrows*). Careful inspection of the solid organs disclosed a small laceration extending to the surface of the right lobe of the liver (*B*, *arrow*).

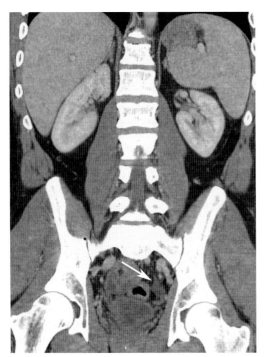

Fig. 17. Coronal reformation from a CT scan of a 28-year-old man who was a passenger in a car involved in a motor vehicle accident. The images show a small pocket of free fluid in the pelvis (*arrow*) as an isolated finding. No evidence suggested trauma to the solid or hollow visceral organs. The mean attenuation of the free fluid was 8 HU. The patient was admitted for observation and was later discharged without the need for laparotomy.

higher volumes of fluid resuscitation.[56] Furthermore, radiologists play an important role through reviewing the images from the trauma scan at the CT scanner, and if a suspicious finding (such as free peritoneal fluid) is noted on the initial portal venous-phase images, the decision to obtain delayed images should be made.

SUMMARY

Delay in diagnosis of a bowel or mesenteric injury that results in hollow viscus perforation leads to significant morbidity and mortality from hemorrhage, peritonitis, or abdominal sepsis. The timely diagnosis of bowel and mesenteric injuries requiring operative repair depends almost exclusively on their early detection by the radiologist on CT examination, because the clinical signs and symptoms of these injuries are not specific and usually develop late. Therefore, the radiologist must be familiar with the often-subtle imaging findings of bowel and mesenteric injury that will allow for appropriate triage of a patient who has sustained blunt trauma to the abdomen or pelvis.

REFERENCES

1. Dauterive AH, Flanchbaum L, Cox EF. Blunt intestinal trauma: a modern-day review. Ann Surg 1985; 201:198–203.
2. Cox EF. Blunt abdominal trauma: a 5-year analysis of 870 patients requiring celiotomy. Ann Surg 1984; 199:467–74.
3. Buck GC III, Dalton ML, Neely WA. Diagnostic laparotomy for abdominal trauma: a university hospital experience. Am Surg 1986;52:41–3.
4. Rizzo MJ, Federle MP, Griffiths BG. Bowel and mesenteric injury following blunt abdominal trauma: evaluation with CT. Radiology 1989;173:143–8.
5. Davis JJ, Cohn I, Nance FC. Diagnosis and management of blunt abdominal trauma. Ann Surg 1976;183:672–8.
6. Killeen KL, Shanmuganathan K, Poletti PA, et al. Helical computed tomography of bowel and mesenteric injuries. J Trauma 2001;51:26–36.
7. Scaglione M, de Lutio di Castelguidone E, Castelguidone EL, et al. Blunt trauma to the gastrointestinal tract and mesentery: is there a role for helical CT in the decision-making process? Eur J Radiol 2004;50:67–73.
8. Hughes TM, Elton C. The pathophysiology and management of bowel and mesenteric injuries due to blunt trauma. Injury 2002;33:295–302.
9. Kim HC, Shin HC, Park SJ, et al. Traumatic bowel perforation: analysis of CT findings according to the perforation site and the elapsed time since accident. Clin Imaging 2004;28:334–9.
10. Hawkins AE, Mirvis SE. Evaluation of bowel and mesenteric injury: role of multidetector CT. Abdom Imaging 2003;28:505–14.
11. Fryer JP, Graham TL, Fong HM, et al. Diagnostic peritoneal lavage as an indicator for therapeutic surgery. Can J Surg 1991;34:471–6.
12. Drost TF, Rosemurgy AS, Kearney RE, et al. Diagnostic peritoneal lavage: limited indications due to evolving concepts in trauma care. Am Surg 1991; 57:126–8.
13. Glazer GM, Buy JN, Moss AA, et al. CT detection of duodenal perforation. AJR Am J Roentgenol 1981; 137:333–6.
14. Jeffrey RB, Federle MP, Stein SM, et al. Case report: intramural hematoma of the cecum following blunt trauma. J Comput Assist Tomogr 1982;6:404–5.
15. Levine CD, Gonzales RN, Wachsberg RH. CT findings in bowel and mesenteric injury. J Comput Assist Tomogr 1997;21:974–9.
16. Hanks PW, Brody JM. Blunt injury to the mesentery and small bowel: CT evaluation. Radiol Clin North Am 2003;41:1171–82.

17. Butela ST, Federle MP, Chang PJ, et al. Performance of CT in detection of bowel injury. AJR Am J Roentgenol 2001;176:129–35.

18. Janzen DL, Zwirewich CV, Breen DJ, et al. Diagnostic accuracy of helical CT for detection of blunt bowel and mesenteric injuries. Clin Radiol 1998;53: 193–7.

19. Tsang BD, Panacek EA, Brant WE, et al. Effect of oral contrast administration for abdominal computed tomography in the evaluation of acute blunt trauma. Ann Emerg Med 1997;30:7–13.

20. Stafford RE, McGonigal MD, Weigelt JA, et al. Oral contrast solution and computerized tomography for blunt abdominal trauma: a randomized study. Arch Surg 1999;134:622–7.

21. Clancy TV, Ragozzino MW, Ranshaw D, et al. Oral contrast is not necessary in the evaluation of blunt abdominal trauma by computed tomography. Am J Surg 1993;166:680–3.

22. Stuhlfaut JW, Lucey BC, Varghese JC, et al. Blunt abdominal trauma: utility of 5-minute delayed CT with a reduced radiation dose. Radiology 2006; 238:473–9.

23. Donohue JH, Federle MP, Griffiths BG, et al. Computed tomography in the diagnosis of blunt intestinal and mesenteric injuries. J Trauma 1987; 27:11–7.

24. Hagiwara A, Yukioka T, Satou M, et al. Early diagnosis of small intestinal rupture from blunt abdominal trauma using computed tomography: significance of the streaky density within the mesentery. J Trauma 1995;38:630–3.

25. Sivit CJ, Eichelberger MR, Taylor GA. CT in children with rupture of the bowel caused by blunt trauma: diagnosis efficacy and comparison with hypoperfusion complex. AJR Am J Roentgenol 1994;163: 1195–8.

26. Mirvis SE, Gens DR, Shanmuganathan K. Rupture of the bowel after blunt abdominal trauma: diagnosis with CT. AJR Am J Roentgenol 1992;159:1217–21.

27. Atri M, Hanson JM, Grinblat L, et al. Surgically important bowel and/or mesenteric injury in blunt trauma: accuracy of multidetector CT for evaluation. Radiology 2008;249:524–33.

28. Stuhlfaut JW, Soto JA, Lucey BC, et al. Blunt abdominal trauma: performance of CT without oral contrast material. Radiology 2004;233:689–94.

29. Hamilton P, Rizoli S, McLellan B, et al. Significance of intra-abdominal extraluminal air detected by CT scan in blunt abdominal trauma. J Trauma 1995; 39:331–3.

30. Brofman N, Atri M, Hanson JM, et al. Evaluation of bowel and mesenteric blunt trauma with multidetector CT. Radiographics 2006;26:1119–31.

31. Malhotra AK, Fabian TC, Katsis SB, et al. Blunt bowel and mesenteric injuries: the role of screening computed tomography. J Trauma 2000;48:991–8.

32. Richardson JD. Treatment of small bowel injuries. In: Cameron JL, editor. Current surgical therapy. 9th edition. Philadelphia: Mosby; 2008. p. 998.

33. Mirvis SE, Shanmuganathan K, Erb R. Diffuse small-bowel ischemia in hypotensive adults after blunt trauma (shock bowel): CT findings and clinical significance. AJR Am J Roentgenol 1994;163:1375–9.

34. Brody JM, Leighton DB, Murphy BL, et al. CT of blunt trauma bowel and mesenteric injury: typical findings and pitfalls in diagnosis. Radiographics 2000;20: 1525–37.

35. Pandey S, Niranjan A, Mishra S, et al. Retrospective analysis of duodenal injuries: a comprehensive review. Saudi J Gastroenterol 2011;17:142–4.

36. Degiannis E, Boffard K. Duodenal injuries. Br J Surg 2000;87:1473–9.

37. Lucas CE, Ledgerwood AM. Factors influencing outcome after blunt duodenal injury. J Trauma 1975;15:839–46.

38. Sriussadaporn S, Pak-art R, Sriussadaporn S, et al. Management of blunt duodenal injuries. J Med Assoc Thai 2004;87:1336–42.

39. Blocksom JM, Tyburski JG, Sohn RL, et al. Prognostic determinants in duodenal injuries. Am Surg 2004;70:248–55.

40. Fraga GP, Biazotto G, Bortoto JB, et al. The use of pyloric exclusion for treating duodenal trauma: case series. Sao Paulo Med J 2008;126:337–41.

41. Cleary RK, Pomerantz RA, Lampman RM. Colon and rectal injuries. Dis Colon Rectum 2006;49:1203–22.

42. Pinedo-Onofre JA, Guevara-Torres L, Sánchez-Aguilar JM. Penetrating abdominal trauma. Cir Cir 2006;74:431–42 [in Spanish].

43. Miki T, Ogata S, Uto M, et al. Multidetector-row CT findings of colonic perforation: direct visualization of ruptured colonic wall. Abdom Imaging 2004;29: 658–62.

44. Livingston DH, Lavery RF, Passannante MR, et al. Free fluid on abdominal computed tomography without solid organ injury after blunt abdominal injury does not mandate celiotomy. Am J Surg 2001;182:6–9.

45. Maxwell RA, Fabian TC. Current management of colon trauma. World J Surg 2003;27:632–9.

46. Miller BJ, Schache DJ. Colorectal injury: where do we stand with repair? ANZ J Surg 1996;66:348–52.

47. Aihara R, Blansfield JS, Millham FH, et al. Fracture locations influence the likelihood of rectal and lower urinary tract injuries in patients sustaining pelvic fractures. J Trauma 2002;52:205–8.

48. Nghiem HV, Jeffrey RB Jr, Mindelzun RE. CT of blunt trauma to the bowel and mesentery. Semin Ultrasound CT MR 1995;16:82–90.

49. Cunningham MA, Tyroch AH, Kaups KL, et al. Does free fluid on abdominal computed tomographic scan after blunt trauma require laparotomy? J Trauma 1998;44:599–602.

50. Breen DJ, Janzen DL, Zwirewich CV, et al. Blunt bowel and mesenteric injury: diagnostic performance of CT signs. J Comput Assist Tomogr 1997; 21:706–12.

51. Brasel KJ, Olson CJ, Stafford RE, et al. Incidence and significance of free fluid on abdominal computed tomographic scan in blunt trauma. J Trauma 1998; 44:889–92.

52. Rodriguez C, Barone JE, Wilbanks TO, et al. Isolated free fluid on computed tomographic tomographic scan in blunt abdominal trauma: a systematic review of incidence and management. J Trauma 2002;53:79–85.

53. Fang JF, Chen RJ, Lin BC, et al. Small bowel perforation: is urgent surgery necessary? J Trauma 1999; 47:515–20.

54. Livingston DH, Lavery RF, Passannante MR, et al. Admission or observation is not necessary after a negative abdominal computed tomographic scan in patients with suspected blunt abdominal trauma: results of a prospective, multi-institutional trial. J Trauma 1998;44:273–80.

55. Drasin TE, Anderson SW, Asandra A, et al. MDCT evaluation of blunt abdominal trauma: clinical significance of free intraperitoneal fluid in males with absence of identifiable injury. AJR Am J Roentgenol 2008;191:1821–6.

56. Yu J, Fulcher AS, Want DB, et al. Frequency and importance of small amount of isolated pelvic free fluid detected with multidetector CT in male patients with blunt trauma. Radiology 2010;256:799–805.

Multi-Detector Row CT of Acute Non-traumatic Abdominal Pain: Contrast and Protocol Considerations

Stephan W. Anderson, MD*, Jorge A. Soto, MD

KEYWORDS

- Acute nontraumatic abdominal pain
- Computed tomography • Intravenous contrast
- Oral contrast

This article discusses the critical protocol considerations in imaging patients with abdominal pain in the emergency department, specifically, the use of oral contrast, intravenous contrast, image post-processing, and radiation dose. The factors that should be evaluated when considering these aspects of computed tomography (CT) protocols in abdominal pain imaging are discussed. The literature regarding the use of oral and intravenous contrast, imaging post-processing, and radiation specific to CT imaging of abdominal pain are reviewed in an evidence-based fashion to familiarize the reader with the current concepts in this area.

ORAL CONTRAST

The use of oral contrast agents in the imaging evaluation of abdominal pain has served to yield a high diagnostic accuracy using CT for the common etiologies of abdominal pain, even with previous generations of CT scanners. For instance, reported accuracy for diagnosing diverticulitis using rectally administered contrast approaches 100% (overall diagnostic accuracy, 99%) using single-detector CT technology.[1] Similarly, excellent diagnostic accuracy for the diagnosis of appendicitis has been described using 4 multi-detector computed tomography (MDCT) technology (sensitivity, 99%; specificity, 95%).[2] However, even in light of the success of positive oral contrast in terms of

diagnostic accuracy in diagnosing the various etiologies of abdominal pain, its use must be reconsidered in light of evidence of its untoward effects as regards emergency department throughput, potential delays in surgical management, and even radiation dose. Specifically, the use of oral contrast has been associated with significant differences in time of patient arrival to the emergency department until physician evaluation, time of CT scan order to CT scan completion, as well as time from emergency department arrival to eventual disposition. The latter was found to increase by more than 4 hours with the use of oral contrast, the differences exceeding the time allotted for the oral contrast preparation.[3] In a separate study comparing length of stay in the emergency department between orally and rectally administered contrast in patients with suspected acute appendicitis, length of stay was found to significantly increase by greater than 1 hour in the oral contrast arm.[4] Gastric emptying time of orally administered contrast has been studied, as the presence of oral contrast may have implications for the induction of general anesthesia in patients requiring operative management of their etiology of abdominal pain. In 1 particular study, 50% of patients were reported to have residual oral contrast in the stomach for greater than 1 hour after administration; 25% of patients were found to have residual oral contrast in the stomach for greater

Department of Radiology, Boston University School of Medicine, 820 Harrison Avenue, Boston, MA 02118, USA
* Corresponding author.
E-mail address: Stephan.Anderson@bmc.org

Radiol Clin N Am 50 (2012) 137–147
doi:10.1016/j.rcl.2011.08.009
0033-8389/12/$ – see front matter © 2012 Published by Elsevier Inc.

than 2 hours, and a single patient was found to have oral contrast in the stomach nearly 3 hours after administration.[5] In light of these findings, the authors advocated waiting at least 3 hours between the administration of oral contrast for CT and the induction of general anesthesia, introducing the potential for delays in management. In a recent large study analyzing the effects of oral contrast, it was found that in nearly 20% of patients with appendicitis, the administration of oral contrast material induced emesis, and nasogastric tubes were place in more than 5% of patients for the administration of oral contrast.[6] Given a similar diagnostic accuracy in diagnosing appendicitis between CT scans performed with or without oral contrast in this particular study, the authors concluded that the rates of emesis and nasogastric tube placement in this patient population support the discontinuation of the use of oral contrast in patients with suspected appendicitis. Finally, a recent study evaluated the radiation dose of abdominopelvic CT scans using automatic exposure control and compared patients administered positive oral contrast versus those administered water as the oral contrast agent.[7] It was found that the use of positive oral contrast increased the volume CT dose index (CTDIvol) by 11% when using automatic exposure control. Thus, given the reported effects on emergency department throughput, a consideration of increasing importance, potential delays in management based on the gastric transit of oral contrast, emesis and nasogastric tube (NGT) placement rates, as well as the potential for increasing radiation, the ongoing use of positive oral contrast deserves reconsideration.

In considering the use of oral contrast material in abdominal pain, the transit time for optimal opacification is a critical factor. If oral contrast is to be administered, an optimal strategy to balance time efficiency and adequate bowel opacification should be sought. In the author's experience using a controlled, 2-hour preparation with 900 mL of barium sulfate suspension, it was found that the distal colon (descending colon and beyond) was opacified in only 35% of patients, and in 30% of patients, no portion of the colon was opacified. As acute diverticulitis and appendicitis are 2 major causes of abdominal pain, a significant proportion of the patient population was not well served with administration of oral contrast but incurred negative implications thereof. However, various oral contrast formulations have been shown to yield dramatically different rates of bowel opacification. For instance, in comparing a 1600 mL water-iodinated contrast mixture with a 2- to 2.5-hour preparation with a polyethylene glycol (PEG)-iodinated contrast mixture with a 1-hour delay, it

was found that the former opacified the cecum in only 18 of 40 patients, while the latter, with only 1 hour of preparation time, resulted in opacification of the cecum in 38 of 40 patients.[8] Thus, if oral contrast agents are to be administered, transit time should be considered, and agents optimizing the transit time, and therefore, bowel opacification, should be administered.

In considering the hypothetical benefits of orally administered contrast in patients with abdominal pain, one may consider the potential benefits for diagnosing 3 common and clinically significant etiologies: appendicitis, diverticulitis, and small bowel obstruction. In the case of appendicitis, the filling of a normal appendiceal lumen with contrast offers the potential for increased confidence in excluding this diagnosis. The absence of oral contrast filling, if specific to acute appendicitis, would be a useful imaging finding. However, oral contrast does not reliably fill the appendiceal lumen in normal patients; in 1 study, 71% of normal appendices were found to opacify to some degree with oral contrast.[9] As a significant number of normal appendices do not fill with oral contrast, this finding is not specific to acute appendicitis, and the absence of oral contrast within the appendiceal lumen is unreliable in diagnosing acute appendicitis. The most useful individual findings in diagnosing acute appendicitis have been reported to be an enlarged appendix, appendiceal wall thickening, periappendiceal fat stranding, and appendiceal wall enhancement (Fig. 1).[10] The conspicuity of these individual imaging findings is unlikely to be affected by the presence of oral contrast, an argument against its administration in cases of suspected appendicitis.

The hypothetical benefits of orally administered contrast in cases of acute diverticulitis include the fact that oral contrast may provide a reliable assessment of the thickness of the bowel wall, assuming that the area of interest is opacified. The accurate assessment of bowel wall thickness is critical in making the diagnosis of acute diverticulitis, as well as other abnormalities of the small and large bowel. In fact, the diagnostic accuracy of the single imaging finding of an abnormally thickened bowel wall has a reported sensitivity of 96% and specificity of 91% in the diagnosis of acute diverticulitis.[11] The use of current MDCT technology, however, offers the distinct advantage of improved temporal resolution, effectively freezing the bowel wall, and limits motion artifact secondary to peristalsis. This improved image quality of the bowel, along with a clear delineation of the enhancing mucosa after intravenous contrast administration, may serve to provide an

A   B

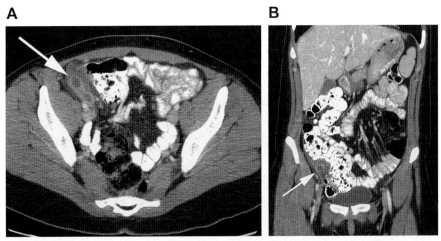

Fig. 1. Axial (*A*) and coronal (*B*) oral and intravenous contrast-enhanced computed tomography images demonstrate an enlarged appendix (*arrows*) with appendiceal wall enhancement and surrounding fat stranding consistent with acute appendicitis. The utility of oral contrast in increasing the conspicuity of these imaging findings is of questionable significance.

accurate assessment of the bowel wall without the need for oral contrast administration.

In the case of small bowel obstruction, there is evidence to suggest that the use of positive oral contrast material may, in fact, be contraindicated. As ischemia is a potential complication of small bowel obstruction, many institutions prefer to evaluate suspected small bowel obstruction without the use of positive oral contrast. The reason for this is the fact that the evaluation of the degree of small bowel mucosal enhancement, a highly specific CT imaging finding of small bowel ischemia, is limited with the use of positive oral contrast (**Fig. 2**). The CT finding of decreased mucosal enhancement has been reported to be the single most specific finding in cases of small bowel ischemia, and the absence of inner layer enhancement has been reported to be associated with significantly increased rates of operative management, bowel resection, bowel necrosis, and patient death.[12,13] Finally, in cases of mechanical small bowel obstruction, given the delayed transit time related to the obstruction, orally administered contrast typically fails to opacify the areas of interest such as the etiology of obstruction or transition point (**Fig. 3**).

With a growing pressure to optimize emergency department throughput as well as significantly improved image quality afforded by the growing implementation of the current generations of MDCT scanners, several studies evaluating the ongoing need for oral contrast material in the emergency department have been published. In an early study, a group of patients presenting to the emergency department with abdominal pain

was imaged both with and without oral contrast material in the absence of intravenous contrast, and the authors concluded that CT imaging, in cases of abdominal pain in the emergency department, should be considered without oral contrast, given a 79% simple agreement, with most disagreement attributable to interobserver variability.[14] Lending further support to a paradigm of imaging abdominal pain without oral contrast, the sensitivity and specificity of diagnosing acute appendicitis in a cohort of patients imaged without oral contrast, using intravenous contrast only, were reported to be 100% and 97%, respectively.[15] In a recent study, patients were randomized to receive or not receive oral contrast to compare the diagnostic accuracy in diagnosing acute appendicitis. In this study, patients were imaged with and without intravenous contrast and standard radiation dose (100 mAs) and simulated low dose (30 mAs) protocols were compared.[16] Adding further support to the lack of need for oral contrast in abdominal pain, the authors found no differences in diagnosing appendicitis with or without oral contrast.

In the author's experience, 303 patients were prospectively enrolled and were randomized to receive oral and intravenous contrast or intravenous contrast only, comparing the diagnostic accuracy for the detecting appendicitis.[17] Using a combined interpretation scheme in which 2 radiologists independently interpreted the images, and a third served as an adjudicator, the author and colleagues found no difference in sensitivity or specificity for the 2 groups of patients (sensitivity, 100% for both arms; specificity, 97.1% for

A   B

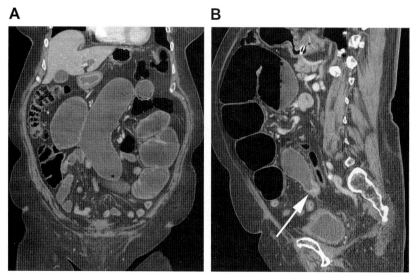

Fig. 2. Coronal (*A*) and sagittal (*B*) intravenous contrast-enhanced computed tomography images without the administration of oral contrast demonstrate enlarged, fluid-filled loops of small bowel with the transition point readily identified (*arrow*, sagittal image). The absence of positive oral contrast material affords an evaluation of the enhancement characteristics of the mucosa of the affected small bowel, a highly specific finding for ischemia, which in this case is found to be normal.

both arms). In this same group of 303 patients, the author and colleagues also analyzed the effect of 2 variables, the presence or absence of oral contrast as well as body habitus as measured by body mass index (BMI) and manual segmentation of intra-abdominal fat on CT, on reader confidence

in diagnosing or excluding appendicitis.[18] The author and colleagues hypothesized that the absence of oral contrast may negatively impact reader confidence in diagnosing appendicitis in patients without oral contrast, and this effect may be amplified in patients with low BMI or

A   B

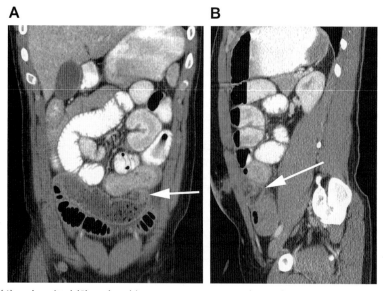

Fig. 3. Coronal (*A*) and sagittal (*B*) oral and intravenous contrast-enhanced computed tomography images with the administration of oral contrast demonstrate enlarged, fluid-filled loops of small bowel with the transition point readily identified (*arrows*). As is common in cases of mechanical small bowel obstruction, the orally administered contrast is seen within the more proximal bowel but does not serve to opacify the areas of interest.

relatively small degrees of intra-abdominal fat. The author found that for only one of the 3 readers, BMI was found to have an impact on reader confidence such that this single reader was more confident in diagnosing or excluding appendicitis in patients with a higher BMI in the group administered oral and intravenous contrast. No further effects on reader confidence in diagnosing appendicitis based on BMI, intra-abdominal fat, or whether or not oral contrast was administered were found for any of the 3 readers. Finally, the author and colleagues also compared appendiceal visualization rates to determine whether variables of oral contrast administration or body habitus may impact this finding, hypothesizing that the lack of oral contrast and lower BMI or intra-abdominal fat may decrease appendiceal visualization rates. The study found no significant impact of body habitus or whether oral contrast was administered on appendiceal visualization rates. These studies lend further credence to the hypothesis that patients with abdominal pain, specifically those with suspected appendicitis, may be successfully imaged without oral contrast in the emergency department setting.

In the author's emergency radiology section, upon the completion and review of the author's studies as well as the relevant literature available at the time, an initial trial period was instituted of administering intravenous contrast only for patients with abdominal pain in the emergency department with BMI greater than 25. While an imperfect measure of intra-abdominal fat, BMI measurements are readily performed in the

emergency department setting and serve as a reasonable surrogate for triaging patients who likely have relatively increased degrees of intra-abominal fat (**Fig. 4**). The author and colleagues felt that the increased degree of intra-abdominal fat would often lead to improved bowel visualization and simplified image interpretation in this patient population. During the initial implementation of this CT protocol in the author's institution, the protocol was only available from 9 a.m. to 5 p.m. on the weekdays, times during which a staff physician was available in the emergency radiology area, as it was felt that the potential decision to reimage a patient based on a limited examination related to the lack of oral contrast should be at the discretion of a staff member. During this initial trial period, these patients were closely monitored for the necessity of repeat imaging, and clinical outcomes were recorded and analyzed. After approximately 6 months of using the protocol, the intravenous only CT protocol was extended to 24 hours per day for all patients with abdominal pain and BMI greater than 25, as the author and colleagues found no evidence of the need for repeat imaging based on the lack of oral contrast or untoward clinical outcomes in this patient population. Since the implementation of this protocol, including its extension to 24 hours per day, the author and colleagues have tracked all patients and found that none required repeat imaging directly related to the absence of oral contrast on the initial CT scan. Two patients are worthy of consideration; both patients presented to the ED with ongoing abdominal pain after being

B

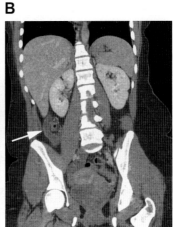

A

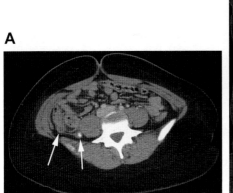

Fig. 4. Axial (A) and coronal (B) intravenous contrast-enhanced CT images without oral contrast administration demonstrate an abnormally dilated, fluid-filled appendix consistent with acute appendicitis (*arrows*). The patient underwent computed tomography imaging without oral contrast per the author's institution's protocol given a body mass index greater than 25. In this case, the degree of intra-abdominal fat was not excessive; the abnormal appendix is nevertheless readily identified.

discharged from the author's institution within 2 weeks after gastrointestinal (GI) surgery. In both cases, the patients had a BMI greater than 25 and were not administered oral contrast during their initial admission CT scan in the emergency department based on the author's revised CT protocol for this patient population. The first patient of note was found to have a small degree of fluid about a distal colonic anastamosis, the differential considerations of which were reported to be normal postoperative findings; however, it was noted that an anastamotic leak could not be definitively excluded. Given the patient's ongoing abdominal pain and these equivocal CT findings, the patient underwent a barium enema to further evaluate for the possibility of an anastomotic leak. While the barium enema was found to be negative, the administration of oral contrast during the initial CT scan may have precluded this second examination, as the absence of extraluminal oral contrast on the CT may have increased the confidence in excluding an anastamotic leak. The second patient was found to have a moderate degree of free intraperitoneal air and simple fluid in the peritoneal cavity (**Fig. 5**). Similar to the first patient, the imaging findings were not entirely unexpected findings relatively recently after GI surgery; however, an anastomotic leak was also considered. This patient was subsequently admitted and after several hours of observation; the patient's abdominal signs and symptoms progressed such that an exploratory laparotomy was undertaken, diagnosing and leading to the repair

of an anastomotic leak. Thus, the absence of oral contrast during the initial CT scan in this case may have led to a delay in management, as an extraluminal leak of oral contrast during the original CT scan, if present, may have led to a more rapid operative intervention. Based on the experience with these 2 patients, the author and colleagues modified the abdominal pain CT protocol at their institution to state that all patients with abdominal pain and a recent GI surgery (within 1 month of emergency department presentation), require an oral contrast preparation, regardless of the BMI.

In addition to the author's work on the influence of measures on body habitus on reader confidence noted previously, several other studies have evaluated the influence of body habitus on diagnostic accuracy and reader confidence in abdominal pain imaging using CT. The first such study compared diagnostic accuracy between oral contrast-enhanced CT examinations and those performed without oral contrast in patients presenting to the emergency department with abdominal pain.[19] No association between diagnostic accuracy and either waist circumference or BMI was found. In another study, the primary aim of which was to compare ultrasound with CT scans performed without oral contrast in patients with suspected appendicitis, no significant differences in diagnostic accuracy of CT scans without oral contrast were found for the diagnosis of appendicitis or appendiceal visualization based on differences in BMI.[20]

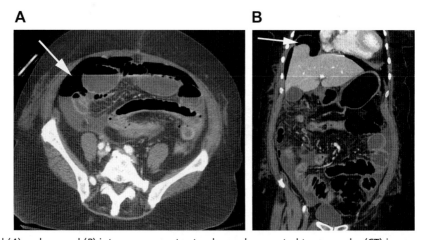

Fig. 5. Axial (*A*) and coronal (*B*) intravenous contrast-enhanced computed tomography (CT) images without oral contrast administration demonstrate moderate degrees of free fluid and air (*arrows*) in a patient with recent gastrointestinal surgery and ongoing pain. As these imaging findings may be seen routinely after surgery, the patient was initially admitted for observation but eventually underwent operative intervention with identification of an anastomotic leak given worsening clinical signs and symptoms. Had oral contrast been administered originally and a leak identified at the time of CT, the patient may not have incurred the delay in surgical management of the postsurgical leak.

INTRAVENOUS CONTRAST

While not associated with a similar potential for a significant decrease in emergency department throughput as in the case of oral contrast, the administration of intravenous contrast carries downsides of risks to the patient, including both nephrotoxicity as well the possibility for allergic reactions. As mentioned previously, in the author's institution, including many others, intravenous contrast is often administered in patients with abdominal pain. The projected benefits include improved delineation of the bowel given mucosal enhancement, as well as improvements in solid visceral organ evaluation, abnormalities of which may be etiologies and complications of certain etiologies of acute abdominal pain (**Fig. 6**). Nevertheless, the question of the ongoing utility of intravenous contrast in this patient population, given the risks of its administration, deserves an evidence-based approach. To date, there are several papers directly evaluating the need for intravenous contrast in patients with abdominal pain, specifically those with suspected appendicitis. In the first paper, the results of which support the use of intravenous contrast, 228 patients (51 cases of appendicitis) underwent focused CT of the right lower quadrant with oral contrast followed by an abdominopelvic CT with oral and intravenous contrast.[21] Three readers diagnosed appendicitis, with a sensitivity ranging from 71% to 83% in the focused CT arm with oral contrast but without intravenous contrast and a sensitivity ranging from 88% to 93% in those patients administered both oral and intravenous contrast. These authors concluded that the primary difference in the sensitivity of diagnosing appendicitis between the 2 CT protocols was related to the increased visualization of the inflamed appendix given the imaging findings of the abnormally enhancing appendiceal mucosa. As noted previously, a recent paper randomized 131 patients to receive or not receive oral contrast, after which all patients were imaged both with and without intravenous contrast. The authors found that the use intravenous contrast did not influence the diagnostic accuracy of CT in diagnosing acute appendicitis whether or not oral contrast was administered.[16] Finally, a recent paper compared a low-dose (30 mAs) oral contrast-enhanced CT protocol with a standard-dose (130 mAs) oral and intravenous contrast-enhanced protocol.[22] This study found no difference in sensitivity (100%) and specificity (98%) for either protocol for patients with BMI greater than 18.5 whether or not intravenous contrast was administered. However, the low radiation dose, oral contrast-enhanced protocol suffered significantly in patients with BMI less

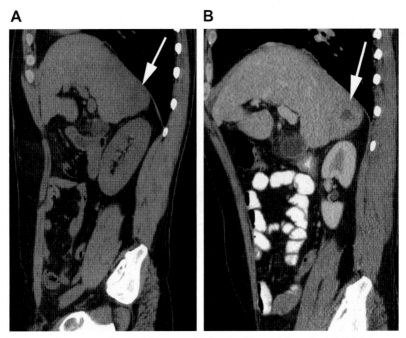

A   **B**

Fig. 6. Sagittal computed tomography (CT) images obtained without (*A*) and with (*B*) intravenous contrast in a patient with abdominal pain demonstrate ill-defined low attenuating areas within the liver parenchyma (*arrows*), the identification of which and characterization as hepatic abscesses are favorably served by the administration of intravenous contrast.

than 18.5, with sensitivity decreasing to 50%. As discussed previously, there is strong evidence to support the use of intravenous contrast in patients with suspected small bowel obstruction given the clinical importance of the CT finding of decrease mucosal enhancement and its association with ischemia. While the literature to date is conflicting and has focused primarily on acute appendicitis, there is evidence to reconsider the general use of intravenous contrast in all patients with acute abdominal pain.

IMAGE RECONSTRUCTION AND POST-PROCESSING

An additional factor in optimizing CT protocols in abdominal pain imaging includes image reconstruction, specifically reconstruction slice thickness. In the case of the appendix, the impact of slice thickness on several factors, including visualization of the appendix, confidence in appendiceal visualization, diagnostic accuracy, and diagnostic confidence in diagnosing appendicitis has been reported for varying CT slice thicknesses.[23] The authors found that the correctness of the diagnosis of appendicitis was not affected by slice thickness using 3 techniques (5 × 5 mm, 3 × 3 mm, and 2 × 1 mm; thickness and interval). However, progressively thinner section thickness was found to be associated with significant increases in the rate of appendiceal visualization and appendiceal visualization confidence. It should be kept in mind that to achieve a thinner slice thickness of comparable noise to that of a thicker slice, increased radiation must be administered, and this must be balanced with any improvements in diagnostic capability. However, thinner slice thickness, even with an increase in image noise, may also provide additional diagnostic capability when compared with an increased slice thickness with improved signal to noise; this area deserves further inquiry. In their own practice, the author and colleagues have anecdotally found that the availability of a 3.75 mm thick axial slice, around which they balance noise and radiation dose, along with a 1.25 mm thick axial slice with a perceptibly higher degree of noise, affords a balance between radiation dose concerns and the availability of a dataset with thinner slice thickness for problem solving and possibly improving diagnostic capability (**Fig. 7**).

Given the availability of volumetric CT datasets with isotropic resolution acquired using the current generations of multidetector CT scanners, high-quality multiplanar reformations are readily available. In the author's institution, for example, coronal and sagittal reformations (2.5 mm × 2.5 mm) are routinely generated for all thoracoabdominal CT examinations. The implications of the availability of multiplanar reformations in abdominal imaging have been studied; coronal reformations, along with the routinely available axial datasets, are found to improve confidence in visualization of the appendix as well as the diagnosis or exclusion of appendicitis.[24] In addition, the use of multiplanar reformations has been demonstrated to increase both the accuracy and reader confidence in identifying transition points in cases of mechanical small bowel obstruction.[25] Finally, in patients with an acute abdomen, axial and coronal datasets have been compared and found to have equal sensitivity and specificity for the diagnosis of the underlying pathology. However, the use of coronal reformations was found to improve diagnostic confidence in this patient population.[26]

RADIATION DOSE

As is the general case with the use of CT, radiation dose is of significant concern in the imaging evaluation of patients with abdominal pain in the emergency department. To date, several studies have evaluated the applications of low-dose imaging protocols to the evaluation of patients with abdominal pain. In a recent study, standard (8.0 mSv) and low-dose (4.2 mSv) protocols were compared, and no differences in diagnostic accuracy for appendicitis, appendiceal visualization rates, or diagnostic accuracy for alternative diagnoses were found.[27] A second study, noted previously, compared low-dose (30 mAs) with standard-dose (180 mAs) examinations and no difference in sensitivity or specificity in the majority of patients, although sensitivity was markedly compromised (sensitivity, 50%) in the low-dose protocol arm in the subset of patients with BMI less than 18.5.[22] In this arm, the absence of intravenous contrast, which was administered in the standard radiation dose arm, may have played a role in decreasing sensitivity, in addition to differences in radiation dose. Finally, as was mentioned previously, a recent paper compared standard (100 mAs) and simulated (30 mAs) examinations, as well as several other factors including the use of oral and intravenous contrast, and found no differences in the diagnostic accuracy for diagnosing appendicitis based on radiation dose.[16]

While these aforementioned low-dose studies suffered from increased levels of noise, a technical development that offers the possibility of lowered radiation without increases in image noise is worthy of mention. The development of iterative

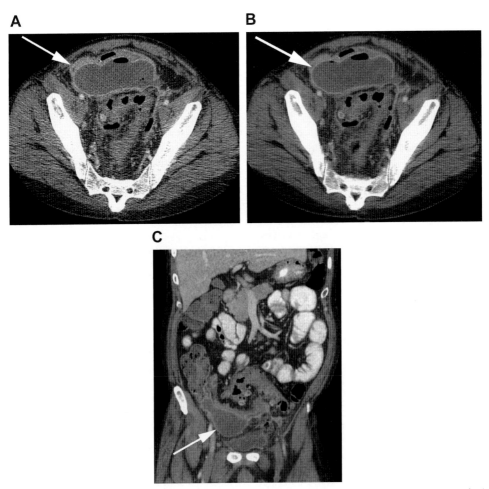

Fig. 7. Axial 1.25 mm (*A*) and 3.75 mm (*B*) intravenous and oral contrast-enhanced computed tomography images demonstrate the differences in image noise between the slice thicknesses. While the thicker dataset is used in the author's practice for routine interpretation, the thinner datasets are available for problem solving. Routinely available coronal (*C*) and sagittal images are also available in all cases for routine interpretation and problem solving. In this case, acute diverticulitis with a large diverticular abscess (*arrows*) was identified.

reconstruction techniques offers the potential for significantly decreasing radiation dose while maintaining noise levels similar to standard radiation levels. Alternatively, iterative reconstruction allows for even further decreases in radiation dose while achieving similar noise levels to the low-dose studies cited previously. Thus, in select patients, unparalleled dose reductions may be possible using iterative reconstruction techniques given early evidence that increased image noise is not found to affect diagnostic accuracy of CT in patients with suspected appendicitis.

SUMMARY

In summary, given mounting evidence of the untoward effects of oral and intravenous contrast, many long-held practices in abdominal CT imaging

deserve further scrutiny. These negative effects include, among others, increased emergency department throughput time, possible delays in diagnosis and management, potential radiation dose increases associated with positive oral contrast agents, and the known risks associated with intravenous contrast, primarily related to nephrotoxicity. In addition, there are numerous studies in which the diagnostic accuracy and reader confidence are similar whether or not oral or intravenous contrast is administered, further demanding a reevaluation of these practices. There is also evidence that low-dose radiation techniques may provide acceptable diagnostic quality in certain populations with abdominal pain, further limiting potential negative effects of CT imaging in this patient population. Advancing CT technology, including the use of iterative reconstruction techniques, may afford further decreases in radiation dose in this imaging application. To date, however, many of the studies on the optimal CT protocol for patients with abdominal pain are relatively small in scale, and there are several areas in which contradictory results have been reported. Thus, these critical aspects of CT protocols in abdominal pain imaging deserve further inquiry on a larger scale to enable the field to come to firm, evidenced-based conclusions regarding the optimal technique.

REFERENCES

1. Rao PM, Rhea JT, Novelline RA, et al. Helical CT with only colonic contrast material for diagnosing diverticulitis: prospective evaluation of 150 patients. AJR Am J Roentgenol 1998;170(6):1445–9.
2. Rhea JT, Halpern EF, Ptak T, et al. The status of appendiceal CT in an urban medical center 5 years after its introduction: experience with 753 patients. AJR Am J Roentgenol 2005;184(6):1802–8.
3. Huynh LN, Coughlin BF, Wolfe J, et al. Patient encounter time intervals in the evaluation of emergency department patients requiring abdominopelvic CT: oral contrast versus no contrast. Emerg Radiol 2004;10(6):310–3.
4. Berg ER, Mehta SD, Mitchell P, et al. Length of stay by route of contrast administration for diagnosis of appendicitis by computed-tomography scan. Acad Emerg Med 2006;13(10):1040–5.
5. Berger-Achituv S, Zissin R, Shenkman Z, et al. Gastric emptying time of oral contrast material in children and adolescents undergoing abdominal computed tomography. J Pediatr Gastroenterol Nutr 2010;51(1):31–4.
6. Laituri CA, Fraser JD, Aguayo P, et al. The lack of efficacy for oral contrast in the diagnosis of appendicitis by computed tomography. J Surg Res 2011; 170(1):100–3.
7. Wang ZJ, Chen KS, Gould R, et al. Positive enteric contrast material for abdominal and pelvic CT with automatic exposure control: what is the effect on patient radiation exposure? Eur J Radiol 2011; 79(2):e58–62.
8. Hebert JJ, Taylor AJ, Winter TC. Comparison of colonic transit between polyethylene glycol and water as oral contrast vehicles in the CT evaluation of acute appendicitis. AJR Am J Roentgenol 2006; 187(5):1188–91.
9. Rao PM, Rhea JT, Novelline RA, et al. Helical CT technique for the diagnosis of appendicitis: prospective evaluation of a focused appendix CT examination. Radiology 1997;202(1):139–44.
10. Choi D, Park H, Lee YR, et al. The most useful findings for diagnosing acute appendicitis on contrast-enhanced helical CT. Acta Radiol 2003; 44(6):574–82.
11. Kircher MF, Rhea JT, Kihiczak D, et al. Frequency, sensitivity, and specificity of individual signs of diverticulitis on thin-section helical CT with colonic contrast material: experience with 312 cases. AJR Am J Roentgenol 2002;178(6):1313–8.
12. Sheedy SP, Earnest F 4th, Fletcher JG, et al. CT of small-bowel ischemia associated with obstruction in emergency department patients: diagnostic performance evaluation. Radiology 2006;241(3):729–36.
13. Chou CK, Wu RH, Mak CW, et al. Clinical significance of poor CT enhancement of the thickened small-bowel wall in patients with acute abdominal pain. AJR Am J Roentgenol 2006;186(2):491–8.
14. Lee SY, Coughlin B, Wolfe JM, et al. Prospective comparison of helical CT of the abdomen and pelvis without and with oral contrast in assessing acute abdominal pain in adult Emergency Department patients. Emerg Radiol 2006;12(4):150–7.
15. Mun S, Ernst RD, Chen K, et al. Rapid CT diagnosis of acute appendicitis with IV contrast material. Emerg Radiol 2006;12(3):99–102.
16. Keyzer C, Cullus P, Tack D, et al. MDCT for suspected acute appendicitis in adults: impact of oral and IV contrast media at standard-dose and simulated low-dose techniques. AJR Am J Roentgenol 2009;193(5):1272–81.
17. Anderson SW, Soto JA, Lucey BC, et al. Abdominal 64-MDCT for suspected appendicitis: the use of oral and IV contrast material versus IV contrast material only. AJR Am J Roentgenol 2009;193(5):1282–8.
18. Anderson SW, Rhea JT, Milch HN, et al. Influence of body habitus and use of oral contrast on reader confidence in patients with suspected acute appendicitis using 64 MDCT. Emerg Radiol 2010;17(6):445–53.
19. Wolfe JM, Smithline H, Lee S, et al. The impact of body mass index on concordance in the interpretation of matched noncontrast and contrast abdominal pelvic computed tomographic scans in ED patients with nontraumatic abdominal pain. Am J Emerg Med 2006;24(2):144–8.
20. Keyzer C, Zalcman M, De Maertelaer V, et al. Comparison of US and unenhanced multidetector row CT in patients suspected of having acute appendicitis. Radiology 2005;236(2):527–34.
21. Jacobs JE, Birnbaum BA, Macari M, et al. Acute appendicitis: comparison of helical CT diagnosis focused technique with oral contrast material versus nonfocused technique with oral and intravenous contrast material. Radiology 2001;220(3):683–90.
22. Platon A, Jlassi H, Rutschmann OT, et al. Evaluation of a low-dose CT protocol with oral contrast for assessment of acute appendicitis. Eur Radiol 2009;19(2):446–54.
23. Johnson PT, Horton KM, Kawamoto S, et al. MDCT for suspected appendicitis: effect of reconstruction section thickness on diagnostic accuracy, rate of appendiceal visualization, and reader confidence

using axial images. AJR Am J Roentgenol 2009; 192(4):893–901.

24. Paulson EK, Harris JP, Jaffe TA, et al. Acute appendicitis: added diagnostic value of coronal reformations from isotropic voxels at multidetector row CT. Radiology 2005;235(3):879–85.

25. Hodel J, Zins M, Desmottes L, et al. Location of the transition zone in CT of small-bowel obstruction: added value of multiplanar reformations. Abdom Imaging 2009;34(1):35–41.

26. Zangos S, Steenburg SD, Phillips KD, et al. Acute abdomen: Added diagnostic value of coronal reformations with 64-slice multidetector row computed tomography. Acad Radiol 2007;14(1): 19–27.

27. Seo H, Lee KH, Kim HJ, et al. Diagnosis of acute appendicitis with sliding slab ray-sum interpretation of low-dose unenhanced CT and standard-dose i.v. contrast-enhanced CT scans. AJR Am J Roentgenol 2009;193(1):96–105.

Imaging of Abdominal Pain in Pregnancy

Douglas S. Katz, MD[a],*, Michele A.I. Klein, MD[a],
George Ganson, MD[a], John J. Hines, MD[b]

KEYWORDS

- Pregnancy • Acute abdomen • Radiation exposure
- Magnetic resonance • Ultrasonography
- Computed tomography

Diagnostic imaging is used frequently for the evaluation of pregnant patients with suspected nonobstetric acute medical and surgical conditions of the abdomen and pelvis, as well as for the evaluation of suspected traumatic injury to the maternal abdomen and pelvis in conjunction with fetal evaluation. Such imaging has been used more liberally in recent years, and there has been increasing attention to this topic, especially in the radiology literature, in conjunction with increased attention to reducing or eliminating exposure of the developing fetus to ionizing radiation when diagnostic imaging procedures are performed.[1–6] Despite this increased attention, there is also some continued controversy and uncertainty regarding the preferred diagnostic imaging examinations for these conditions, and how they should be best performed to minimize risk while achieving the highest possible diagnostic accuracy.

Regardless of the actual risks to the fetus from maternal abdominal and pelvic computed tomography (CT), in this situation imaging modalities that do not use ionizing radiation—sonography and magnetic resonance (MR)—are strongly preferable whenever possible for a variety of reasons, assuming diagnostic capability is not compromised. Unfortunately, the limitations of sonography in this setting, particularly for suspected appendicitis and suspected urolithiasis, are substantial. Although there was a 90% increase in the use of abdominal and pelvic CT in pregnant women requiring diagnostic imaging for acute abdominal and pelvic conditions (150–285 examinations) in a second 5-year period (2002–2006) compared with the first 5-year period (1997–2001) at one institution,[7] and although surveys published in 2007[8] and 2008[9] found substantial radiologist/institutional/practice preference for CT for suspected appendicitis compared with other cross-sectional imaging, especially in the later stages of gestation, in the last few years there has been an apparent substantial shift to the routine use of MR imaging for evaluation of appendicitis in pregnancy. MR imaging has played an increasingly important role in the past several years in general for evaluation of the acute abdomen and pelvis in pregnant patients, although there are still some challenges to MR imaging implementation and interpretation in these patients.

A theoretical risk of fetal carcinogenesis exists from exposure to ionizing radiation from diagnostic imaging, although at current levels of exposure this is controversial. In addition, there is no documented risk of congenital malformations or mental retardation in fetuses exposed to such imaging.[10] However, regardless of what the actual risks are, if ionizing radiation truly needs to be used for imaging the acute abdomen and pelvis in pregnant patients, the principle of ALARA (As Low As Reasonably Achievable) must be adhered to after an appropriate risk/benefit discussion with the patient, in the nontrauma setting. Imaging of the pregnant patient is a unique situation whereby the American College of Radiology's (ACR) "Image Gently" and "Image Wisely" campaigns need to be applied in concert.

[a] Department of Radiology, Winthrop-University Hospital, 259 First Street, Mineola, NY 11501, USA
[b] Department of Radiology, Long Island Jewish Medical Center, 270-05 7th Avenue, New Hyde Park, NY 11040, USA
* Corresponding author.
E-mail address: dkatz@winthrop.org

Radiol Clin N Am 50 (2012) 149–171
doi:10.1016/j.rcl.2011.08.001

radiologic.theclinics.com

This article reviews the evolving radiology and clinical literature on imaging of suspected common and relatively common maternal non-obstetric conditions of the abdomen and pelvis, including appendicitis, urolithiasis, and biliary disease, as well as literature on trauma to the maternal abdomen and pelvis and to the fetus. The authors also propose recommendations for imaging these conditions, based on the literature to date and on their experiences at two tertiary-care institutions with busy obstetric services. The potential and theoretical fetal and maternal risks from such imaging are also reviewed.

GENERAL CONSIDERATIONS
Determination of Pregnancy Status

The pregnancy status of all women of childbearing age should be determined before using ionizing radiation, if a patient's condition permits. The patient's menstrual history should be elicited, and ideally a urine (or if needed, blood) pregnancy test for β–human chorionic gonadotropin (β-hCG) should be performed. If indicated, sonography of the pelvis can be used to check for pregnancy beyond several weeks, as well as to check on the status of the pregnancy.

Effect of Ionizing Radiation on the Fetus

The estimated approximate threshold for induction of anomalies and/or growth retardation during organogenesis, at 2 to 8 weeks, is greater than 200 mGy. Similarly, fetuses are at risk for severe mental retardation at 8 to 15 weeks of development if exposed to greater than 500 mGy, with an estimated 25 IQ points lost per Gy, and are at risk at greater than 250 mGy at 16 to 25 weeks of development.[1] By contrast, common values for estimated absorbed fetal dose from a single abdominal and pelvic CT examination are in the range of 17 to 25 mGy. The estimated average fetal dose was 17.15 mGy, for 435 CT examinations performed over a 10-year period at one institution,[7] and 24.8 mGy for 86 examinations performed over a 7-year period at another institution.[11]

The risk of inducing anomalies is considered to be very low at less than 5 mGy compared with the other "risks" of pregnancy, which include baseline incidences of 3% of birth defects, 15% of spontaneous abortion, 4% of prematurity, and 1% of mental retardation.[10] It should also be realized that the estimated natural background fetal "dose" in pregnancy is approximately 1 mGy. In addition, if CT is being considered for maternal evaluation of the acute abdomen and pelvis, it should be understood that "inaccurate, missed,

or delayed diagnosis may represent a more significant risk to the patient [ie, the fetus and the mother] than the radiation risk."[12]

The most substantial area of controversy is whether there is an increased risk of childhood cancer following fetal radiation from abdominal and pelvic CT.[13] One study estimated the fetal doses during early gestation, using a 16-detector CT for suspected appendicitis and urolithiasis, may double the theoretical risk of subsequent development of childhood cancer.[14] Another publication estimated a theoretical risk of inducing one childhood cancer per 500 fetuses exposed to 30 mGy.[15] Yet McCollough and colleagues[16] concluded that "the risk to the conceptus from radiation doses of less than 50 mGy is negligible." Moreover, recently Ray and colleagues[17] completed a population-based study of 1.8 million maternal-child pairs in the province of Ontario, Canada, from 1991 to 2008. There were 5590 mothers exposed to "major radiodiagnostic testing" in pregnancy (3 per 1000). After a median duration of follow-up of 8.9 years, only 4 childhood cancers arose in the exposed group, and 2539 cancers in the unexposed group, with essentially no difference in risk between the two groups.

Regardless of the actual risk to the fetus from abdominal and pelvic CT, as with nonpregnant patients radiation reduction should be used whenever possible, so long as diagnostic accuracy is not compromised. The authors believe that in general, CT doses can be somewhat further decreased compared with previously reported estimated fetal doses already mentioned, without compromising diagnostic accuracy, especially in earlier stages of gestation and/or in suspected renal colic, although this becomes more problematic later in pregnancy, when the patient's cross-sectional area is larger and the anatomy becomes more crowded and more difficult to evaluate. A variety of strategies can be used as in nonpregnant patients, including reducing the mAs through auto-mA, z-axis modulation, and other newer strategies such as iterative reconstruction in combination with other dose reduction techniques.[18]

Use of Iodinated Contrast

Iodinated intravenous (IV) contrast crosses the placenta, but there is no known teratogenicity or mutagenicity. It is a United States Food and Drug Administration (FDA) category B drug, which should be used only after assessing the potential risk/benefit ratio.[1] Depression of fetal thyroid function is possible, due to exposure to free iodine.[19] One small study that assessed this specific issue showed no ill effects on subsequent neonatal thyroid function in fetuses exposed to iodinated contrast material in utero, based on thyroid-stimulating hormone levels.[20] Regardless, thyroid function is routinely checked in all United States newborns.

MR Imaging in Pregnancy

MR imaging has been used to evaluate obstetric disease for more than 20 years without any documented harmful effects, at 1.5 T or lower magnetic field strength, based on numerous clinical and laboratory studies.[21] Some concerns linger regarding heating effects of radiofrequency pulses and effects of acoustic noise on the fetus.[22] MR imaging may be used on pregnant patients if considered necessary by the referring physician and attending radiologist, regardless of gestational age. Written informed maternal consent prior to MR imaging is recommended, to "document maternal understanding of risk/benefit ratio and alternative diagnostic options, if any."[23]

Pulse sequences should be limited to those truly necessary. There is lack of experience at greater field strengths, and magnets of 3 T or higher should be avoided at present. For all abdominal and pelvic MR examinations performed on pregnant women, in general close radiologist input and monitoring is advised.[23]

IV gadolinium administration in pregnancy is considered an FDA category C drug. In animal laboratory studies with gadolinium compounds, growth retardation and congenital malformations were identified at relative doses of 2 to 7 times larger than those typically used in humans. However, there are no known adverse effects to human fetuses documented to date from maternal IV gadolinium administration, either inadvertently or for diagnostic purposes.[24,25] In a series of 26 pregnant women exposed to IV gadolinium during the first trimester, there were no identifiable adverse effects on the pregnancies or on neonatal outcomes.[26] The ACR's white paper on MR imaging safety recommends the need for "documented, in-depth analysis of the potential risks and benefits to that patient and her fetus", to justify the clinical advisability of gadolinium use in pregnancy.[23] The authors essentially never use IV gadolinium in their practices in conjunction with abdominal and pelvic MR imaging.

Sonography in Pregnancy

There are no documented adverse effects on the developing human fetus from diagnostic sonography. The FDA has proposed an upper limit of 720 mW/cm^2 for spatial-peak temporal-average intensity for obstetric sonography.[27] Doppler sonography can produce high intensities and therefore time exposure should be limited, and acoustic output should also be limited to the lowest level possible.[28]

General Maternal Abdominal and Pelvic Imaging Principles

The general principle for imaging the acute abdomen and pelvis in pregnant patients is that if an imaging examination is required for evaluation, a modality that does not use ionizing radiation, namely ultrasound—also known as ultrasonography (US)—or MR imaging should, if possible, be the first procedure performed. If US and MR imaging is neither feasible nor desirable, or is nondiagnostic, and ionizing radiation, particularly CT, is used, the radiation dose to the fetus and mother should be kept ALARA.

APPENDICITIS IN PREGNANCY
General Considerations

Acute appendicitis is the most common nonobstetric emergency requiring surgery in pregnancy. It is associated with premature labor, fetal morbidity and mortality, and a higher rate of appendiceal perforation—upwards of 43% for the latter—although exactly to what extent these occur is controversial.[29–31] In one study there was a 6% rate of fetal loss and an 11% early delivery rate in complicated appendicitis, compared with 2% and 4%, respectively, in simple appendicitis.[30] It is more difficult to clinically assess pregnant patients with suspected appendicitis than nonpregnant women, which is in part related to the inflamed appendix located outside of the right lower quadrant in a substantial percentage of patients, and also because of the presence of leukocytosis in many otherwise normal pregnant patients. There is a tendency for the appendiceal base to be located above the L4 vertebral body level later in gestation, although the position of the appendix is variable in the individual patient.[32,33] Delays in diagnosis contribute to a higher perforation rate, which lowers the threshold for imaging, leading to the vast majority of examinations showing no evidence of appendicitis.[34] On the other hand there is a high negative appendectomy rate (NAR) if no preoperative imaging is used—upwards of 23% to 33% in recent surgical series.[30,35] The goal of imaging pregnant patients with suspected appendicitis is therefore to make an accurate and timely diagnosis in the pregnant patient, minimizing risk to both the mother and the fetus, and to reduce the NAR and the appendiceal perforation rate.

Ultrasonography

The initial imaging test for suspected appendicitis in pregnancy remains ultrasound at many practices/institutions, despite its major limitations, because of the absence of ionizing radiation and the identification of alternative diagnoses, particularly of gynecologic origin. These limitations are primarily related to the body habitus in the later stages of gestation, including overlying bowel gas and uterus/fetus, but also reflect the difficulty in accurately imaging the appendix in adults in general with US (**Figs. 1–3**). A technique similar to that carried out in nonpregnant individuals, graded compression with a linear transducer, is used. An attempt is made by the technologist/radiologist to find a normal or abnormal appendix, or an alternative cause for pain. As in nonpregnant patients, appendicitis is identified as a noncompressible fluid-filled appendix, measuring greater than 6 mm in diameter. Doppler imaging can be used to assist in identification and characterization of the appendix.[1–4,6] There was improved appendiceal visualization with left lateral decubitus positioning in an early report.[36]

In that early series of 42 pregnant patients there were 16 positive cases, with 100% sensitivity, 96% specificity, and 98% accuracy on US. Very few patients were in the third trimester.[36] Unfortunately, no subsequent study has been able to reproduce these results, which more recently have been rather poor. In the publications that followed the initial report by Lim and colleagues,[36] in one series of 22 patients there was 95% specificity but only 66% sensitivity for ultrasound.[37] Confident identification of the appendix occurred in only 1 of 12 patients in another series, compared with 3 abnormal and 7 normal appendices on MR imaging.[38]

In a more recent series of 33 pregnant patients, the sensitivity of MR imaging for acute appendicitis was 80%, versus 20% for US. Most disturbingly, the appendix could not be identified in 29 patients, including in 3 with proven appendicitis.[39] Similarly, in the largest series reported to date to the authors' knowledge, from Pedrosa and colleagues,[34] of 140 patients imaged with both US and MR imaging, US had a sensitivity of 36% (5 of 14), and a normal appendix was identified on US in only 2 of 126 patients without appendicitis (<2%). In the series by Israel and colleagues,[39] multiple problems and limitations of US were noted as possible explanations for its poor performance in this setting: variable operator skill, multiple operators, after-hours scanning, and the difficulty in identifying the appendix in the later stages of pregnancy. This experience with US in pregnancy has also anecdotally been that of the authors: low yield, a time-consuming procedure, and a frustrating examination for the patient, technologist, radiologist, and referring physician, although a substantial percentage of their pregnant patients still undergo initial right lower quadrant sonography.

MR Imaging

If neither a normal or abnormal appendix can be confidently identified on sonography—as noted, the case in the vast majority of pregnant patients—and no clear alternative diagnosis is identifiable on US, then MR imaging is the next

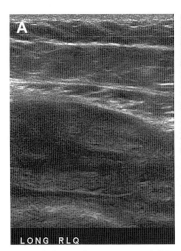
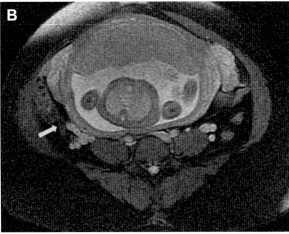

Fig. 1. Acute abdomen in pregnancy. (*A*) Representative image from nondiagnostic abdominal ultrasound of a 32-year-old woman, 6 months pregnant, with acute right lower quadrant pain. (*B*) Axial 2-dimensional (2D)-weighted FIESTA (fast imaging employing steady-state acquisition) MR image shows a normal appendix (*arrow*).

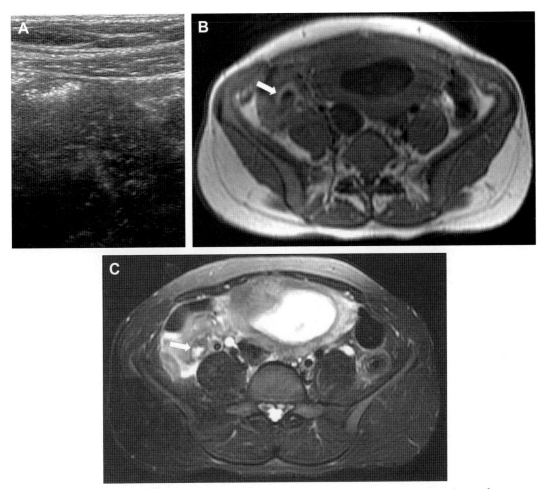

Fig. 2. Acute abdomen in pregnancy, with surgically proven appendicitis. (*A*) Representative image from a non-diagnostic abdominal ultrasound of a 26-year-old woman, 11 weeks pregnant, presenting with acute right lower quadrant pain. (*B*) Axial T1-weighted MR image shows a thickened appendix and adjacent edema (*arrow*) consistent with acute appendicitis. (*C*) Axial T2-weighted FS (fat-suppressed) MR image shows an enlarged, thickened, and edematous appendix (*arrow*), consistent with acute appendicitis.

ideal imaging test (see **Figs. 1–3**; **Figs. 4–8**). MR imaging to date has shown high sensitivity and specificity for appendicitis and alternative diagnoses in pregnant women.[36,39–47] At both of the authors' institutions, MR imaging has emerged over the past few years as the predominant cross-sectional imaging examination for suspected appendicitis in pregnancy, and the use of CT has essentially been eliminated in this situation, although there is a learning curve for interpretation of MR examinations for suspected appendicitis in pregnancy; in particular, sorting out the right lower quadrant anatomy may be somewhat difficult, especially in the later stages of gestation.

In general, although specific protocols differ, multiplanar T2-weighted sequences (eg, single-shot fast spin echo, HASTE, and so forth) with or without fat suppression, are used. Findings of appendicitis on MR imaging include a distended appendix with a hyperintense lumen, a slightly hyperintense wall, and periappendiceal inflammatory changes. T2-weighted sequences are supplemented by sequences such as time-of-flight gradient recalled-echo or balanced steady-state free precession, to differentiate right lower quadrant vessels from the appendix, as well as T1-weighted gradient recalled-echo images. The protocol of Pedrosa and colleagues[34] includes a mixture of oral iron oxides and barium sulfate, to reduce susceptibility artifacts from right lower quadrant bowel gas and to improve visualization of an abnormal, fluid-filled and obstructed appendix, if present. If normal, using this protocol the appendix will negatively opacify and/or demonstrate susceptibility artifacts on T2* images. Oral contrast adds time and minor additional

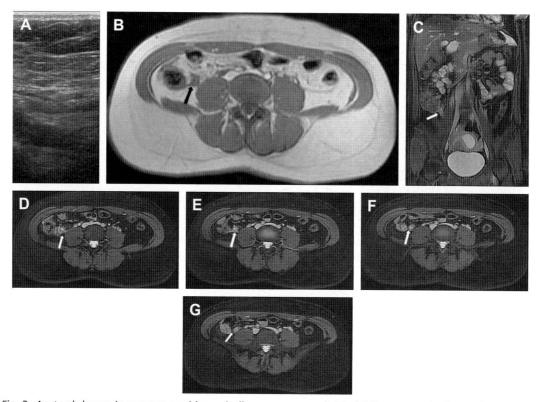

Fig. 3. Acute abdomen in pregnancy with surgically proven appendicitis. (*A*) Representative image from a non-diagnostic abdominal ultrasound of a 29-year-old pregnant woman presenting with right lower quadrant pain. (*B*) Axial T1 in-phase MR image shows an enlarged, thickened, and edematous appendix (*arrow*) consistent with acute appendicitis. (*C*) Coronal 2D FIESTA MR image shows a thickened appendix and adjacent edema (*arrow*). (*D–G*) Sequential images from an axial 2D FIESTA FS MR sequence demonstrating a 9 mm appendix with mild edema of the appendiceal wall at its base, slight adjacent fat infiltration, and fluid in the lumen of the proximal to mid appendix (*arrow*).

effort, inconvenience, and expense, but yields the highest reported rate of identification of a normal appendix. Oto and colleagues[40] used no oral contrast, nor have others,[39,48] and oral contrast is not widely used in clinical practice to the authors' knowledge.

It is also unclear as to whether there is a role for diffusion-weighted imaging in pregnant patients with suspected appendicitis. As already noted, at present IV gadolinium is almost never given for appendicitis, although its potential utility in selected problematic cases has not been studied to the authors' knowledge. Regardless of the specific protocol used, ideally these examinations should be checked by a radiologist before concluding the examination.

Of the first of the two largest reported series to date, there were 118 patients with abdominal and/or pelvic pain who underwent MR imaging in the report by Oto and colleagues,[40] although not all of these patients necessarily had suspected appendicitis. There were 9 confirmed cases of

appendicitis that were correctly interpreted on MR imaging, 2 cases consistent with appendicitis on MR imaging who improved without surgery, and 1 "false-negative" case (equivocal on MR imaging but positive at surgery), with an overall sensitivity of 90% and specificity of 98%. In the series described by Pedrosa and colleagues,[34] of the 148 pregnant patients with suspected appendicitis, 14 ended up with the diagnosis, 3 of whom had perforation. There were no false-negative MR imaging examinations, and there were 9 false positives (2 read as positive, 7 read as inconclusive), for a sensitivity of 100% and a specificity of 93%. Only 4 patients underwent CT, and only 27 (18%) underwent surgery; of the 27 who underwent surgery, only 8 ended up having no surgical or histopathological evidence for appendicitis, and for 5 of these 8 patients the MR examinations were correctly interpreted prospectively as negative for appendicitis. Final alternative diagnoses that were correctly identified prospectively on MR imaging included a prolapsed

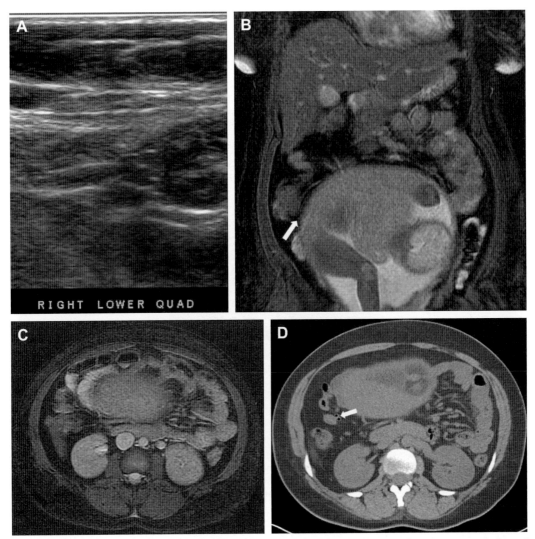

Fig. 4. Acute abdomen in pregnancy, with negative imaging for appendicitis. (*A*) Representative image from the non-diagnostic abdominal ultrasound of a 29-year-old woman, 30 weeks pregnant, presenting with acute right lower quadrant pain. (*B*) Coronal 2D FIESTA FS MR image does not demonstrate any primary or secondary findings of appendicitis (*arrow*). (*C*) Axial 2D FIESTA FS MR image does not demonstrate any primary or secondary findings of appendicitis. (*D*) Representative axial image from the subsequent non-enhanced CT scan, performed at the insistence of the referring clinicians, demonstrates a normal caliber air-filled appendix (*arrow*). The patient was then managed conservatively.

ureterocele in 1 patient, ovarian torsion in 4 patients, and an ectopic pregnancy in 1 patient. If the decision to avoid surgery had been based on a negative MR imaging interpretation, the NAR would have been only 7%.[34]

The cost of MR imaging is somewhat greater than CT or US; however, this represents a relatively minor expense compared with a negative appendectomy. It should also be realized that the specific positive findings of appendicitis on any imaging modality can be used as a surgical roadmap, as in nonpregnant patients. In addition, further research is needed on the optimal MR imaging protocol and the accuracy of MR in early appendicitis. Other issues—which appear to be diminishing over time—include the availability of emergency MR imaging (performance and interpretation) and the lower comfort level of radiologists. Also, the question becomes: should MR imaging become the *initial* imaging test of choice for right lower quadrant pain in pregnant patients?[49,50]

Computed Tomography

If MR imaging cannot be performed, due to the occasional contraindication or if not available

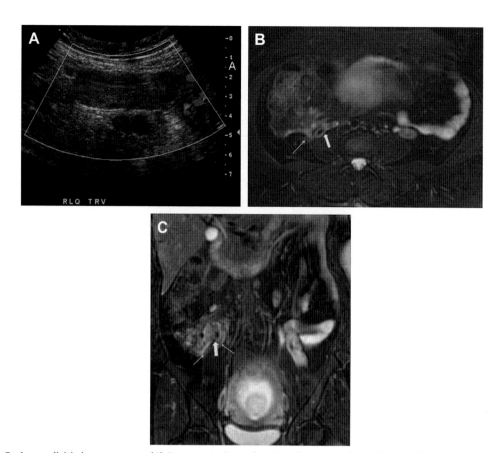

Fig. 5. Appendicitis in pregnancy. (*A*) Representative color Doppler image from the nondiagnostic abdominal sonogram of a 39-year-old woman with right lower quadrant pain. (*B*) Axial T2 FS MR image demonstrating an enlarged, edematous appendix (*thick arrow*) with infiltrative changes of the adjacent fat (*thin arrow*). (*C*) Coronal T2 fast-relaxation fast spin echo (FRFSE) FS MR image demonstrating an enlarged, edematous appendix (*thick arrow*) with inflammatory changes of the adjacent fat (*thin arrows*).

emergently, CT can be used as a second-line or third-line examination. Most of the small series reported on the utility of CT for appendicitis in pregnancy were with oral and IV contrast, although rectal contrast has been used exclusively or in combination with other contrast material.[51,52] Positive CT findings are the same as in nonpregnant patients, although as with MR imaging, particularly in the later stages of gestation, prominent but normal adnexal vessels, or collapsed bowel loops, may be confused with an abnormal appendix. As already noted, a low-radiation-dose technique should ideally be used, but is more problematic later in pregnancy, as image noise increases with lower radiation dose and increased abdominal circumference.

To the authors' knowledge, the largest reported series of CT examinations for suspected appendicitis in pregnancy was that of 55 patients by Lazarus and colleagues.[53] Sensitivity was 92% and specificity was 99%. Fifty-two of these patients underwent US, which was negative in 46, yet 14 of these 46 were abnormal on CT, and

of these 9 patients required surgery, including 6 with proven appendicitis. A recent series of 27 patients who underwent CT for suspected appendicitis in pregnancy, 23 of whom had initial US, yielded 5 positive cases for appendicitis and 2 alternative diagnoses (tubal torsion and ovarian torsion).[54] CT had 100% sensitivity, compared with 46% for US.

If used selectively, in practices without either availability of MR imaging or an acceptable comfort level for MR imaging performance and interpretation, the risks of misdiagnosis without accurate imaging, particularly that of perforation, and of an unnecessary surgical exploration, outweigh the small potential risk of ionizing radiation from CT, although ALARA should be used and nonchalant CT imaging avoided.

Alternative Diagnosis

In pregnant patients with suspected appendicitis, as already noted alternative diagnoses can be

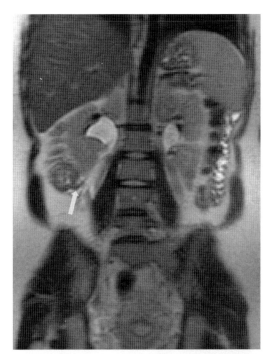

Fig. 6. Appendicitis in pregnancy. Coronal T2 single-shot fast spin echo (SSFSE) FS MR image of a 29-year-old woman in her third trimester of pregnancy with right lower quadrant pain. The image shows a 6-mm structure extending medially from the cecal base representing the appendix (*arrow*). There is no definitive periappendiceal inflammatory change or fluid, and the MR findings were interpreted prospectively as equivocal for appendicitis. Appendicitis was then confirmed at surgery.

identified on all cross-sectional imaging modalities. On initial US, for example, alternative diagnoses including adnexal masses (eg, hemorrhagic ovarian cyst, dermoid, degenerating fibroid, and ovarian torsion), and bowel pathology can be found, with much higher accuracy for the former category. On CT, as in nonpregnant patients a wide variety of alternative diagnoses can be identified. Of the 355 CT examinations performed for abdominal/pelvic pain over a 10-year period at one institution, there was a 24% positive rate: 44 had urinary tract calculi, 25 had appendicitis, and there were multiple alternative diagnoses.[53] Similarly, MR imaging also has high accuracy for demonstrating a wide range of alternative diagnoses in patients with right lower quadrant or other sites of abdominal and pelvic pain in pregnancy (**Figs. 9–13**). Gynecologic etiology, bowel obstruction, biliary and pancreatic disease, and pyelonephritis, among others, have been reported in the imaging literature using MR imaging.[39–45] In a recent publication, Maselli and colleagues[45] reported on 40 patients with inconclusive US and

an acute abdomen in pregnancy. There were a variety of final diagnoses, for which MR imaging had a prospective accuracy of 100%.

UROLITHIASIS
General Considerations

The most common painful nonobstetric maternal abdominal and pelvic conditions in pregnancy are urolithiasis (1 in 200–3300 deliveries) and urinary tract infection, and the two may be concurrent. Not surprisingly, therefore, the most common nonobstetric indication for hospitalization of pregnant patients is urolithiasis.[55] Increased urinary filtration and stasis are implicated. As with appendicitis, history and physical examination are not reliable.[56] Right urinary tract dilatation in the later stages of pregnancy is very common and problematic. Seventy-five percent to 80% of ureteral calculi in pregnant patients reportedly pass spontaneously. If misdiagnosed or inadequately treated, urolithiasis can be complicated by premature labor, with or without concurrent infection—and infection is also a frequent clinical mimicker of urolithiasis.[55,56]

Ultrasonography

The sensitivity of US for urolithiasis in pregnancy, particularly for identification of an obstructing ureteral stone, has a wide reported range, between 34% and 95%. The authors' experience is on the lower end of this range (**Figs. 14–16**). Employing resistive indices and ureteral jet analysis can be helpful, in addition to analysis of gray-scale images. The resistive index (RI) of intrarenal arteries should not be elevated by normal pregnancy alone.[57] RI elevation usually occurs within 6 hours of acute obstruction. A difference of greater than or equal to 0.04 in RI between the kidney on the symptomatic side and the opposite kidney was 99% accurate, and RI greater than or equal to 0.70 on the symptomatic side was 87% accurate, in 22 pregnant women with acute unilateral obstruction.[58] Absence of the ureteral jet on the symptomatic side had 100% sensitivity and 91% specificity for obstruction in another series.[59] However, in a third study, 15% of asymptomatic pregnant women had unilateral absent ureteral jets, and Wachsberg[60] recommended that imaging in a contralateral decubitus position should be performed to decrease false positives. Patient hydration helps to improve diagnostic accuracy, by distending the bladder and optimizing determination of ureteral jet status. In addition, transvaginal US assists in the identification of distal ureteral calculi if transabdominal US is inconclusive or normal, in the face of continued suspicion for

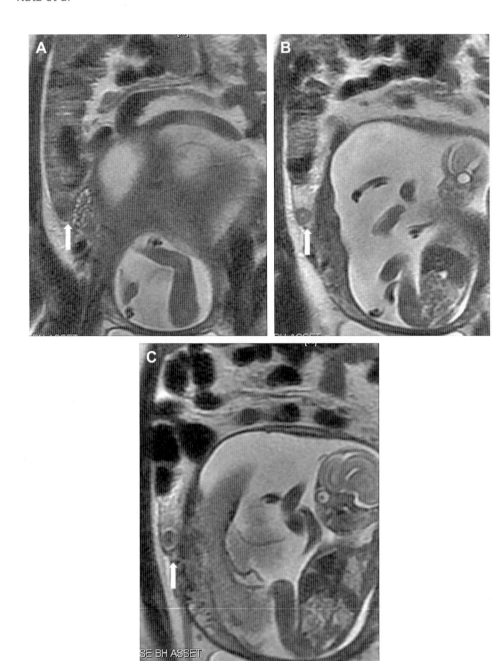

Fig. 7. Appendicitis in pregnancy. Imaging of a 29-year-old woman, 20 weeks pregnant, with right lower quadrant pain. (*A–C*) Coronal T2 SSFSE FS MR images show a hyperintense lumen, slightly hyperintense wall, and periappendiceal inflammatory changes, representing acute appendicitis (*arrows*), which was subsequently proved at surgery.

stone disease,[61] although it is unclear whether transvaginal US is actually being used in current practice for this reason.

The authors performed a retrospective analysis of transabdominal renal and bladder US reports of 77 women who underwent 113 examinations during a total of 84 pregnancies over a 5-year period at one of their institutions.[62] There was

mild to moderate bilateral renal pelvic dilatation in 21 patients and right-sided dilatation in another 20. Only 3 definitive ureteral calculi were identified. The only alternative diagnosis identified was pyelonephritis in 3 patients. Fewer than 5% of the patients had a definitive diagnosis of urolithiasis directly established on US, and fewer than 5% had an alternative diagnosis established. The

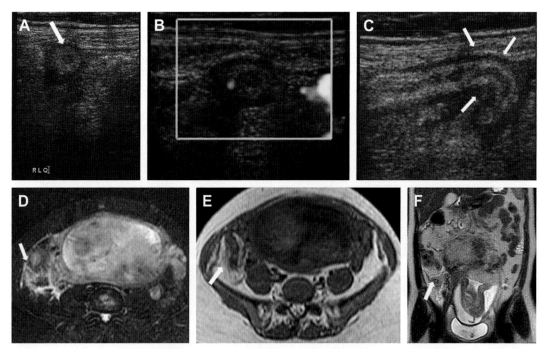

Fig. 8. Appendicitis in pregnancy. Imaging of a 33-year-old pregnant woman with acute right lower quadrant pain. (*A*) Transverse, (*B*) transverse power Doppler, and (*C*) sagittal ultrasound images show a tubular noncompressible structure compatible with appendicitis versus terminal ileitis (*arrows*). (*D*) Axial T2 FS image shows an enlarged edematous appendix with adjacent inflammatory changes (*arrow*). (*E*) Axial T1 MR image shows an enlarged edematous appendix with adjacent inflammatory changes (*arrow*). (*F*) Coronal T2 FS MR image shows an enlarged and edematous appendix with adjacent inflammatory changes (*arrow*).

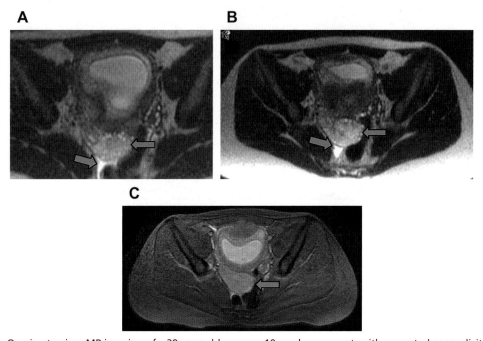

Fig. 9. Ovarian torsion. MR imaging of a 29-year-old woman, 10 weeks pregnant, with suspected appendicitis. (*A*) Axial T2 SSFSE image shows a mildly enlarged and edematous posterior right ovary with peripheral follicles and trace free fluid in the cul-de-sac (*arrows*). The appendix is not identified. (*B*) Axial T2 SSFSE image further demonstrates a mildly enlarged and edematous posterior right ovary with peripheral follicles and trace free fluid (*arrows*). (*C*) Axial FIESTA image shows a mildly enlarged and edematous posterior right ovary with peripheral follicles (*arrow*). The diagnosis of ovarian torsion was confirmed at subsequent surgery.

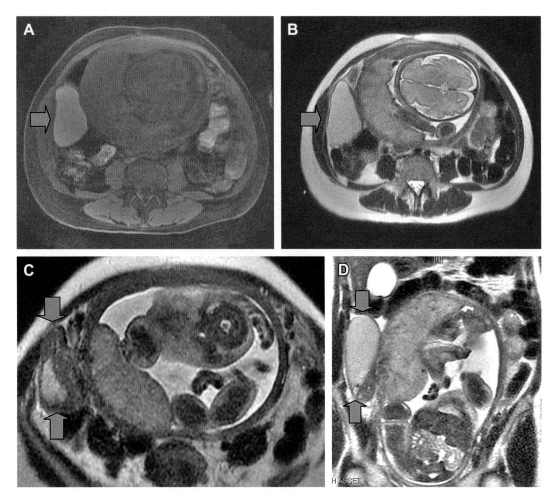

Fig. 10. Torsed hemorrhagic cyst. MR imaging of a 37-year-old woman, 32 weeks pregnant. (*A*) Axial T1 FS image shows a hemorrhagic cystic right ovarian mass (*arrow*), which was subsequently proved to be infarcted and torsed at surgery. (*B*) Axial T2 SSFSE image shows a hemorrhagic cystic right ovarian mass (*arrow*). (*C*) Axial T1 SSFSE image further demonstrates the hemorrhagic cystic right ovarian mass (*arrows*). (*D*) Coronal T2 SSFSE image shows the hemorrhagic right ovarian mass (*arrows*).

limitations of this study included its retrospective nature, that the true incidence of ureteral stones was not known, and that evaluation of RI and ureteral jets was inconsistent.

In a recent study of 262 pregnant patients with suspected urolithiasis—the largest such study to date—the accuracy of US improved from 56% to 72%, when ureteral jet and RI analysis was added to interpretation of gray-scale images.[56]

US can be used to guide ureteral stent placement and nephrostomy tube placement, eliminating or reducing the need for fluoroscopy.

MR Imaging

US is still considered the usual initial test of choice for suspected urolithiasis in pregnancy, despite its substantial limitations. MR imaging, particularly

MR urography (MRU) (ie, heavily T2-weighted multiplanar images, similar to what is performed in suspected appendicitis), is a supplemental examination. But as with appendicitis, should MR imaging be used to replace US as the initial examination for suspected urolithiasis? MRU reportedly had high accuracy for identification of the side and site of obstruction in pregnancy in early reports,[63] but to the authors' knowledge there are no large or even medium-sized series replicating these findings.

It can be difficult to determine, especially in the middle to later stages of gestation, if there is just physiologic urinary tract dilatation on US, especially on the right, or if there is abnormal dilatation related to urolithiasis. MRU appears to be helpful in this situation. In a series of 24 pregnant patients studied with MRU, renal enlargement

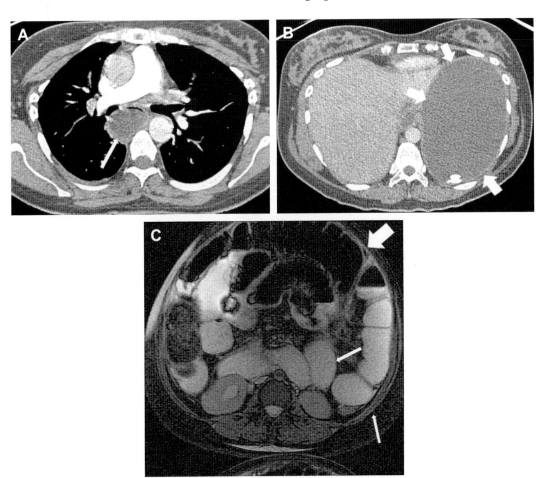

Fig. 11. Small and large bowel obstruction. CT and MR imaging of a 34-year-old woman, 27 weeks pregnant, presenting with tachycardia, back pain, and shortness of breath. (A, B) Representative images from a CT pulmonary angiogram demonstrate no evidence of pulmonary embolism, but there is esophageal distention and gastric distention (*arrows*). (C) Axial 2D FIESTA FS image shows diffuse dilatation of the proximal small bowel through to the distal small bowel (*thin arrows*), consistent with obstruction. The mid transverse colon is mildly dilated (*thick arrow*), measuring 5.5 cm in diameter. The more distal colon is collapsed. An appendix is not identified. There is no specific evidence for appendicitis or complications of appendicitis. At surgery, the patient was found to have a perforated right colon with no clear etiology.

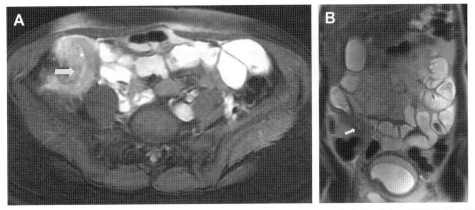

Fig. 12. Small bowel obstruction and thickening of the terminal ileum (*arrows*). (A) Axial 2D FIESTA FS MR image of a 37-year-old woman, 11 weeks pregnant, with a history of Crohn disease and prior appendectomy, presenting with abdominal pain. (B) Coronal T2 SSFSE MR image demonstrating thickening of the terminal ileum (*arrow*) and dilated loops of small bowel.

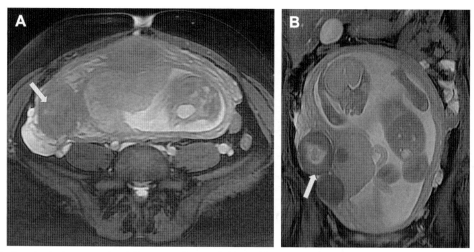

Fig. 13. Exophytic degenerating leiomyoma (*arrows*). (*A*) Axial 2D FIESTA FS MR image of a 37-year-old woman with right abdominal pain demonstrates normal venous/adnexal structures, and an adjacent exophytic uterine fibroid. (*B*) Coronal 2D FIESTA FS MR image demonstrates two exophytic fibroids. The more superior of the two fibroids has increased T2 signal centrally, characteristic of cystic degeneration.

and perinephric edema were absent in physiologic dilatation, and physiologic dilatation often tapered at the middle third of the ureter because of the mass effect from the uterus.[64]

Limitations of MRU include difficulty in directly identifying stones, especially when small, and the restriction to noncontrast sequences only, as well

as flow artifacts that may be confused with calculi.[65] A recent article highlighted the potential advantages and disadvantages of using MRU on a more regular basis for imaging patients in general (in nonpregnant as well as pregnant patients).[65] However, anecdotally the authors have found the identification of secondary MR findings of an

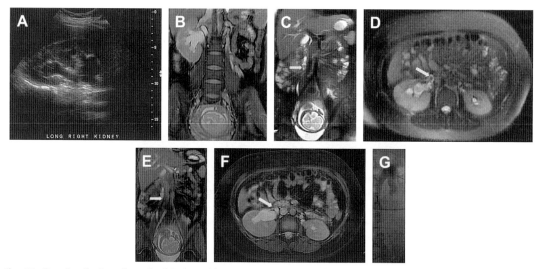

Fig. 14. Renal colic. Imaging of a 29-year-old pregnant woman with a history of renal stones. (*A*) Sagittal sonographic image through the right kidney demonstrates hydronephrosis. (*B*) Coronal 2D FIESTA FS MR image taken the following day also shows right hydronephrosis. (*C*) Coronal T2 SSFSE FS and (*D*) axial T2 SSFSE FS MR images through the proximal right ureter show a low-signal-intensity oval structure in the proximal right ureter (*arrows*), which may represent a ureteral stone or flow-related artifact. (*E*) Coronal 2D FIESTA FS and (*F*) axial 2D FIESTA FS MR images through the proximal ureter do not demonstrate this low-signal-intensity focus, raising the possibility that this is a flow-related artifact (*arrows*). (*G*) Fluoroscopic spot image from the subsequent right nephrostogram shows no stone.

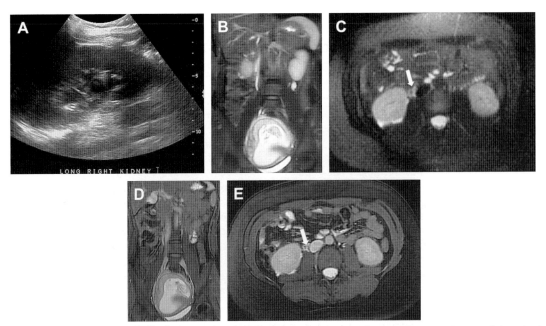

Fig. 15. Renal colic. Imaging of a 16-year-old woman, 14 weeks pregnant, with a history of renal stones. (*A*) Sagittal sonographic image through the right kidney demonstrates hydronephrosis. (*B*) Coronal T2 SSFSE FS and (*C*) axial T2 SSFSE FS MR images through the proximal to mid right ureter show a low-signal-intensity oval structure at the transition from dilated to normal-caliber ureter (*arrow*), which is consistent with a stone. (*D*) Coronal 2D FIESTA FS and (*E*) axial 2D FIESTA FS MR images through the proximal to mid right ureter confirm this finding (*arrow*).

obstructing ureteral stone—or findings consistent with urinary tract infection—to be very helpful in confirming a urinary tract source of the patient's pain, although much poorer success has been achieved in actually identifying ureteral calculi on MR imaging. Moreover, as with imaging for appendicitis, MR imaging may be less readily available than US or CT, and has relatively higher cost.

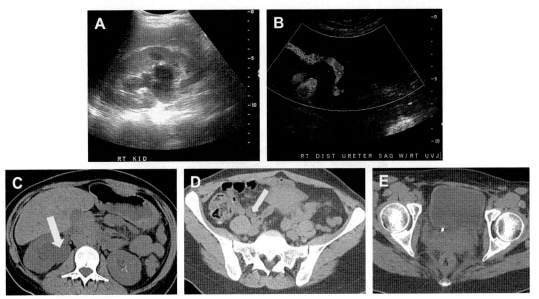

Fig. 16. Renal colic. Imaging of a 35-year-old woman in her third trimester presenting with right flank pain. (*A*) Sagittal ultrasound image of the right kidney shows hydronephrosis. (*B*) Sagittal ultrasound image of the right distal ureter shows hydroureter; however, a stone is not directly identified. (*C*) Axial CT images following delivery show continued obstruction, with significant hydronephrosis (*arrow*), and (*D*) Hydroureter (*arrow*), (*E*) Secondary to a stone at the right ureterovesical junction (*arrow*).

Computed Tomography

Low-radiation-dose noncontrast CT, using a variety of strategies, has been validated in non-pregnant patients for the diagnosis of urolithiasis in multiple publications, some of which are by the authors.[66–68] The estimated fetal dose at 0 and 3 months of gestation with relatively low tube current technique using a 16-detector CT scanner (160 mA and 150 kVp) was 8 to 12 mGy and 4 to 7 mGy, respectively.[14] In a series of 20 pregnant patients with refractory flank pain, the average estimated fetal dose, using a low-radiation-dose CT technique, was 7 mGy.[69]

Because CT appears to have high accuracy in the limited reported literature to date, analogous to in nonpregnant patients, in the authors' opinion the threshold is somewhat decreased for using CT as a supplemental test, particularly in patients with continued suspected renal colic and without a definitive answer on US and/or MR, although in their practices the authors generally still attempt to avoid CT if at all possible.

SUSPECTED BILIARY TRACT DISEASE

Symptomatic biliary tract disease in pregnancy is uncommon, but gallstones are more prevalent in pregnancy (up to 12%).[70] Sonography is clearly the initial imaging test of choice for evaluation of suspected biliary tract disease, particularly gallstones and complications of gallstones (**Fig. 17**). Obstructive jaundice and gallstone pancreatitis are associated with high maternal and fetal morbidity, as well as mortality. Management is somewhat controversial, but more recent evidence favors surgical management, ie, cholecystectomy, especially with gallstone pancreatitis, as there is a high rate of recurrence with nonoperative management.[71,72]

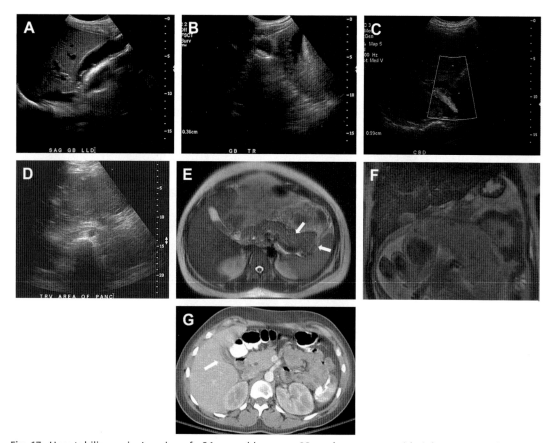

Fig. 17. Hepatobiliary pain. Imaging of a 24-year-old woman, 33 weeks pregnant, with right upper quadrant pain. (*A*) Sagittal ultrasound image of the gallbladder shows multiple gallstones. (*B*) Transverse ultrasound image of the gallbladder shows mild wall thickening. (*C*) Sagittal ultrasound image of the common duct shows a dilated duct measuring approximately 1 cm. (*D*) Transverse ultrasound image in the region of the pancreas is limited. (*E*) Axial T2 SSFSE MR image shows gallstones versus sludge in the gallbladder and an enlarged pancreas (*arrows*). (*F*) Coronal T2 SSFSE MR image shows gallstones versus sludge and mild infiltrative changes adjacent to the pancreas. (*G*) Axial CT image through the gallbladder performed after delivery shows pericholecystic fluid and a contracted gallbladder (*arrow*).

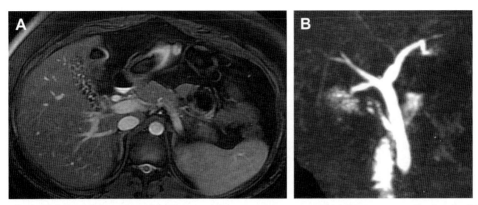

Fig. 18. Cholelithiasis. MR imaging of a 28-year-old pregnant woman with right upper quadrant pain. (*A*) Axial 2D FIESTA FS image of the right upper quadrant shows cholelithiasis without evidence of cholecystitis. (*B*) Three-dimensional MR cholangiopancreatography image shows no evidence of a common duct stone.

MR imaging, namely magnetic resonance cholangiopancreatography (MRCP), which consists of heavily T2-weighted multiplanar sequences, similar to MRU, has significant utility for evaluating patients with suspected common duct stones, as well as patients with pancreatitis, as in nonpregnant patients (see **Fig. 17**; **Figs. 18** and **19**). MR imaging demonstrates findings of pancreatitis and its complications, although gadolinium is not administered. MR imaging should be used in lieu

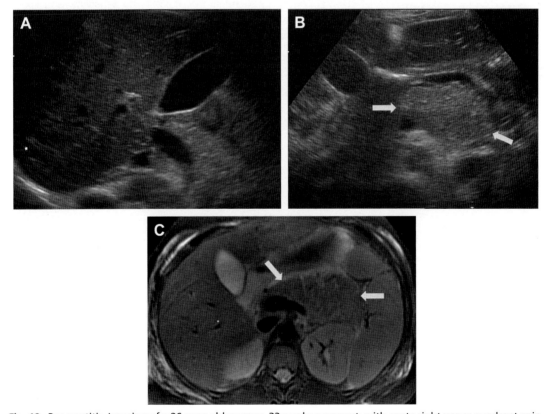

Fig. 19. Pancreatitis. Imaging of a 26-year-old woman, 33 weeks pregnant, with acute right upper quadrant pain. (*A*) Sagittal ultrasound image of the right upper quadrant shows a normal liver, gallbladder, and common duct. (*B*) Axial ultrasound image through the pancreas shows diffuse pancreatic enlargement representing pancreatitis (*arrows*). (*C*) Axial T2 SSFSE FS image through the abdomen shows inflammatory changes adjacent to an enlarged pancreas (*arrows*), confirming pancreatitis.

of fluoroscopic techniques, namely endoscopic retrograde cholangiopancreatography (ERCP), for diagnosis, with ERCP reserved for therapy only. As in nonpregnant patients, MR imaging is noninvasive, involves no ionizing radiation, and there is no risk of inducing pancreatitis when evaluating for common duct stones.

In a series of 18 pregnant patients reported by Oto and colleagues,[73] various types of biliary pathology were demonstrated on MRCP in 4 patients despite negative US (specifically, ductal stones in 2, a choledochal cyst in 1, and Mirizzi syndrome in 1). MRCP was also particularly helpful in this series if US showed only biliary dilatation without an identifiable cause.

Fetal radiation exposure during ERCP is reportedly within safe limits, if performed by experienced operators.[74] However, common duct stones can be removed and sphincterotomy performed without fluoroscopy, with or without a choledochoscope, or with endoscopic ultrasound/intraductal ultrasound.[75,76]

IMAGING OF ABDOMINAL AND PELVIC TRAUMA IN PREGNANCY
General Considerations

Trauma is the leading nonobstetric cause of maternal death. Upwards of 6% to 7% of pregnant women sustain trauma, most commonly from motor vehicle collisions, but also from falls as well as nonaccidental trauma. Physiologic changes during pregnancy can mask the seriousness of injuries to both fetus and mother. Pregnant patients with suspected blunt abdominal and pelvic trauma, especially if unconscious or with decreased mental status, are particularly difficult to reliably evaluate. Fetal death can occur with both major and minor trauma—from 3% to 38%—secondary to placental abruption, maternal death, or shock.[77]

There is a need for accurate and rapid imaging of the abdomen and pelvis following trauma to the pregnant woman. Concerns regarding fetal radiation exposure should neither deter nor delay radiologic evaluation. However, if CT is used, as always the ALARA principle should be adhered to.

Ultrasonography

US is the appropriate initial imaging examination for rapid patient triage, if available. Abdominal and pelvic sonography should be considered positive if substantial peritoneal fluid and/or evidence of solid organ injury are identified. However, free fluid isolated to the pelvis is less specific than abdominal free fluid.[78] The sensitivity and specificity of US for detection of abdominal injury in pregnant women ranges from 61% to 86% and 98% to 100%, respectively.[79,80] When the mother is stabilized, a rapid fetal sonogram should be performed, including assessment of fetal heart rate/ viability, evaluation of the placenta (although the accuracy for identification of placental abruption

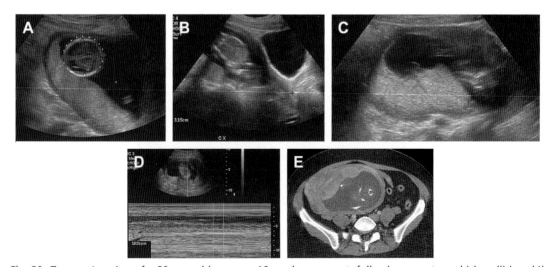

Fig. 20. Trauma. Imaging of a 29-year-old woman, 16 weeks pregnant, following a motor vehicle collision. (*A*) Pelvic ultrasound image through the fetal head and placenta is negative for traumatic injury. (*B*) Pelvic ultrasound image shows a closed cervix measuring 3.15 cm. (*C*) Pelvic ultrasound image shows no evidence of traumatic injury to the placenta. (*D*) Pelvic ultrasound image through the fetal heart obtained in M-mode shows a fetal heart rate of 162 beats per minute. (*E*) Representative axial CT image through the pelvis shows no evidence of traumatic injury to the placenta, fetus, or mother.

is only approximately 50%), and estimation of gestational age. Mothers in the third trimester should be placed in the left lateral decubitus position if possible during evaluation.

Other Imaging

What should be done if the US of the abdomen and pelvis is negative: 24-hour follow-up US, or immediate CT, or even MR imaging? In general CT is performed, either following US or initially, although to the authors' knowledge there is no large-scale study supporting the use of abdominal and pelvic CT in all or a substantial subset of pregnant women with blunt trauma, with or without initial US (Fig. 20).

As with nonpregnant patients, CT is more sensitive for the detection of abdominal and pelvic injury, including organ and retroperitoneal injury.[81,82] CT, performed with IV contrast only, shows maternal as well as placental, and even rarely fetal, injuries.[83] However, placental injuries, particularly abruption, may not be recognized prospectively as with US, and the CT appearance of such injuries is variable (Fig. 21).[84,85]

To the authors' knowledge there is no literature supporting the use of MR imaging for emergency imaging of the abdomen and pelvis in pregnancy following trauma, instead of CT, although this is theoretically possible. Challenges include obtaining immediate MR scanner access, and difficulty

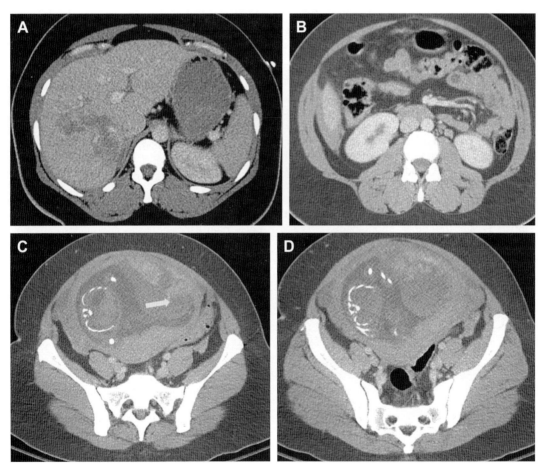

Fig. 21. Trauma. Imaging of a 36-year-old woman, 24 weeks pregnant, following a motor vehicle collision. On examination by the obstetricians, there was a poorly heard fetal heart beat on Doppler. (A) Axial CT image through the liver, using a liver window, shows a liver laceration with associated hemoperitoneum. (B) Axial CT image through the liver using an abdominal window shows a collection of blood at the right hepatic edge. (C) Axial CT image through the uterus and placenta shows an abrupted and partially devascularized placenta, with a focus consistent with active bleeding (arrow). (D) Axial CT image through the placenta shows discontinuous hypervascular regions in the placenta and interspersed lower density, with an abnormal large associated collection consistent with contained hemorrhage. The fetus could not be saved at emergency cesarean section. The mother was successfully managed conservatively.

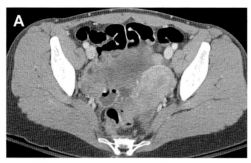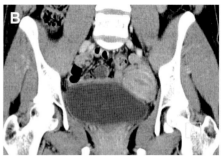

Fig. 22. Unanticipated pregnancy. Images from a CT pulmonary angiogram and concurrent CT of the abdomen and pelvis performed for chest and abdominal pain in a 29-year-old woman. The examination did not show a pulmonary embolism or other acute pathology; however, the patient was found to be 6 weeks pregnant. (*A*) Axial CT image shows a small amount of fluid in the endometrial cavity. (*B*) Coronal CT image through the pelvis shows a small amount of fluid in the endometrial cavity.

monitoring patients and performing resuscitations if needed during the examination.

PATIENT COUNSELING

Counseling the pregnant patient is important to decrease anxiety and for legal purposes.[1] Terms should be used that can be understood by patients. Patients should be informed that for most diagnostic procedures the risk of birth defects, miscarriage, and mental retardation is negligible, and that although the risk of development of subsequent childhood malignancy exists at least in theory, it seems to be small or very small compared with the other spontaneous "risks" associated with pregnancy, and when balanced against the risk of incorrect or delayed diagnosis

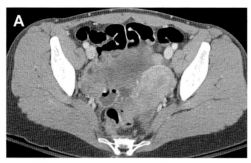

Fig. 23. Unanticipated pregnancy. Axial CT image of a woman following a motor vehicle collision. Note the round shape of the endometrial cavity. This unanticipated early pregnancy was first identified by the interpreting radiologist, based on CT findings.

in the mother. Imaging options available should be described, and the consequences of delaying or refusing imaging must also be explained.[1]

Occasionally, particularly in the trauma setting whereby a β-hCG level may not be checked, the radiologist may be the first to suggest that a patient is pregnant, based on the round, oval, and/or complex appearance of the endometrial cavity on CT (**Figs. 22** and **23**).[86]

SUMMARY

In a pregnant patient with acute abdominal and/or pelvic pain, if the necessary information can be obtained using imaging without ionizing radiation, that is, by US and particularly MR imaging, it should be used as a first-line examination. If it is necessary to use an imaging examination that will irradiate the fetus, the radiation dose should be kept as low as possible, without compromising diagnostic accuracy. If radiation dose-reduction principles are followed when performing CT on women of childbearing age in general, the occasional exposure during a previously unknown pregnancy can also be minimized. The potential risks and benefits of doing or not doing an imaging examination should be communicated with each patient. Documentation of the estimated radiation dose to the fetus, if the fetus is in the field of view, is recommended. Although this is an evolving topic with some continued controversies, this article has attempted to summarize the current literature on imaging of the acute abdomen and pelvis in pregnancy, illustrated by recent case material from the authors' two institutions. An attempt has also been made to shed light on this problematic topic with personal insight from the authors' busy clinical practices.

REFERENCES

1. Patel SJ, Reede DL, Katz DS, et al. Imaging the pregnant patient for nonobstetric conditions: algorithms and radiation dose considerations. Radiographics 2007;27:1705–22.
2. Wieseler KM, Bhargava P, Kanal KM, et al. Imaging in pregnant patients: examination appropriateness. Radiographics 2010;30:1215–33.
3. McGahan JP, Lamba R, Coakley FV. Imaging nonobstetrical causes of abdominal pain in the pregnant patient. Appl Radiol 2010;10–25.
4. Beddy P, Keogan MT, Sala E, et al. Magnetic resonance imaging for the evaluation of acute abdominal pain in pregnancy. Semin Ultrasound CT MR 2010; 31:433–41.
5. Glanc P, Maxwell C. Acute abdomen in pregnancy: role of sonography. J Ultrasound Med 2010;29:1457–68.
6. Long SS, Long C, Lai H, et al. Imaging strategies for right lower quadrant pain in pregnancy. AJR Am J Roentgenol 2011;196:4–12.
7. Lazarus E, DeBenedectis C, North D, et al. Utilization of imaging in pregnant patients: 10-year review of 5270 examinations in 3285 patients—1997-2006. Radiology 2009;251:517–24.
8. Jaffe TA, Miller CM, Merkle EM. Practice patterns in imaging of the pregnant patient with abdominal pain: a survey of academic centers. AJR Am J Roentgenol 2007;189:1128–34.
9. Thomas J, Rideau AM, Paulson EK, et al. Emergency department imaging: current practice. J Am Coll Radiol 2008;5:811–6.
10. Brent RL, Mettler FA. Pregnancy policy. AJR Am J Roentgenol 2004;182:819–22.
11. Goldberg-Stein S, Liu B, Hahn PF, et al. Body CT during pregnancy: utilization trends, examination indications, and fetal radiation doses. AJR Am J Roentgenol 2011;196:146–51.
12. Srirangam SJ, Hickerton B, Van Cleynenbreugel B. Management of urinary calculi in pregnancy: a review. J Endourol 2008;22:867–75.
13. DeSantis M, DiGianantonio E, Straface G, et al. Ionizing radiations in pregnancy and teratogenesis: a review of literature. Reprod Toxicol 2005;20:323–9.
14. Hurwitz LM, Yoshizumi T, Reiman RE, et al. Radiation dose to the fetus from body MDCT during early gestation. AJR Am J Roentgenol 2006;186:871–6.
15. Wagner LK, Huda W. Question/answer. When a pregnant woman with suspected appendicitis is referred for a CT scan, what should a radiologist do to minimize potential radiation risks? Pediatr Radiol 2004; 34:589–90.
16. McCullough CH, Schueler BA, Atwell TD, et al. Radiation exposure and pregnancy: when should we be concerned? Radiographics 2007;27:909–18.
17. Ray JG, Schull MJ, Urquia ML, et al. Major radiodiagnostic imaging in pregnancy and the risk of childhood malignancy: a population-based cohort study in Ontario. PLoS Med 2010;7:1–9.
18. Jaffe TA, Yoshizumi TT, Toncheva GI, et al. Early first-trimester fetal radiation dose estimation in 16-MDCT without and with automated tube current modulation. AJR Am J Roentgenol 2008;190:860–4.
19. Webb JA, Thomsen HS, Morcos SK. The use of iodinated and gadolinium contrast media during pregnancy and lactation. Eur Radiol 2005;15:1234–40.
20. Atwell TD, Lteif AN, Brown DL, et al. Neonatal thyroid function after administration of IV iodinated contrast agent to 21 pregnant patients. AJR Am J Roentgenol 2008;191:268–71.
21. Shellock FG, Crues JV. MR procedures: biologic effects, safety, and patient care. Radiology 2004; 232:635–52.
22. De Wilde JP, Rivers AW, Price DL. A review of the current use of magnetic resonance imaging in pregnancy and safety implications for the fetus. Prog Biophys Mol Biol 2005;87:335–53.
23. Kanal E, Barkovich AJ, Bell C, et al. ACR guidance document for safe MR practices: 2007. AJR Am J Roentgenol 2007;188:1447–74.
24. Katzberg RW, McGahan JP. Science to practice: will gadolinium-enhanced MR imaging be useful in assessment of at-risk pregnancies? Radiology 2011;258:325–6.
25. Lee I, Chew FS. Use of IV iodinated and gadolinium contrast media in the pregnant or lactating patient: self-assessment module. AJR Am J Roentgenol 2009;293(Suppl 6):S70–3.
26. DeSantis M, Straface G, Cavaliere AF, et al. Gadolinium periconceptional exposure: pregnancy and neonatal outcome. Acta Obstet Gynecol Scand 2007;86:99–101.
27. Barnett SB. Routine ultrasound scanning in first trimester: what are the risks? Semin Ultrasound CT MR 2002;23:387–91.
28. Abramowicz JS, Kossoff G, Marsal K, et al. Safety statement, 2000 (reconfirmed 2003). International Society of Ultrasound in Obstetrics and Gynecology (ISUOG). Ultrasound Obstet Gynecol 2003;21:100.
29. Brown JJ, Wilson C, Coleman S, et al. Appendicitis in pregnancy: an ongoing diagnostic dilemma. Colorectal Dis 2009;11:116–22.
30. McGory ML, Zingmond DS, Tillou A, et al. Negative appendectomy in pregnant women is associated with a substantial risk of fetal loss. J Am Coll Surg 2007;205:534–40.
31. Freeland M, King E, Safcsak K, et al. Diagnosis of appendicitis in pregnancy. Am J Surg 2009;198:753–8.
32. Oto A, Srinivasan PN, Ernst RD, et al. Revisiting MRI for appendix location during pregnancy. AJR Am J Roentgenol 2006;186:883–7.
33. Lee KS, Rosfky NM, Pedrosa I. Localization of the appendix at MR imaging during pregnancy: utility of the cecal tilt angle. Radiology 2008;249:134–41.

34. Pedrosa I, Lafornara M, Pandharipande PV, et al. Pregnant patients suspected of having acute appendicitis: effect of MR on negative laparotomy rate and appendiceal perforation rate. Radiology 2009;250:749–57.

35. Lemieux P, Rheaume P, Levesque I, et al. Laparoscopic appendectomy in pregnant patients: a review of 45 cases. Surg Endosc 2009;23:1701–5.

36. Lim HK, Bae SH, Seo GS. Diagnosis of acute appendicitis in pregnant women: value of sonography. AJR Am J Roentgenol 1992;159:539–42.

37. Barloon TJ, Brown P, Abu-Yousef MM, et al. Sonography of acute appendicitis in pregnancy. Abdom Imaging 1995;20:149–51.

38. Cobben LP, Groot I, Haans L, et al. MRI for clinically suspected appendicitis during pregnancy. AJR Am J Roentgenol 2004;183:671–5.

39. Israel GM, Malguria N, McCarthy S, et al. MRI vs. ultrasound for suspected appendicitis during pregnancy. J Magn Reson Imaging 2008;28:428–33.

40. Oto A, Ernst RD, Ghulmiyyah LM, et al. MR imaging in the triage of pregnant patients with acute abdominal and pelvic pain. Abdom Imaging 2009;34:243–50.

41. Eyvazzadeh AD, Pedrosa I, Rofsky NM, et al. MRI of right-sided abdominal pain in pregnancy. AJR Am J Roentgenol 2004;183:907–14.

42. Birchard KR, Brown MA, Hyslop WB, et al. MRI of acute abdominal and pelvic pain in pregnant patients. AJR Am J Roentgenol 2005;184:452–8.

43. Pedrosa I, Levine D, Eyvazzadeh AD, et al. MR imaging evaluation of acute appendicitis in pregnancy. Radiology 2006;238:891–9.

44. Oto A, Ernst RD, Shah R, et al. Right-lower-quadrant pain and suspected appendicitis in pregnant women: evaluation with MR imaging—initial experience. Radiology 2005;234:445–51.

45. Maselli G, Brunelli R, Casciani E, et al. Acute abdominal and pelvic pain in pregnancy: MR imaging as a valuable adjunct to ultrasound? Abdom Imaging 2010. [Epub ahead of print].

46. Barger RL, Nandalur KR. Diagnostic performance of magnetic resonance imaging in the detection of appendicitis in adults: a meta-analysis. Acad Radiol 2010;17:1211–6.

47. Blumenfeld YJ, Wong AE, Jafari A, et al. MR imaging in cases of antenatal suspected appendicitis: a meta-analysis. J Matern Fetal Neonatal Med 2011;24:485–8.

48. Singh AK, Desai H, Novelline RA. Emergency MRI of acute pelvic pain: MR protocol with no oral contrast. Emerg Radiol 2009;16:133–41.

49. Katz DS, Merunka V, Hines JJ, et al. Invited commentary. Radiographics 2007;27:743–9.

50. Pedrosa I, Zeikus EA, Levine D, et al. MR imaging of acute right lower quadrant pain in pregnant and nonpregnant patients. Radiographics 2007;27:721–53.

51. Mullins ME, Rhea JT, Greene MF, et al. Diagnostic imaging of suspected appendicitis in pregnant women: comparison of CT to ultrasonography. Emerg Radiol 2001;8:262–6.

52. Castro MA, Shipp TD, Castro EE, et al. The use of helical computed tomography in pregnancy for the diagnosis of acute appendicitis. Am J Obstet Gynecol 2001;184:954–7.

53. Lazarus E, Mayo-Smith WW, Mainiero MB, et al. CT in the evaluation of nontraumatic abdominal pain in pregnant women. Radiology 2007;244:784–90.

54. Shetty MK. Abdominal computed tomography during pregnancy: a review of indications and fetal radiation exposure issues. Semin Ultrasound CT MR 2010;31:3–7.

55. McAleer SJ, Loughlin KR. Nephrolithiasis and pregnancy. Curr Opin Urol 2004;14:123–7.

56. Andreoiu M, MacMahon R. Renal colic in pregnancy: lithiasis or physiological hydronephrosis? Urology 2009;74:758–61.

57. Hertzberg BS, Carroll BA, Bowie JD, et al. Doppler US assessment of maternal kidneys: analysis of intrarenal resistivity indexes in normal pregnancy and physiologic pelvicaliectasis. Radiology 1993;186:689–92.

58. Shokeir AA, Mahran MR, Abdulmaaboud M. Renal colic in pregnant women: role of renal resistive index. Urology 2000;55:344–7.

59. Deyoe LA, Cronan JJ, Breslaw BH, et al. New techniques of ultrasound and color Doppler in the prospective evaluation of acute renal obstruction: do they replace the intravenous urogram? Abdom Imaging 1995;20:58–63.

60. Wachsberg RH. Unilateral absence of ureteral jets in the third trimester of pregnancy: pitfall in color Doppler US diagnosis of urinary obstruction. Radiology 1998;209:279–81.

61. Laing FC, Benson CB, DiSalvo DN, et al. Distal ureteral calculi: detection with vaginal US. Radiology 1994;192:545–8.

62. Hsu C, Meiner EM, Katz DS. Utility of sonography for the evaluation of suspected urolithiasis in pregnancy. Scientific poster, the annual meeting of the American College of Emergency Physicians. October, San Francisco (CA), 2004.

63. Roy C, Saussine C, LeBras Y, et al. Assessment of painful ureterohydronephrosis during pregnancy by MR urography. Eur Radiol 1996;6:334–8.

64. Spencer JA, Chahal R, Kelly A, et al. Evaluation of painful hydronephrosis in pregnancy: magnetic resonance urographic patterns in physiological dilatation versus calculous obstruction. J Urol 2004;171:156–60.

65. Kalb B, Sharma P, Salman K, et al. Acute abdominal pain: is there a potential role for MRI in the setting of the emergency department in a patient with renal calculi? J Magn Reson Imaging 2010;32:1012–23.

66. Diel J, Perlmutter S, Venkataramanan N, et al. Unenhanced helical CT using increased pitch for suspected renal colic: an effective technique for radiation dose reduction? J Comput Assist Tomogr 2000;24:795–801.

67. Katz DS, Venkataramanan N, Napel S, et al. Can low-dose unenhanced multidetector CT be used for routine evaluation of suspected renal colic? AJR Am J Roentgenol 2003;180:313–5.

68. Tack D, Sourtzis S, Delpierre I, et al. Low-dose unenhanced multidetector CT of patients with suspected renal colic. AJR Am J Roentgenol 2003;180:305–11.

69. White WM, Zite NB, Gash J, et al. Low-dose computed tomography for the evaluation of flank pain in the pregnant population. J Endourol 2007; 21:1255–60.

70. Lu EJ, Curet MJ, El-Sayed YY, et al. Medical versus surgical management of biliary tract disease in pregnancy. Am J Surg 2004;188:755–9.

71. Date RS, Kaushal M, Ramesh A. A review of the management of gallstone disease and its complications in pregnancy. Am J Surg 2008;196:599–608.

72. Eddy JJ, Gideonsen MD, Song JY, et al. Pancreatitis in pregnancy. Obstet Gynecol 2008;112:1075–81.

73. Oto A, Ernst R, Ghulmiyyah L, et al. The role of MR cholangiopancreatography in the evaluation of pregnant patients with acute pancreaticobiliary disease. Br J Radiol 2009;82:279–85.

74. Kahaleh M, Hartwell GD, Arseneau K, et al. Safety and efficacy of ERCP in pregnancy. Gastrointest Endosc 2004;60:287–92.

75. Shelton J, Linder JD, Rivera-Alsina ME, et al. Commitment, confirmation, and clearance: new techniques for nonradiation ERCP during pregnancy. Gastrointest Endosc 2008;67:364–8.

76. Moon JH, Cho YD, Cha SW, et al. The detection of bile duct stones in suspected biliary pancreatitis: comparison of MRCP, ERCP, and intraductal US. Am J Gastroenterol 2005;100:1051–7.

77. Baerga-Varela Y, Zietlow SP, Bannon MP, et al. Trauma in pregnancy. Mayo Clin Proc 2000;75: 1243–8.

78. Richards JR, Ormsby EL, Romo MV, et al. Blunt abdominal injury in the pregnant patient: detection with US. Radiology 2004;233:463–70.

79. Goodwin H, Holmes JF, Wisner DH. Abdominal ultrasound examination in pregnant blunt trauma patients. J Trauma 2001;50:689–94.

80. Brown MA, Sirlin CB, Farahmand N, et al. Screening sonography in pregnant patients with blunt abdominal trauma. J Ultrasound Med 2005;24:175–81.

81. Lowdermilk C, Gavant ML, Qaisi W, et al. Screening helical CT for evaluation of blunt traumatic injury in the pregnant patient. Radiographics 1999;19: S243–55.

82. Goldman SM, Wagner LK. Radiologic ABCs of maternal and fetal survival after trauma: when minutes may count. Radiographics 1999;19:1349–57.

83. Siddall KA, Rubens DJ. Multidetector CT of the female pelvis. Radiol Clin North Am 2005;43: 1097–118.

84. Wei SH, Helmy M, Cohen AJ. CT evaluation of placental abruption in pregnant trauma patients. Emerg Radiol 2009;16:365–73.

85. Elsayes KM, Trout AT, Friedkin AM, et al. Imaging of the placenta: a multimodality pictorial review. Radiographics 2009;29:1371–91.

86. Shin DS, Poder L, Courtier J, et al. CT and MRI of early intrauterine pregnancy. AJR Am J Roentgenol 2011;196:325–30.

Diagnosis of Acute Gastrointestinal Hemorrhage and Acute Mesenteric Ischemia in the Era of Multi-Detector Row CT

Jamlik-Omari Johnson, MD

KEYWORDS
- Gastrointestinal hemorrhage • Mesenteric ischemia • MDCT
- Bleeding • Bowel ischemia

ACUTE GASTROINTESTINAL HEMORRHAGE

Acute gastrointestinal (GI) hemorrhage is a commonly encountered symptom in both the primary care and emergency care settings. Acute GI hemorrhage is classified as upper or lower depending on the location of the source of the bleed in reference to the ligament of Treitz.[1] Upper GI hemorrhage is more common than lower GI hemorrhage. The annual incidence of upper GI hemorrhage ranges from 40 to 150 episodes per 100,000 persons, and the annual incidence of lower GI hemorrhage ranges from 20 to 27 episodes per 100,000 persons.[2]

Although most GI hemorrhages cease spontaneously, recurrent bleeding occurs in approximately 25% of patients.[3] Over the past 3 decades, the estimated overall mortality rate from acute GI hemorrhage decreased from 10% to 3%–5%.[4] Despite the improved survival for this common problem, mortality rates can reach up to 23% in the settings of massive hemorrhage or recurrent bleeding after hospital discharge.[5] A thorough understanding of the initial management of GI hemorrhage is important because prompt and aggressive diagnostic and therapeutic interventions are required. Managing acute GI hemorrhage involves 3 phases: resuscitation, diagnosis, and therapy. This section briefly discusses presentation, resuscitation, and therapy; a more detailed discussion of diagnosis ensues.

Presentation

The clinical presentation of GI hemorrhage depends on several factors, including the source of the hemorrhage, rate of hemorrhage, and amount of blood loss. Black or tarry stool or melena is associated with an upper GI hemorrhage. Often patients are unaware that this presentation reflects a GI source of bleeding. Consequently, patients may present later in the process with more severe symptoms, such as volume depletion. Although red rectal bleeding or hematochezia is associated with a lower GI hemorrhage and is more readily identified as alarming by patients, this symptom actually more accurately reflects the rate of blood loss and duration of blood within the GI tract. For example, a patient with a cecal hemorrhage and slow colonic transit may present with melena, whereas a patient with a brisk upper

Division of Emergency Radiology, Department of Radiology and Imaging Sciences, Emory University Hospital Midtown, 550 Peachtree Street NE, Atlanta, GA 30308, USA
E-mail address: jamlik.johnson@emoryhealthcare.org

Radiol Clin N Am 50 (2012) 173–182
doi:10.1016/j.rcl.2011.09.001
0033-8389/12/$ – see front matter © 2012 Elsevier Inc. All rights reserved.

radiologic.theclinics.com

GI hemorrhage and rapid transit may present with hematochezia.[6,7]

Resuscitation

Volume depletion leads to decreased cardiac output that causes insufficient tissue oxygenation. In the acute setting, the complications from GI hemorrhage result form hypoperfusion rather than from the loss of hemoglobin. Thus, volume resuscitation is paramount. Intravenous (IV) access is essential. Clinicians should establish immediate IV access with large bore lines. Isotonic solutions are preferable. In most cases, the average adult can receive a bolus of 500 to 1000 mL without complications. Elderly patients or patients with heart disease may need more cautious hydration with a close evaluation of the fluid status. In the acute setting, fluid overload is less dangerous than volume depletion. Although transfusions are often necessary, hematocrit and hemoglobin levels are poor reflections of blood loss. Decisions to transfuse should be individualized. Ongoing monitoring is essential during the stabilizing period.[4]

Diagnosis

The differential diagnosis of acute GI hemorrhage is wide; **Box 1** outlines the more common causes. Multiple diagnostic modalities are used to confirm the presence of, and to establish the cause of, an acute GI hemorrhage.

Endoscopy

Esophagogastroduodenoscopy (EGD) and colonoscopy remain the first-line diagnostic modalities for upper and lower GI hemorrhage.[8] Endoscopic evaluation is relatively safe. It allows direct visualization of hemorrhagic foci within the upper GI tract or colon and distal ileum. Many investigators report the sensitivity and specificity of EGD for GI hemorrhage between 92% and 98% and 30% and 100%, respectively.[9,10] Endoscopy can also serve as the means for therapeutic interventions in many patients with acute GI hemorrhage. The main limitation of EGD is the very poor visualization of the distal duodenum and the inability to evaluate the majority of the jejunum and the ileum. Complications are relatively low among experienced operators; however, perforation, aspiration pneumonia, and hemorrhage are known risks.[9] Endoscopy relays prognostic information as well. Variceal hemorrhage is associated with a mortality rate of 30%, much higher than other causes. The characteristics of ulcerations are used to estimate the likelihood of recurrent hemorrhage. A visible vessel, sentinel clot, or oozing ulcer is more likely to rebleed (**Fig. 1**). If the ulcer base is clean, only an estimated 10% rebleed.[4] Investigators have reported successful management of GI hemorrhage with injection therapy, thermal coagulation, and laser therapy.[11–13] An important limitation of emergency colonoscopy in the setting of acute GI hemorrhage is that blood clots and fecal material

---

Box 1
Differential diagnoses of GI hemorrhage

Common causes of upper GI hemorrhage

- Duodenal/gastric ulcers or erosions
- Esophageal varices
- Mallory-Weiss tears

Common causes of lower GI hemorrhage

- Diverticular disease
- Colonic neoplasm
- Ulcerative or ischemic colitis
- Angiodysplasia

Less common causes of GI hemorrhage

- Esophagitis
- Crohn's disease
- Radiation colitis
- Hemorrhoids

Data from Lee EW, Laberge JM. Differential diagnosis of gastrointestinal bleeding. Tech Vasc Interv Radiol 2004;7:112–22.

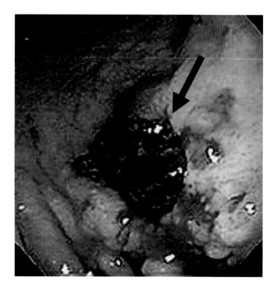

Fig. 1. Endoscopic view of GI mucosa demonstrates fresh blood at the base of the ulceration (*arrow*).

may obscure visualization of hemorrhagic sites in unprepared patients.

Capsule Endoscopy

Capsule endoscopy has a reported sensitivity varying between 42% and 80% among patients with obscure intestinal bleeding (negative upper and lower endoscopic examination results). Capsule endoscopy is more appropriately used in a select group of patients with obscure GI bleeding (no source identified on upper and lower endoscopic evaluation) assumed to originate from small bowel. This modality is time consuming and not appropriate in the acute care setting. In addition, it only visualizes mucosal surfaces. Capsule retention is the major known risk (**Fig. 2**), and up to 20% of examinations are incomplete.[14]

Diagnostic Imaging

In the setting of acute GI hemorrhage, abdominal radiographs seldom yield useful information and should be avoided because they delay diagnosis and treatment.

Nuclear Imaging

Technetium 99m (Tc 99m)-labeled red blood cell (RBC) or Tc 99m sulfur colloid scintigraphy can detect and localize GI hemorrhage (**Fig. 3**). Tc 99m RBC is 93% sensitive and 95% specific for detecting active GI hemorrhage at rates as low as 0.2 mL/min. Uptake of radiolabeled colloid by the liver and spleen minimizes the application in upper GI hemorrhage. Compared with Tc-99m sulfur colloid, labeled RBC scintigraphy allows patient evaluation for 24 hours after injection to detect rebleeding. However, scintigraphy is a time-consuming method with only limited sensitivity. The high false-positive localization rate (approximately 22%) limits the diagnostic value of this modality.[15,16]

Mesenteric Angiography

Angiography detects GI hemorrhages greater than 0.5 mL/min (**Fig. 4**). Scintigraphy can help guide selective contrast injections. Therapeutic intervention via embolization is a potential advantage of this diagnostic tool. However, angiography is only 40% to 86% sensitive.[17] Complications include groin hematomas, vascular injuries at puncture sites, and distal embolization and occur in up to 2.2% of patients.[18]

Multidetector Computed Tomography

Over the past decade, multidetector computed tomography (MDCT) angiography emerged as a promising first-line modality for the time-efficient evaluation of GI hemorrhage. CT scanners are readily available in most acute care settings. The examination can be quickly performed with reproducible results and minimal invasiveness. MDCT is sensitive and accurately diagnoses or excludes active GI hemorrhage (**Figs. 5** and **6**). A meta-analysis published in 2010 demonstrated a pooled sensitivity of 89% and specificity of 85%. The initial experience of MDCT suggests the strong diagnostic capability of this modality.[19] Investigators report detection of hemorrhage with MDCT in animal models at a rate of 0.3 mL/min.[20] In addition, MDCT often diagnoses hemorrhagic foci when angiography fails to identify the source.[21,22] MDCT can detect hemorrhagic foci within the small bowel unlike upper or lower endoscopy. MDCT risks include ionizing radiation dose, IV contrast allergy, and contrast-induced nephropathy.

MDCT Techniques

The techniques and phases vary among institutions and individual radiologists. One example is provided. Images are acquired with the following parameters: detector configuration, 64 × 0.625 mm; section thickness, 0.9 mm; section increment, 0.45 mm; 120 kV; 405 mA; pitch, 0.923; and rotation time, 0.75 seconds. One hundred milliliters of IV contrast material is delivered at 4 mL/s. Automatic bolus-triggering software with use of a circular region of interest is placed on the abdominal aorta at the level of the diaphragm with a trigger threshold of 150 HU. Twenty-five seconds after the bolus trigger, data acquisition commences from the xyphoid process through the pubic symphysis. Continuous 3-mm axial, sagittal, and coronal sections are generated and

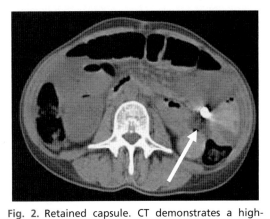

Fig. 2. Retained capsule. CT demonstrates a high-density metallic artifact (*arrow*) in the in the left upper quadrant in a patient who recently underwent capsule endoscopy. After 4 days, the capsule did not pass.

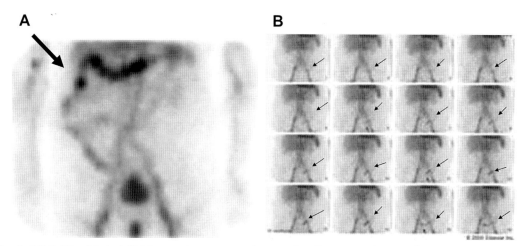

A

B

Fig. 3. (A) Tc-99m–labeled RBC image demonstrates increased radiotracer activity in the right and transverse colon consistent with acute GI hemorrhage (*arrow*). (B) Tc-99m–labeled bleeding scan demonstrates increased radiotracer activity in the sigmoid colon consistent with acute GI hemorrhage (*arrows*).

sent to picture archiving and communication system (PACS) for interpretation.

An unenhanced computed tomographic (CT) scan may be obtained immediately before CT angiography to identify any preexisting hyperattenuating areas within the bowel lumen that could be confused with hemorrhage at CT angiography. The technical parameters used to acquire the unenhanced data are as follows: detector configuration, 64 × 0.625 mm; section thickness, 3 mm; section increment, 3 mm; 120 kV; 150 mA; pitch, 0.891; and rotation time, 0.5 seconds. Contiguous 3-mm axial sections are then reconstructed and transferred to the PACS with CT angiographic data for interpretation.

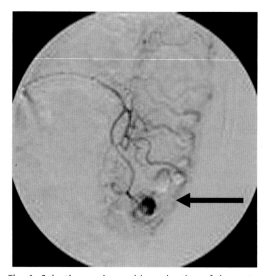

Fig. 4. Selective angiographic evaluation of the rectosigmoid region demonstrates pooling of contrast consistent with active colonic hemorrhage (*arrow*).

MDCT Findings

The increased spatial and temporal resolution provided by newer-generation MDCT technology, depicts active extravasation of IV contrast during the arterial and portal venous phases. The diagnosis of active GI bleed is made when hyperattenuating extravasated contrast material is identified within the bowel lumen. The extravasated contrast material may appear as jetlike, swirled, linear, ellipsoid, or pooled hyperattenuating foci or may fill the entire bowel lumen, resulting in a hyperattenuating loop. Varied approaches exist in evaluating patients with acute GI bleeds with MDCT. Some investigators apply attenuation thresholds as criteria for the diagnosis of acute bleeding.[23,24] Other investigators prefer to compare sequentially acquired unenhanced CT scans and CT angiograms without adherence to attenuation analysis. Most acutely extravasated contrast material into the bowel lumen will exceed 90 HU. It is conceivable that small amounts of bleeding may not reach this threshold because of volume averaging. Comparison with unenhanced images distinguishes active hemorrhage from other high-attenuation material within the GI tract. However, acquisition of both unenhanced and enhanced images increases the overall radiation dose in the patient. In either case, care must be taken to distinguish intraluminal contrast material extravasation from mucosal enhancement.

Therapy

As noted earlier, endoscopy and mesenteric angiography allow for both the detection and treatment of GI hemorrhage. Benefits, limitations, and risks are discussed.

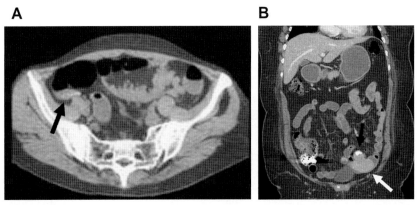

Fig. 5. (*A*) Delayed postcontrast image through the pelvis demonstrate pooling contrast in the right lower quadrant (*black arrow*) in a patient with bloody stools and anemia. Findings correlated to focus of hemorrhage at endoscopy. (*B*) Gastrointestinal hemorrhage. Coronal reformatted CT image through the bowel with focal high-attenuation focus in the sigmoid colon (*black arrow*). Intermediate-density hemorrhagic material pools in the colonic lumen (*white arrow*).

Summary

Acute GI hemorrhage commonly presents in the acute care setting. Potentially dire consequences necessitate rapid resuscitation, identification of the bleeding source, and treatment. Historically, the first-line approach used endoscopy. The advantages include the ability to both identify and treat the hemorrhagic source. The radiologic imaging choices in this setting include nuclear scintigraphy, angiography, and MDCT angiography. The previous sections outlined the strengths and weaknesses of these modalities. Although CT is not widely used as a first-line modality for the evaluation of acute GI hemorrhage, it is gaining popularity. CT is a noninvasive, rapid, readily available tool that accurately identifies GI hemorrhage and can provide useful information to guide subsequent therapeutic intervention.

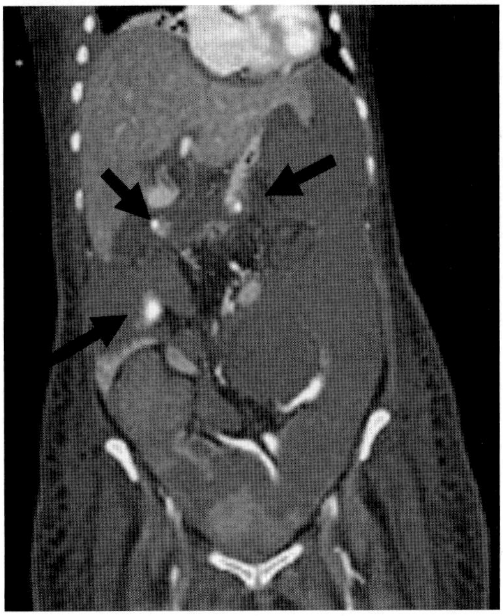

ACUTE MESENTERIC ISCHEMIA

Although bowel ischemia is a complex disease with many manifestations, it is essentially caused by a significant reduction in the blood supply to the mesenteric circulation. Acute bowel ischemia represents one of the most dangerous abdominal conditions presenting in the acute care setting.[25,26] Investigators suggest that only 1% of acute abdomen hospitalizations are secondary to acute bowel ischemia.[27] Although acute bowel ischemia is an uncommonly encountered entity in the emergency department, the increase in average life expectancy of the population and the associated increase in vascular disease may lead to more frequent encounters in clinical practice.[28]

Despite the recognition and growing interest in this entity, identification and early diagnosis is challenging. Early diagnosis is essential because the consequences for acute bowel ischemia that progresses to bowel infarction are associated with extremely high mortality. In various case series, the mortality rate ranges from 60% to 90%.[29,30] In the mid-twentieth century, very few tools existed to diagnose this condition.[31] Patients were generally surgically explored, or the

Fig. 6. Coronal reformatted image of the abdomen after IV contrast administration in a patient with clinical infectious (pseudomembranous) colitis. Focal high densities (*arrows*) in the right colon are consistent with active colonic hemorrhages.

diagnosis was made at autopsy. Over the past 60 years, the development of imaging technology expanded diagnostic possibilities.[32]

Radiographic evaluation of acute bowel ischemia in the initial phases is not optimal. At best, the findings in advanced stages are nonspecific and may represent several other entities with varying degrees of severity. Angiography provides the possibility to both identify the vascular lesion and to treat it; however, this service is often unavailable in the immediate acute care setting. In addition, angiography remains an invasive, labor-intensive, and expensive screening tool. CT is gaining popularity in evaluating patients suspected of acute bowel ischemia. Advances in CT imaging have improved the sensitivity and specificity of this modality. Investigators claim 92% specificity and 64% sensitivity.[28]

Etiology

The causes of mesenteric ischemia can be divided into 2 categories. In the overwhelming majority (approximately 80% of cases), the cause is secondary to occlusive or thromboembolic sources.[28] The remaining 20% are secondary to non-occlusive states (**Box 2**).

Box 2
Causes of acute mesenteric ischemia

Mesenteric arterial occlusion
- Thrombosis
- Embolism
- Dissection
- Stent placement
- Vasculitis
- Small vessel disease

Mesenteric venous occlusion
- Thrombosis
- Phlebitis
- Bowel obstruction or strangulation

Nonocclusive ischemia
- Shock
- Cardiac dysfunction
- Cardiac bypass
- Dehydration
- Vasoconstrictive drugs

Data from Wiesner W, Khurana B, Hoon J, et al. CT of acute bowel ischemia. Radiology 2003;226:635–50.

Occlusive Mesenteric Ischemia

Intestinal ischemia secondary to occlusive causes is due to blockage of either the arterial or venous system. The vast majorities of occlusions are arterial and may be either embolic or thrombotic in nature. Up to 50% of mesenteric infarctions are secondary to embolic obstruction of the superior mesenteric artery. These patients usually have cardiac arrhythmias such as atrial fibrillation or valvular vegetative disease that predisposes to arterial thrombi. In the remaining 50% of cases of bowel ischemia, arterial thrombosis causes ischemia. These patients usually suffer from atherosclerotic disease and develop atheromas at the level of the splanchnic arteries. Progressive narrowing of the lumen leads to mesenteric ischemia.

Venous thrombosis is responsible for about 10% of cases of mesenteric ischemia. Venous occlusion leads to blood stasis, decreased capillary circulation, and diminished cellular oxygen exchange. The ensuing cascade includes hemorrhagic distention of the intestinal wall, necrosis, and perforation. Venous ischemia and infarction are commonly associated with closed-loop obstruction. In rare cases, hypercoagulable states and vasculitis cause mesenteric ischemia.

Nonocclusive Mesenteric Ischemia

Nonocclusive causes account for approximately 20% of mesenteric ischemia. In this setting, the arterial and venous systems are patent, but the common pathway of drastically diminished perfusion exists for different reasons. Hypovolemic shock, cardiac failure, severe anemia, neurogenic vasodilatation, or splanchnic vasoconstriction can cause nonocclusive mesenteric ischemia and, if not corrected, lead to mesenteric infarction.

Anatomy, Physiology, and Pathology

Three main arteries supply the small bowel and colon. The celiac trunk, superior mesenteric artery, and inferior mesenteric artery arise from the abdominal aorta. The celiac trunk supplies the GI tract from the distal esophagus to the descending duodenum. The superior mesenteric artery supplies the distal duodenum, jejunum, ileum, and colon, generally to the splenic flexure. The inferior mesenteric artery supplies the colon from the splenic flexure to the rectum. Several rich vascular safety nets in the form of anastomoses exist in the mesenteric circulation. The gastroduodenal artery, usually the first branch of the common hepatic artery, connects the celiac trunk and the superior mesenteric artery. The marginal artery of Drummond and the arcade of Riolan provide important collateral pathways between the superior mesenteric artery and the inferior mesenteric artery. The anastomotic connections between the inferior mesenteric artery and the lumbar branches of the aorta, sacral artery, and internal iliac arteries form up to 4 arcades. Several peripheral mesenteric vascular circuits run in series and in parallel. The 3 main parallel circuits supply the muscularis propria, submucosa, and mucosa. The 5 series vascular circuits include the arterioles, capillary complexes, and venous complexes. The superior mesenteric and inferior mesenteric veins run parallel to their similarly named arteries and drain the bowel in a similar manner. The inferior mesenteric vein flows into the splenic vein that joins the superior mesenteric vein to form the portal vein. A network of shared collateral pathways connects the mesenteric and systemic venous drainage allowing gastric and esophageal connections to communicate with renal, lumbar, and pelvic veins.[33,34] In cases of acute occlusions, collateral pathways provide essential means for perfusion and drainage. Distal vessels provide end organ perfusion and have fewer associated collateral pathways. Distal occlusions can be more damaging for this reason. Similarly, fewer patent collateral pathways exist in diffuse occlusive disease states.

Under normal circumstances, the mesenteric circulation receives approximately 25% of the cardiac output, of which two-thirds supplies the intestinal mucosa. These levels vary depending on physiologic needs. During periods of extreme stress, such as occurs with the fight-or-flight phenomenon, as little as 10% of the cardiac output may be diverted to the bowel. After a large carbohydrate meal, the mesentery may receive up to 35% of the cardiac output.[35] Under normal conditions, local and systemic autoregulation ensure adequate perfusion. In cases of hypovolemia, systemic autoregulation overrules the local mechanism in an attempt to protect the brain and heart.

The initial ischemic damage to the mesentery results in mild or superficial necrosis involving the mucosa. If ischemia is not corrected, the necrosis extends to submucosa. If ischemia continues, necrosis of the deep submucosal and muscular layers occurs. Fibrotic strictures secondary to local reparative changes may develop. In severe cases, partial mural bowel ischemia progresses to transmural bowel wall necrosis. This degree of infarction is a surgical emergency because it is associated with high mortality rates. Edema and hemorrhage follow partial-thickness necrosis. The inflammatory response that follows releases several mediators, such as cytokines and platelet-activating factor, into the mesenteric circulation. These mediators damage the already susceptible bowel. The mucosal barrier weakens. The bowel is more prone to bacterial invasion that can lead to bacterial enteritis or colitis that can lead to sepsis. Bleeding, intestinal perforation, abscess formation, and peritonitis can occur.[36]

CT of Mesenteric Ischemia

The changes at the cellular level contribute to the CT appearance of a mesentery during acute ischemic episodes.[32] **Box 3** outlines some of the common CT findings associated with mesenteric ischemia. Acute bowel ischemia may present as focal or diffuse, segmental or focal, and superficial or transmural changes. It can mimic many other mesenteric conditions encountered in the acute care setting. A high level of suspicion must exist.

Bowel Wall Thickening

Bowel wall thickening is the most commonly cited finding in acute mesenteric ischemia (**Fig. 7**). Investigations report bowel wall thickening in 26% to 96% of cases. Although the thickness of the normal bowel wall depends on the degree of distention and the presence of spasmodic contractions, ranges from 3 to 5 mm are generally accepted. Wall thickening is secondary to mural edema, hemorrhage, and/or superinfection of the bowel. However, bowel wall thickening is the least specific CT finding of mesenteric ischemia, as it is observed in a host of nonischemic entities affecting the bowel.

Dilatation

Bowel lumen dilation is associated with mesenteric ischemia in 56% to 91% of reported cases. Interruption of normal intestinal peristalsis is a direct result of ischemic damage to the bowel wall (**Fig. 8**).

Box 3
CT findings in mesenteric ischemia

- Bowel wall thickening
- Bowel dilation
- Abnormal or absent wall enhancement after IV contrast administration
- Mesenteric stranding/ascites
- Vascular engorgement
- Pneumatosis
- Portal venous gas

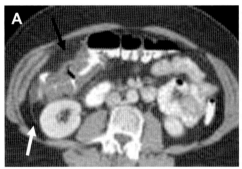 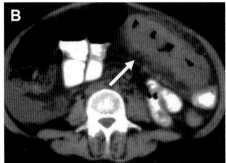

Fig. 7. Mesenteric ischemia. (*A*) Focal thickening of the ascending colon and a portion of the transverse colon (*black arrow*) spares the left colon. Minimal mesenteric stranding is noted along the right conal fascia (*white arrow*). (*B*) Focally thickened transverse colon involving the transverse colon and splenic flexure (*arrow*). Ischemic changes continued into descending colon.

Abnormal Enhancement

Ischemic bowel may demonstrate hypoenhancing or hyperenhancing walls. Poorly enhancing walls are usually homogenous secondary to wall edema. Hyperattenuating walls are associated with intramural hemorrhage or increased enhancement secondary to hyperemia or hyperperfusion.

Mesenteric Stranding/Ascites

Standing of the mesenteric fat, mesenteric fluid, and ascites are nonspecific CT findings of mesenteric ischemia. The presence of these findings depends on the cause of the ischemia, location, and severity. Investigators report the sensitivity and specificity of these 3 factors as 58%, 88%, and 75% and 79%, 90%, and 76%, respectively. If 2 of the 3 findings are present, the specificity increases to 94%.

Venous Engorgement

In cases of mesenteric venous occlusion and subsequent outflow obstruction, venous engorgement may be identified.

Pneumatosis and Portal Venous Gas

Pneumatosis and portomesenteric venous gas are less common but more specific findings of acute mesenteric ischemia. Investigators report these findings between 6% and 28% and 3% and 14%, respectively. Pneumatosis and portomesenteric venous gas may be focally or diffusely present (**Fig. 9**). When present in the liver, portomesenteric venous gas distributes to the periphery of the liver (**Fig. 10**).

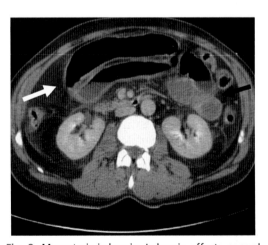

Fig. 8. Mesenteric ischemia. Ischemia affects normal peristalsis. Multiple loops of dilated small bowel (*white arrow*) and thickened loops of small bowel (*black arrow*) are noted. Mesenteric stranding is present.

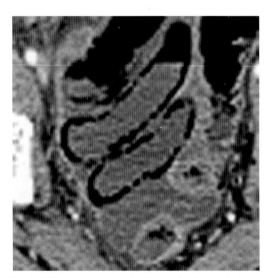

Fig. 9. Diffuse pneumatosis. Coronal reformatted post contrast image of the small bowel demonstrates diffuse pneumatosis.

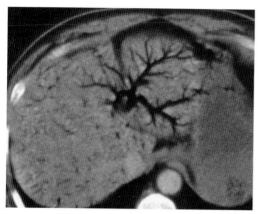

Fig. 10. Portal venous gas. Portal venous gas extends to the periphery of the liver.

SUMMARY

Although mesenteric ischemia is not one of the most commonly encountered entities in the acute care setting, it is associated with a high mortality rate. Thus, rapid and accurate diagnosis is imperative. The variable clinical and radiologic presentations and appearances of mesenteric ischemia pose a challenge to both clinicians and radiologists. Strong clinical-imaging communication and correlation is important to detect, diagnose, and treat this entity in the appropriate time course. CT is becoming an important tool in the evaluation of patients with mesenteric ischemia in the acute care setting. CT can not only aid in the rapid evaluation and diagnosis of mesenteric ischemia but also evaluate other abdominal conditions that may present in a similar manner. As the technology continues to mature, that is, higher speed, improved resolution, and multiplanar/multidimensional reformatting, CT is poised to play an increasingly important role in evaluating patients with suspected mesenteric ischemia.[37]

REFERENCES

1. Culter JA, Mendeloff AI. Upper gastrointestinal bleeding: nature and magnitude of the problem in the U.S. Dig Dis Sci 1981;26(Suppl 7):90S–6S.
2. Manning-Dimmitt LL, Dimmitt SG, Wilson GR. Diagnosis of gastrointestinal bleeding in adults. Am Fam Physician 2005;71:1339–46.
3. Imdahl A. Genesis and pathophysiology of lower gastrointestinal bleeding. Langenbecks Arch Surg 2001;386:1–7.
4. Hilsden RJ, Shaffer EA. Management of gastrointestinal hemorrhage. Can Fam Physician 1995;41: 1931–41.
5. Longstreth GF. Epidemiology and outcomes of patients hospitalized with acute lower gastrointestinal hemorrhage: a population-based study. Am J Gastroenterol 1997;92:419–24.
6. Daniel WA, Egan S. The quantity of blood required to produce a tarry stool. JAMA 1939;113:2232.
7. Jensen DM, Machicado GA. Diagnosis and treatment of severe hematochezia. Gastroenterology 1988;95:1569–74.
8. Walker TG. Acute gastrointestinal hemorrhage. Tech Vasc Interv Radiol 2009;12:80–91.
9. Gilbert DA, Silversetin FE, Tedesco FJ, et al. The national ASGE survey on upper gastrointestinal bleeding; endoscopy in upper gastrointestinal bleeding. Gastrointest Endosc 1981;27:94–102.
10. Barnert J, Messmann H. Diagnosis and management of lower gastrointestinal bleeding. Nat Rev Gastroenterol Hepatol 2009;6:637–46.
11. Lin HJ, Perng CL, Lee FY, et al. Endoscopic injection for the arrest of peptic ulcer hemorrhage: final results of a prospective, randomized comparative trial. Gastrointest Endosc 1993;39:15–9.
12. Lain L. Multipolar electrocoagulation in the treatment of active upper gastrointestinal tract hemorrhage. N Engl J Med 1987;316:1613–7.
13. O'Brien JD, Day SJ, Burnham WR. Controlled trial of small bipolar probe in bleeding peptic ulcers. Lancet 1986;1:464–7.
14. Huprich JE, Fletcher JG, Fidler JL, et al. Prospective blinded comparison of wireless capsule endoscopy and multiphase CT enterography in obscure gastrointestinal bleeding. Radiology 2011;260:744–51.
15. Fallah MA, Prakash C, Edmundowicz S. Acute gastrointestinal bleeding. Med Clin North Am 2000; 84:1183–208.
16. Zuckier LS. Acute gastrointestinal bleeding. Semin Nucl Med 2003;33:297–311.
17. Cohn SM, Moller BA, Zieg PM, et al. Angiography for preoperative evaluation in patients with lower gastrointestinal bleeding: are the benefits worth the risks? Arch Surg 1998;133:50–5.
18. Waugh JR, Sacharias N. Angiographic complications in the DSA era. Radiology 1992;182:243–6.
19. Lian-Ming W, Jian-Rong X, Yan Y, et al. Usefulness of CT angiography in diagnosing acute gastrointestinal bleeding: a meta-analysis. World J Gastroenterol 2010;16(31):3957–63.
20. Kuhle WG, Sheiman RG. Detection of active colonic hemorrhage with use of helical CT: findings in a swine model. Radiology 2003;228:743–52.
21. Hyare H, Desigan S, Nicholl H, et al. Multi-section CT angiography compared with digital subtraction angiography in diagnosing arterial hemorrhage in inflammatory pancreatic disease. Eur J Radiol 2006;59:295–300.
22. Ettore GC, Francioso G, Garribba AP, et al. Helical CT angiography in gastrointestinal bleeding of

obscure origin. AJR Am J Roentgenol 1997;168: 727–31.

23. Tew K, Davies RP, Jadun CK, et al. MDCT of acute lower gastrointestinal bleeding. AJR Am J Roentgenol 2004;182(2):427–30.

24. Yoon W, Jeong YY, Shin SS, et al. Acute massive gastrointestinal bleeding: detection and localization with arterial phase multi–detector row helical CT. Radiology 2006;239(1):160–7.

25. Jrvinen O, Larika J, Salenius C, et al. Acute intestinal ischemia: a review of 214 cases. Ann Chir Gynaecol 1994;83:22–5.

26. Levine JS, Jacobson ED. Intestinal ischemic disorders. Dig Dis 1995;13:3–24.

27. Brandt L, Boley S, Goldberg L, et al. Colitis in the elderly. Am J Gastroenterol 1981;76:239–45.

28. Angelelli G, Scardapane A, Memeo M, et al. Acute bowel ischemia: CT findings. Eur J Radiol 2004;50: 37–47.

29. Ruotolo RA, Evan SR. Mesenteric ischemia in the elderly. Clin Geriatr Med 1999;15:527–57.

30. Inderbitzi R, Wagner HE, Seiler C, et al. Acute mesenteric ischemia. Eur J Surg 1992;158:123–6.

31. Boley SJ, Sprayregen S, Veith FJ, et al. An aggressive roentgenologic and surgical approach to acute mesenteric ischemia. Surg Annu 1973;5:355–78.

32. Wiesner W, Khurana B, Hoon J, et al. CT of acute bowel ischemia. Radiology 2003;226:635–50.

33. Geobes K, Geobes KP, Maleux G. Vascular anatomy of the gastrointestinal tract. Baillieres. Best Pract Res Clin Gastroenterol 2001;15:1–14.

34. Fisher DF, Fry WJ. Collateral mesenteric circulation. Surg Gynecol Obstet 1987;164:487–92.

35. Gallavan RH, Parks DA, Jacobson ED. Pathophysiology of the gastrointestinal system. Bethesda (MD): American Physiological Society; 1989. p. 1713–32.

36. Chambert S, Porcheron J, Balique JG. Management of acute intestinal arterial ischemia. J Chir 1999;136:130.

37. Horton KM, Fishman EK. Multi-detector row CT of mesenteric ischemia: can it be done? Radiographics 2001;21:1463–73.

Index

Note: Page numbers of article titles are in **boldface** type.

Radiol Clin N Am 50 (2012) 183–189
doi:10.1016/S0033-8389(11)00227-2
0033-8389/12/$ – see front matter © 2012 Elsevier Inc. All rights reserved.

Moving?

Make sure your subscription moves with you!

To notify us of your new address, find your **Clinics Account Number** (located on your mailing label above your name), and contact customer service at:

Email: journalscustomerservice-usa@elsevier.com

800-654-2452 (subscribers in the U.S. & Canada)
314-447-8871 (subscribers outside of the U.S. & Canada)

Fax number: 314-447-8029

Elsevier Health Sciences Division
Subscription Customer Service
3251 Riverport Lane
Maryland Heights, MO 63043

ELSEVIER